TEXAS SOCIETY OF PATHOLOGISTS
75th
1921 ANNIVERSARY 1996

OUT OF THE MIST

by
Harold M. Malkin

The Foundation of Modern Pathology and Medicine during the Nineteenth Century

Publisher:Vesalius Books
250 The Uplands, Berkeley, CA 94705
Printed in the United States of America
Second Printing 1995

Photo credits: Parke, Davis & Company
Editor: Editorial Services$_{Plus}$

Library of Congress Catalog Card Number: 93-061028

Malkin, Harold M.
The Foundation of Modern Pathology and Medicine

Bibliography: p.
Includes index.

ISBN 0-9637689-0-5

IT MIGHT WELL BE SAID OF ME THAT HERE I HAVE MERELY MADE UP A BUNCH OF OTHER MEN'S FLOWERS, AND PROVIDED NOTHING OF MY OWN BUT THE STRING TO BIND THEM.

— MICHAEL DE MONTAIGNE (1533-1592)

This book is dedicated to my heroes, Louis Pasteur, Paul Ehrlich, William Osler and William Henry Welch, whose humanism shone as brightly as their accomplishments.

TABLE OF CONTENTS

Introduction

Man as a Machine 1
Reductionism 2
Man as a Happening 5
Definition of Pathology 8

Chapter I

Pathology from Prehistoric Times to the Nineteenth Century 17
The Earliest Ideas on Disease 17
Stagnation of Thought during the Middle Ages (450A.D.–1400A.D.) 18
Science and Medicine during the Renaissance (1400A.D.–1600A.D.) 19
Andreas Vesalius 22
Science and Medicine during the Seventeenth Century — The Age of Reason 25
William Harvey 26
The "Invisible Colleges" 29
Minerva Medica Contemplates Moving from Italy to Holland 29
Science and Medicine during the Eighteenth Century — The Age of Enlightenment 31
Hermann Boerhaave 31
The Old Vienna School of Medicine 31
Giovanni Battista Morgagni 32

Chapter II

The Disease Taxonomists 39
Thomas Sydenham 40
Francois Boissier de Sauvages and Carl von Linné 41

William Cullen 42
Philippe Pinel 43
The Taxonomists versus the Anatomical Pathologists 43

Chapter III

The Paris School of Anatomical Pathology 47
Medicine in France Prior to 1800 47
Medicine in France during the First Half of the Nineteenth Century 51
Marie Francois Xavier Bichat 52
Rene Theophile Hyacinthe Laennec 54
Jean Nicolas Corvisart 58
Other Eminent French Physicians during the Nineteenth Century 61

Chapter IV

The Progress of Pathology and Medicine in Great Britain during the First Half of the Nineteenth Century 73
The Fragmentation of Medical Care 73
Medicine in Scotland 78
The Edinburgh Influence 81
The School of William and John Hunter 81
Guy's Hospital School 86
Astley Cooper 86
Richard Bright 87
Thomas Addison 91
Thomas Hodgkin 95
The Dublin School 97
Later Developments in Scotland 101

Chapter V

The Progress of Pathology and the Organization of Science in the Germanic Countries during the Nineteenth Century 107

Chapter VI

Vienna, Karl Rokitansky, and Neohumoralism 113
- Karl Rokitansky — The Early Years 113
- The Attack by Rudolf Virchow 118
- The Declining Years of Rokitansky 125

Chapter VII

The Advancement of Normal and Pathological Histology 129
- The Evolution of the Microscope 129
- The School of Johannes Müller in Berlin 135
- Later Developments in Microtechniques 136

Chapter VIII

The Contributions of Rudolf Virchow to Pathology 143

Chapter IX

François Magendie and the Beginnings of Pathological Physiology 159

Chapter X

Pathological Physiology Moves to Germany 173

Chapter XI

Julius Cohnheim: From Anatomic Pathology to Pathological Physiology 179

Chapter XII

The Great Pus Cell Controversy at the Berlin Institute of Pathology 189

Chapter XIII

Microbiology and Its Revolutionary Effect on Pathology 199
- Early Ideas on Contagion 199
- Louis Pasteur 202
- Anthrax 214
- The Micrococci 214
- Typhoid Fever 225
- Discovery of the Organisms Responsible for Leprosy, Gonorrhea, and Meningitis 226
- Plague 227
- Tuberculosis 228
- Cholera 230
- Diphtheria 234
- David Bruce and Malta Fever 236
- Tetanus, Bacillary Dysentery, and the Japanese Influence 238
- Salmonella Pathogens 240

Chapter XIV

Pasteur and the Prevention of Disease 249

Chapter XV

Animal Parasites ln Pathology 263
- Trichinosis 264
- Schistosomiasis 268
- Hookworm 270
- Filariasis 272
- Malaria and Ronald Ross 275
- African Trypanosomiasis 284

Chapter XVI

The Cellular and Humoral Immunity Debate 295

Chapter XVII

The Pathology of the Blood 307
- Normal Physiology of the Blood 307
- Chemical Analysis of the Blood 308
- Studies of the Cellular Elements 309
- The Development of the Blood Count 310
- Determination of the Hemoglobin and Packed Cell Volume 311
- Blood Cell Morphology 313
- Paul Ehrlich 314
- The Platelets 320
- Clinical Applications of the New Knowledge and Techniques 320

Chapter XVIII

Tumors 327
- Antiquity to 1800 327
- 1800–1839 329
- 1839–1855 332
- The Problem of Metastatic Cancer 333
- The Question of the Origin of Cancer and the Specificity of the Cancer Cell 335
- Inflammatory Tumors 336
- The Definitive Studies of Wilhelm Waldeyer 337
- Nineteenth Century Ideas on the Etiology of Cancer 338

Chapter XIX

The Beginnings of the Study of Pathology in the United States 343

Chapter XX

Renaissance in Medicine in Baltimore at Johns Hopkins Hospital and Medical School 351

William Henry Welch 357

Henry Newell Martin 361

William Councilman 363

Later Major Figures 364

William Osler 364

William Stewart Halsted 371

Howard A. Kelly 373

The Basic Scientists 376

Franklin Paine Mall 376

John Jacob Abel 378

William Henry Howell 378

Harvey Cushing 379

Inspiration for the Establishment of The Rockefeller Institute for Research 383

Chapter XXI

The Conquest of Yellow Fever and the Influence of the Johns Hopkins 387

Epilogue 401

Plate Index

LAVOISIER — OXYGEN, COMBUSTION, AND RESPIRATION	3
VESALIUS AND THE ANATOMY OF MAN	23
HARVEY AND THE CIRCULATION OF BLOOD	27
MORGAGNI AND PATHOLOGIC ANATOMY	35
LAENNEC AND THE STETHOSCOPE	55
THE EARLY NINETEENTH CENTURY PARISIANS	59
HUNTER: FOUNDER OF SCIENTIFIC SURGERY	83
THE MEN OF GUY'S HOSPITAL	89
THE DUBLIN TRIAD	99
KARL ROKITANSKY	115
LEEUWENHOEK AND THE "LITTLE ANIMALS"	131
JOHANNES MÜLLER AND HIS STUDENTS	139
VIRCHOW AND CELLULAR PATHOLOGY	149
FRANÇOIS MAGENDIE	161
CLAUDE BERNARD	167
JULIUS COHNHEIM	181
PASTEUR: THE CHEMIST WHO TRANSFORMED MEDICINE	203
LISTER INTRODUCES ANTISEPSIS	211
KOCH AND HIS DISCIPLES	215
PASTEUR AND HIS DISCIPLES	231
PASTEUR WITH RABIES VICTIMS	253
FAMOUS PARASITOLOGISTS	265
ELIE METCHNIKOFF	297
EHRLICH IN HIS STUDY	315
EHRLICH WITH HIS TEST-TUBE EXPERIMENTS	315
THE HOPKINS: A REVOLUTION IN MEDICAL EDUCATION	353
WILLIAM OSLER	365
HARVEY CUSHING AND NEUROSURGERY	381
THE CONQUEST OF YELLOW FEVER	397

> The moral law of the universe is progress. Every generation that passes idly over the earth without adding to that progress remains uninscribed upon the register of humanity, and the succeeding generation tramples its ashes as dust.
>
> — Mazzini

Introduction

The nineteenth century properly has been called the scientific century, because it was the first time in which Man began to implement in a systematic manner the idea promoted during the eighteenth century (the period of Enlightenment) that the only valid manner in which he could achieve truth and knowledge about the physical and biological world was through the inductive experimental method. This approach promised to lift scientific knowledge out of the mist of human ignorance and was in contradistinction to the prior method, dating back to the time of Aristotle and Galen, in which knowledge was expected to be gained by making valid deductions on the bases of few and superficial observations. There had been knowledge accumulated, of course, and through the centuries progress was made, but discoveries, particularly in biology, were haphazard. In medicine the use of quinine for malaria, opiates for pain, digitalis for heart disease, and metallic salts for syphilis were essentially accidental discoveries rather than planned in a laboratory.

Man as a Machine

With regard to modern scientific biology, it is fair to state now that the foundations for this field were laid by Lavoisier and Laplace during the years 1777–1785. They conclusively showed that respiration in man and other animals was simply a combustion of carbon and hydrogen in foodstuffs with the combination of breathed oxygen in the air and the production of heat. They also found that

> this combustion (did not) evolve perceptible light, because the substance of the fire thus liberated is immediately absorbed by the moisture of the lungs; the heat developed in this combustion is

communicated to the blood . . . and is dispersed in the whole body system.[1]

This work confirmed the earlier deductive ideas of René Descartes[2] (1596–1650) and later Julien O. La Mettrie (1709–1791)[3] that Man is basically a machine. With this principle established in the last decades of the eighteenth century, the stage was set for the scientific study of biology without the inhibiting concept of a unique "vital force" in living organisms, which was not explainable in terms of the laws of chemistry and physics. This idea was constantly recurring during the nineteenth century and only during the twentieth century did it lose its popularity. Its widespread belief was best explained by Joseph Needham, who used the quotation of Columbus's mapmaker who was supposed to have said, "where unknown, there places terrors."[4]

Reductionism

It is the thesis of the author that progress in biology and medicine and the refutation of a "vital force" has occurred because scientists since 1800 have been able to explain normal and abnormal living phenomena at lower and lower levels of the organisms, starting with organ systems and ultimately being able to discuss life in terms of cell membranes and even molecules themselves. This method has been called reductionism by philosophers of science, and this approach has been eminently successful.

On occasion, when reductionism seemed to have arrived at an impasse, and the vitalists would attempt to claim victory, superior individuals with innovative ideas and techniques would give new life and direction to the reductionist methodology. Fermentation was historically a mystery, and spontaneous generation was accepted almost as fact, until Pasteur performed his classic experiments on bacteria and clarified both mysteries. A more recent example was the nature of gene action, which was solved by the elucidation of the structure of DNA by Watson and Crick[5] followed by the work of many others showing the functions of the various types of RNA in the synthesis of specific proteins in cells.[6] The result has been that, from a semantic point of view, all explanations of biological phenomena have ended up being a more detailed description of what is occurring at the molecular level. It is also clear that modern

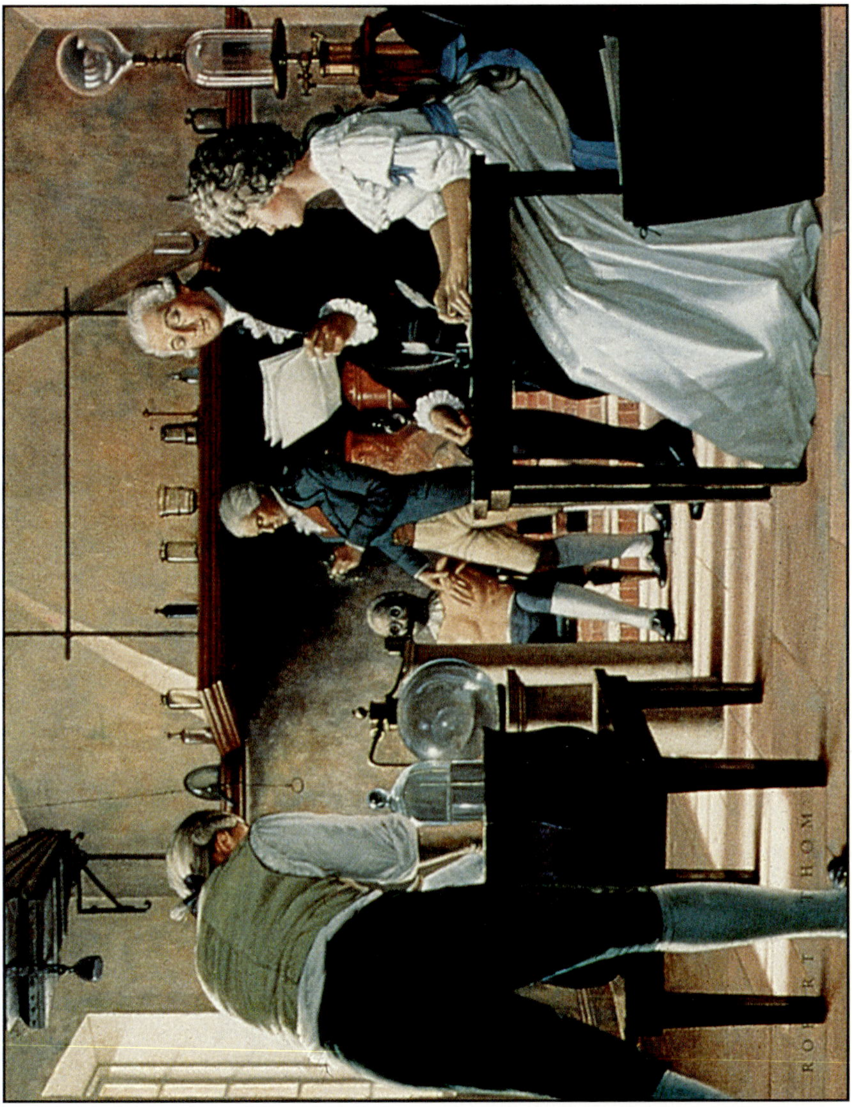

LAVOISIER — OXYGEN, COMBUSTION, AND RESPIRATION

biologists (using reductionist methodology with such diverse techniques as enzymological procedures, chromatography, electrophoresis, differential centrifugation of cell organelles, isotopic and immunologically active tracer molecules, electron microscopy, and DNA splicing during the twentieth century) have reached the level where the classical subjects of anatomy and physiology have come together because they are both dealing with the same macromolecules.

Perhaps the last frontier in biology is the Mind–Body Problem; the unresolved debate that essentially started at the time of Descartes as to whether the mind (or even the "soul") or thought processes can be explained in terms of the function of molecular action. The different points of view were aptly argued by a reductionist and a "boggled sceptic" in a book review recently.[7] Pathology, which can draw so greatly on the vast amount of knowledge in the basic sciences, has already, of course, gone a long way in explaining organic disease processes in molecular terms.

Man as a Happening

As a result of progress made during the past two hundred years, it appears that the concept of Man as a machine should be modified to perhaps the more sophisticated idea that Man is a happening, although his body continues to obey the laws of chemistry and physics.[8] The difference is that inanimate machines, such as an automobile, can be stationary or moving and therefore structures and function can indeed be considered separately, and the molecules of which it is made remain the same until it goes to the junkyard. But in an organism there are continual orderly processes that never cease from the time a sperm and ovum come together to form a zygote until death occurs as the natural result of the longevity program built into the genome. Attributes that we describe as structures in an organism or individual are actually slow processes of long duration; what we commonly call functions are rapid processes of short duration. This idea was expressed by Plato over two thousand years ago in this manner:

> Even during the period for which a living being is said to live and retain its identity — as a man for example, is called the same man from boyhood to old age — he does not in fact retain the same attributes, although he is called the same person; he is always in the process of becoming a new being by undergoing loss and restora-

tion which affects his hair, his flesh, his bones, his blood and his whole body.[9]

Five hundred years later the great Roman Emperor, Marcus Aurelius (121–180 AD), also saw the life of man in a similar way when he wrote in his diaries:

> Observe how all things are continually being born of change. . . . Nature's highest happiness lies in changing the things that are, and forming new things after their kind. . . . Time is a river, the resistless flow of all created things. One thing no sooner comes in sight than it is hurried past and another is borne along, only to be swept away in its turn. . . . Observe in short, how transient and trivial is all mortal life; yesterday a drop of semen, tomorrow a handful of ashes. . . . In the life of a man, his time is but a moment, his being an incessant flux, his senses a dim rushlight, his body a prey of worms, his soul an inquiet eddy, his fortune dark, and his fame doubtful. In short, all that is the body is as coursing waters, all that is of the soul as dreams and vapors; life is a warfare, a brief sojourning in an alien land; and after repute, oblivion. . . . I consist of a formal element and material. Neither of these ever pass away into nothing anymore than either of them come into being from nothing. Consequently every part of me will one day be refashioned by a process of transition into some other portion of the universe, which in its turn will be changed into another part, and so onward into infinity. It is the same process by which I myself was brought into existence, and my parents before me, and so backward once more to infinity. [10]

In 1938, this idea was restated by Benninghoff as follows:

> Thus while within the body the components are in a state of flux, the body itself seems to persist. But also the individual represents a series of events that starts with fertilization and ends with death. . . . What is in a slow flow, and is relatively persistent and quasi-stationary, is impressive as an organic form, the quicker flow of events is the function maintaining that form. If I look from the lower levels to the higher, then forms are apparent. The higher system acts as the form into which all subordinate events are integrated. Looking the other way, travelling down through the various levels, the forms are resolved one after the other into processes whose speed increases with decreasing size of a system.[11]

The proof for this idea came when Rudolf Schoenheimer and his group at Columbia University during the years 1938–1941 were the first to give experimental evidence of the dynamic state of the body with the use of amino acids labelled with the isotope N^{15}.[12] The group found

> that nitrogenous groupings of tissue proteins are constantly involved in chemical reactions; peptide linkages open, the amino acids liberated mix with others of the same species of whatever source, diet or tissue. This mixture of amino acid molecules while in the free state, takes part in a variety of chemical reactions; some reenter directly into vacant positions left open by the rupture of peptide linkages; others transfer their nitrogen to deaminated molecules to form new amino acids. These in turn continuously enter the same chemical cycles which render the source of the nitrogen indistinguishable. Some body constituents like glutamic acid and aspartic acid and some proteins like those of liver, serum and other organs are more actively involved than others in this general metabolic pool originating from interaction of dietary nitrogen from the relatively larger quantities of reactive tissue nitrogen.[13]

This rapid turnover of molecules (especially proteins, both large and small), which in many cases were thought to be structural and essentially inert, was confirmed many times using other isotopes such as amino acids labeled with C^{14}. Specifically, although some metabolites such as glycogen in muscle or liver have a half-life of 0.5–1.0 days, even structural proteins such as those in muscle have a half-life of only 60 days. This means that although muscle visually maintains its form, over a comparatively short period of time it has completely changed its atomic and molecular composition.[14] Finally the method by which the chemical energy stored in foodstuffs is actually used by the organism for its energy requirements for such functions as secretion and motion has been elucidated during the past sixty years with the finding of how the muscle protein, myosin, contracts by working in conjunction with high-energy phosphate bonds, such as ATP which were produced during the metabolism of food molecules such as glucose and amino and fatty acids.

Thus essentially, Man, as a happening rather than a machine, is in a continuous chemical steady state with the environment; old atoms or molecules are constantly and rapidly being replaced, leaving the body primarily through the kidneys and lungs, and new molecules are formed from those molecules taken into the body through respiration or intestinal absorption. This process is regulated and monitored through a system of homeostatic mechanisms initially proposed by Claude Bernard in his ideas about an "interieur and exterieur milieu."[15] Bernard's ideas were extended by the work of L. J. Henderson,[16] Walter Cannon,[17] J. Barcroft,[18] Bayliss and Starling,[19] and Sherrington [20] in the twentieth century as the nature of buffers, hemoglobin, and the endocrine, autonomic, and central nervous systems were elucidated. It became clear during the twentieth century that Man proceeds through life in delicate balance with his environment, both of which undergo changes but his body is always in a constant steady state. Any disturbance, due to external or internal factors that disrupt this steady state, produces illness. This is the study of pathology.

Using the above historical factors in biology, this book will attempt to show how knowledge about disease evolved during the nineteenth century and the social and scientific milieu that enabled certain individuals to produce these advancements. And because scientific medicine evolved from and usually developed parallel to the study of pathology, which caused William Osler to say late in the nineteenth century "as is our pathology, so is our practice," [21] it is important to view its history in light of a modern definition and its variations.

Definition of Pathology

What is pathology? One definition is that it is that branch of natural science that studies the cause and mechanism of disease and includes: (1) structural changes in the cells, tissues, and organs, both gross and microscopic; (2) disturbances of function at the cell, tissue, or organ level; (3) the relationship of the signs and symptoms of the patient to both the structural and functional changes; (4) methods used to detect both structural and functional abnormalities; and (5) identification of external and internal factors initiating structural or functional changes. But what then is disease? Actually it is an abstract term that can have different meanings depending on the point of view of the beholder. The practicing physician sees disease as a combination of signs (factors that he can determine or measure with his senses or instruments during his physical examination using classical visualization, palpation, percussion and auscultation) and the symptoms related by the patient such as pain, nausea, dyspnea, vertigo, or itching. The well-trained physician on the basis of evaluating these signs and symptoms should be able to understand what is occurring in the patient's body, both from the standpoint of deviations of structure and function from normal. Then, hopefully, he will be able to intervene to hasten the return of his patient to normal. The anatomical pathologist on the other hand, although understanding the point of view of the clinician, is trained to see disease more in terms of structural changes, which he interprets basically in terms of Rokitansky's gross and Virchow's cellular pathology.

At the present time, it is generally agreed that disease is produced by either external or internal factors or a combination of both. The external factors are (l) infections by microorganisms (bacteria, protozoans, fungi, rickettsia, viruses), (2) larger animal parasites (tapeworms, roundworms, hookworms, ticks, fleas, and other insects), (3) physical irritants (heat, cold, electricity, trauma, radiation, and (4) chemical poisons (arsenic, lead, mercury, phosphorus, acids, alkalies, solvents, gases, medication). The internal factors are (l) neoplasia (tumors, benign or malignant), (2) metabolic or functional changes in one of the bodily systems (digestive, endocrine, circulatory, respiratory, excretory, reproductive, muscular, nervous, skeletal, skin and blood forming, and immunological), (3) food deficiencies, (4) degenerative, and (5) genetic.

Perhaps the author's idea that disease is a failure of the organism to maintain a molecular steady state or a failure of the homeostatic mechanisms in the body as a result of one or more of the extrinsic or intrinsic factors listed is as valid as any of the above definitions of disease, but it is too broad to be of pragmatic value in discussing specific pathological changes.

Historically, because only some of the extrinsic factors listed above were known before 1800, there was a progression of only three major methods that could be used in studying disease. The first was the defining of disease by specific signs and symptoms of the patient, which was used by the disease "taxonomists" such as Thomas Sydenham. This method had limited success for identifying some of the acute infectious diseases, especially during an epidemic when there was a uniform pattern of disease in many individuals, but produced great confusion in the presence of chronic disease when there was great variability in the signs and symptoms. The second method was looking for the "seats of disease" by identifying gross lesions, which was used first by Morgagni, then Bichat, and later Rokitansky. This method was expanded when the compound microscope was developed in 1830 and continued to be perhaps the most successful research method until the end of the century. It was soon obvious to the anatomic pathologists that structural lesions were not always identifiable and when they were present, the lesions did not seem to be specific and such conditions as tuberculosis, pneumonia, and malignancy of the lungs could not be differentiated until late in the nineteenth century. The third method was the study of abnormalities in function or pathological physiology. Athough it was championed by Magendie, Wunderlich, Traube, and Virchow, it had to await the accumulation of knowledge about normal organ, tissue, and cell function until it was practiced, primarily by Julius Cohnheim during the period 1868–1884.

It is of interest that the greatest knowledge about pathology during the last century resulted from work in an almost completely unrelated field of research, that carried out by the French chemist Louis Pasteur, who found that specific microorganisms were responsible for various types of fermentation in the production of wine and beer. This genius found that when particular bacteria grew in large numbers in the wine vats in France, the normal yeasts were overwhelmed and a "disease" of wine resulted with the production of lactic and acetic acid. On the basis of these studies and those he made on the diseases of silk worms, Pasteur's intuition told him that specific microorganisms could produce specific diseases in animals and by the late 1870s, along with Robert Koch, he proved this was the case with anthrax.

During the last twenty years of the century there were many discoveries that identified bacteria as the extrinsic factors or etiologies in the production of the following diseases: tuberculosis, plague, tetanus, diphtheria, cholera, pneumonia, glanders, meningitis, gonorrhea, leprosy, typhoid, some types of dysenteries, and Malta and relapsing fevers. Submicroscopic organisms, later called viruses, were suspected of producing rabies, yellow fever, foot and mouth disease, and smallpox. Certain types of fungi were found to produce superficial diseases such as ringworm, and some like actinomycoses could produce deep-tissue infections. Protozoans were found to be responsible for malaria and were soon found to be responsiblefor sleeping sickness as well. Thus the identity of the extrinsic factors for most of the severe diseases of Mankind were discovered during the nineteenth century. Soon there were studies of the immunological reactions to these organisms, which in many cases would lead to their prevention. Diseases produced by the metazoas, or those animals higher on the phylogenetic scale, had also been identified and the nature of infection by tapeworm, ascaris, schistosome, hookworm, liver and lung flukes, and trichina had been studied. By the beginning of the twentieth century however, the number of diseases whose etiologies were attributable to bacteria and protozoans began to diminish in number. Viruses were suspected in some diseases but were difficult to prove and had to await the development of new techniques of isolation and growth. In the meantime, diseases that would eventually be found to be due to intrinsic factors, such as neoplasia and dysfunction of the various organ systems, also had to wait until the normal physiology and biochemistry of these essential parts of the body were determined.

The result was that the frontier of pathology shifted from anatomic pathology and microbiology to return to pathological physiology where it was hoped that such conditions as diabetes, Grave's disease, Addison's disease, beri-beri, scurvy, anemia, and acidosis could be pathologically understood and treated. Although there were many microbiologists recruited from the early anatomic pathologists, the new frontier became the realm of physiologists, biochemists, or clinicians who were well trained in those disciplines. After 1900 there was a progressive drift of those individuals trained in anatomic pathology away from research and toward clinical service. The surgeon and internist needed such people to help them in diagnosis and therapy, and by the second quarter of the twentieth century, most anatomic pathologists were working in community hospitals performing autopsies and examining surgical specimens for evidence of malignancy. It is fair to say that during the twentieth century, Osler's dictum regarding pathology could be extrapolated to "as is our physiology and biochemistry, so is our pathology."

The difficulty in writing a history of pathology was the necessity of having to make arbitrary selections of discoveries and events that appeared to be the most important in bringing the state of knowledge of pathology and medicine to its high level near the end of the twentieth century. So many experiments and observations were occurring in biology and medicine in so many different places and times during the past two hundred years that only retrospective evaluations enable the historian to determine the significant discoveries that have survived the test of time and were used by other investigators as foundations on which to build. Although there was an explosion of research and discoveries after 1900 in pathology, nevertheless the groundwork was established during the nineteenth century; therefore this book is primarily about the period 1800-1900. Claude Bernard, in addition to saying "We stand upon the intellectual shoulders of those mental giants of bygone days, and because of the help they afford us, we are able to see a little more clearly than they were able to do," also said "while recognizing the superiority of great men, I think that the influence, particular or general they exert on science is always and by necessity a product of their time."[22]

Nevertheless there were some individuals, particularly during the nineteenth century, whose discoveries or leadership greatly influenced the study of pathology for later generations. These scientists give the historian focal points around which to produce a comprehensive matrix of the times and give continuity to the narrative.

At the risk of having this book criticized as simply a compilation of comments and writings of contemporary scientists and physicians, it is the author's belief that a book on history should present the reader with primary sources where possible so that no misinterpretation or subjectivity could change the meaning or emphasis of the individuals who lived during the periods under discussion. It is virtually impossible for a modern person with his outlook, knowledge, and value system to give a completely objective interpretation of people, their thoughts, and events that occurred one hundred to two hundred years before. The medical historian Lester King calls this "presentism," or attempting to interpret the past through meanings and values of today and considers it a "cardinal sin" in writing history.[23] Additionally, Michel de Montaigne, the famous sixteenth century essayist stated, "I quote others only the better to express myself."[24] This is still true today. Also, the author has attempted at times to humanize some of the famous scientists by quoting anecdotes written about them by contemporaries, because the personality of individuals sometimes gives a clue to their success. The book also will be cognizant of the fact that the progress in the study of pathology has not occurred in a geographically uniform manner, and different parts of the Western World made different contributions at different times often due to nonmedical reasons. William Osler in 1907 expressed this fact in his typical poetic manner by writing:

> Minerva Medica has never had her chief temples in any one country for more than a generation or two. For a long period at the Renaissance she dwelt in Northern Italy, and from all parts of the world men flocked to Padua and to Bologna. Then for some reason of her own she went to Holland where she set up her chief temple at Leyden with Boerhaave as her high priest. Uncertain for a time she flitted here [Vienna] with Boerhaave's pupils, van Sweiten and de Haën, and could she have come to terms about a

temple, she doubtless would have stayed permanently in London, where she found in John Hunter a great high priest. In the first four decades of the nineteenth century she lived in France, where she built a glorious temple to which all flocked. Why she left Paris, who can say? But suddenly she appeared here, and Rokitansky and Skoda rebuilt for her the temple of the new Vienna school, but she did not stay long. She had never settled in Northern Germany for though she loves art and science she hates with a deadly hatred philosophy and all philosophical systems applied to her favorite study. Her stately Grecian shrines, her beautiful Alexandrian home, her noble Roman temples, were destroyed by philosophy. Not until she saw in Johannes Müller and in Rudolf Virchow true and loyal disciples did she move to Germany, where she stays in spite of the tempting offers from France, from Italy, from England and from Austria. In an interview most graciously granted to me, as a votary of long standing, she expressed herself very well satisfied with her present home [Germany], where she has much honor and is everywhere appreciated. I boldly suggested that it was perhaps time to think of crossing the Atlantic and setting up her temple in the new world for a generation or two. I spoke of the many advantages, of the absence of tradition — here she visibly weakened, as she has suffered so much from this poison — the greater freedom, the enthusiasm; and then I spoke of missionary work. At these words she turned on me sharply and said: "That is not for me. We gods have but one motto — those that honor us we honor. Give me the temples, give me the priests, give me the true worship, the old Hippocratic service of the art and of the science of ministering to man, and I will come. By the eternal law under which we gods live, I would have to come. I did not wish to leave Paris, where I was so happy and where I was served so faithfully by Bichat, by Laennec and by Louis" and tears filled her eyes and her voice trembled with emotion "but where the worshipers are the most devoted, not, mark you, where they are most numerous; where the clouds of incense rise highes, there must my chief temple be, and to it from all quarters will the faithful flock. As it was in Greece, in Alexandria, in Rome, in northern Italy, in France, so it is now in Germany, and so it may be in the new world I long to see". Doubtless she will come, but not till the present crude organization of our medical clinics is changed, not until there is a fuller realization of internal medicine as a science as well as an art.[25]

That Minerva Medica moved to the United States shortly after Osler wrote this passage from Vienna in 1907, and has remained here for most of the twentieth century, is certainly a fact. During this time knowledge about disease has been exponential in growth. The reasons for her delay in coming to the new world were basically a function of our American value system, and the author discusses his reasons why there is danger that Minerva Medica will go elsewhere in the next century.

Bibliography

1. Lavoisier, A.L., and De La Place, P.S., *De la combustion et la respiration. Oeuvres de Lavoisier*, Volume 11, Article I, p. 331. Imprimerie Imperiale, Paris, 1854.
2. Descartes, R., De Homine, 1664, in Suner, A.D., *Classics of Biology*, p. 286. Philosophical Library, N.Y., 1955.
3. La Mettrie, J.O., *Man, A Machine* (1748). The Open Court Publishing Co., La Salle, Illinois, 1961.
4. Needham, J., Mechanistic Biology and the Religious Consciousness, p. 249, in *Science, Religion, and Reality*. George Brazilier, Inc., N.Y., 1955.
5. Watson, J.D., and Crick, F., A Structure for Deoxyribose Nucleic Acid. *Nature*, **171**, p. 737, 1953.
6. Lehninger, A.L., *Principles of Biochemistry*, Chapter 29. Work Publishing Co., N.Y., 1982.
7. Stent, G.S., Book Review of Neurophilosophy, by P.S. Churchland, *Science*, **236**, p. 990, 1987.
8. von Bertalanffy, L., *Problems of Life*, p. 124. John Wiley and Sons, Inc. London, 1952.
9. Plato, in Symposia, quoted from Florkin, M., *History of Biochemistry in Comprehensive Biochemistry*, Vol. 30, p. 97. Elsevier Pub. Co., Amsterdam, 1972.
10. Staniforth, M., *Marcus Aurelius Meditations*. Dorset Press, N.Y., 1964.
11. Benninghoff, A., Über Einheiten und Systembildungen im Organismus. *Dtsch. Med. Wschr.* quoted in Ref. 8, page 135.
12. Schoenheimer, R., *The Dynamic State of the Body Constituents*. Harvard Univ. Press, Cambridge, Mass., 1949.
13. Schoenheimer, R., Ratner, S., and Rittenberg, D., Studies in protein metabolism, *J. Biol. Chem.*, **130**, p. 703.
14. Ref. 6, p. 352.
15. Bernard, C., *Leçons sur les propriétés physiologiques et les alterations pathologiues des liquides de l'organisme*. Vol. I, p. 42. J.B. Baillière, Paris, 1859.
16. Henderson, L. J., *Blood, A Study in General Physiology*. Yale Univ. Press, New Haven, 1928.
17. Cannon, W. B., Organization for Homeostasis. *Physiol. Rev.* **9**, 399, 1929.

18. Barcroft, J., *Features in the Architecture of Physiological Function.* Univ. Press, Cambridge, England, 1934.
19. Starling, E.H., Croonian Lectures on the Chemical Correlation of the Functions of the Body. *Lancet*, **2**, pp. 339. 423, 501, 579, 1905.
20. Sherrington, C.S., *The Integrative Action of the Nervous System.* Yale Univ. Press. New Haven, 1906.
21. Osler, W., Quoted in Boyd, *Textbook of Pathology,* p. 4, 7th Edition. Lea and Febiger, 1961.
22. Bernard, Claude, *An Introduction to the Study of Experimental Medicine*, p. 224. Dover Publications, N.Y., 1957.
23. King, L., *Transformations in American Medicine*, p. 18. Johns Hopkins Univ. Press, Baltimore, 1991.
24. Montaigne, M., in Tyron Edwards, *Useful Quotations.* Grosset and Dunlap, N.Y., 1933.
25. Osler, W., Vienna after Thirty-Four Years, *J.A.M.A.*, May 9, p. 1523, 1908.

CHAPTER I

Life can only be understood backwards, but it must be lived forwards.

—Kierkegaard

Pathology from Prehistoric Times to the Nineteenth Century

The Earliest Ideas on Disease

A history of the development of Man's understanding of the diseases that affect him, particularly those of a pestilent nature, in many ways parallels the history of human thought, primarily because both are so directly related to his ultimate questions regarding life and death. Because of Man's delusion of self-importance, it was natural that the earliest explanations for pestilences were similar to those for other catastrophes such as famine, droughts, floods, and earthquakes — simply that it was the result of the actions of angry gods or evil spirits who would either project something noxious into the bodies of the victims or remove something vital. Meteorological conditions or positions of the celestial bodies were also sometimes blamed. Because of these beliefs, priests, magicians, or medicine men would be called upon to restore health through incantations or the giving of potions.

Although they obtained some of their knowledge from the Egyptians, Babylonians, Cretans, and Hebrews, the Greeks produced the first famous physicians. The greatest ones were Hippocrates (460–370 B.C.) and Galen (131–201 A.D.). Hippocrates did not perform dissections or experiments and had little faith in theories about disease, but he did stress the importance of making detailed observations on patients throughout their illnesses. In this manner he was able to diagnose and make accurate prognoses for many diseases. His description of tuberculosis, puerperal fever, epilepsy, mumps, and the various forms of malarial fevers are still, for the most part, valid today. Galen, on the other hand, dissected many animals (including apes), and wrote extensive treatises on anatomy, physiology, and pathology. Many of his findings were correct, but his theories on physiology and pathology were, in retrospect, worthless. Galen's concept of disease was essentially that of the Humoral Doctrine, which had been passed on from antiquity. This theory was based on the belief that there were four humors in the body, blood, phlegm, and yellow and black bile, which were supposed to be in perfect balance during health. When an individual became ill, his case was diagnosed according to which of the four humors might temporarily be in excess. The individual's natural healing powers would then endeavor with the help of the physician to restore the ideal balance. Imbalances were thought to occur during illness because of the observations of the various quantities, colors, and consistencies of the discharges from the nose and mouth in diseases of the respiratory tract, the vomitus and feces in diseases of the digestive tract, the type of suppuration of abscesses in the various parts of the body, together with the character and quantity of urine excreted. The concept of imbalance of the humors together with other theories of Galen were accepted as gospel until the middle of the seventeenth century, and remnants of these ideas were not completely eliminated from Western medical thought until the middle of the nineteenth century.

Stagnation of Thought during the Middle Ages (450 A.D.–1400 A.D.)

Why did these theories last so long? Historians are almost unanimous in their explanations for the stagnation of scientific and medical knowledge for more than one thousand years. The problem was that, with the decline of the Roman civilization, the Christian church became stronger both religiously and politically, and its officials and monks became the dominating factor in the life of all the communities throughout Europe. In spite of the fact that the churches and monasteries contained for a time the books and relics of learning of the Greco-Roman civilization, they ignored them. Concern or interest in the material world and particularly curiosity about the human body, which was regarded as only the temporary container of the all-important soul, was censured. Any attempts at systematic observations of nature or experimentation was condemned as sinful meddling. Worldly things were regarded as unworthy of pure Christian thought, and only prayer and preparation for eternal life was considered important. As a result, ideas about and knowledge of art, science, philosophy, and medicine were essentially lost.

As evidence for this fact, one of the mysteries in the history of art is the nonprogressive, stereotypical, often grotesque and primitive portrayal of the human being in paintings during the Christian Era for almost a thousand years. There were certainly examples of painting and sculpture from the times of the Romans, who copied the great art of the Greeks, that portray the human figure and face in a natural and ideal way that has never been surpassed. If they could not be improved upon by the Christian artists, they could have at least been copied. The answer to the mystery is most likely that it was deliberate; this was expressed by the ninth century theologian, Johannes Scotus Erigena, who feared that portraying the human figure as beautiful and an object of admiration in sacred pictures might lead the faithful toward an appreciation of the seen rather than the unseen world, toward false rather than true beauty. With this philosophy it is not surprising that human anatomy was not studied for a thousand years. However, there were times when discussions of a biological nature by the church hierarchy could not be avoided, and when this occurred the authorities referred to the works of Galen or Aristotle. Galen, who was primarily concerned with medicine, wrote in a dogmatic manner and essentially closed the book on every subject he studied. Although he did not propose a God that created everything in the universe, he teleologically came to many conclusions based upon his own notions of a preconceived design in all of nature. This approach, together with his leaving no open questions about the human in health and disease, posed no threat to the church; eventually his ideas were considered infallible, and to doubt their truth was deemed a sacrilege.

Science and Medicine during the Renaissance (1400 A.D.–1600 A.D.)

The advent of the Renaissance in 1400 in western Europe was like an explosion of human activity. The seeds of these endeavors had been planted primarily by the contacts over the centuries with the Moslem world where the great works of the Greek scholars had been preserved and translated from Greek to Arabic. From the second half of the eighth to the end of the eleventh century, Arabic had become the scientific language of Mankind, although the scholars of that time were primarily Persians, Jews, or Spaniards. Although these individuals spent most of their time simply translating, in certain areas of knowledge they made valuable contributions of their own, particularly in the precursor of chemistry, known as alchemy, where they developed the processes of extraction, distillation, sublimation, precipitation, and production of pure metals and their salts.

There were two major pathways in which this knowledge was passed to the Christian world. The first was through the endeavors of the North African Christian monk Constantine (1015–1087), who came to the struggling medical school at Salerno in the eleventh century where he translated many works of Hippocrates from Arabic to Latin. The more important source was through the Latin translators in Spain, of whom the most important was Gerard (1115–1185). His successors continued this work until the middle of the thirteenth century. Then in 1450 Gutenberg developed the printing press, and, with the new mills producing cheap paper to replace vellum, as many as twenty million volumes of books were produced during the following hundred years to an increasingly literate population.

The years 1400-1495 saw the greatest achievement in art and architecture, and daring mariners with their new compasses and knowledge of heavenly bodies sailed out into the unknown seas with the result that Columbus discovered the New World and Magellan's crew circled the earth. The result of all these activities soon came into conflict with the dogma and asceticism of the Catholic church. The result was the monumental breaking out of the Reformation throughout Europe. However, in biology and medicine the advancements were minimal. The famous Arabic physicians Avicenna (980–1037), Hali Abbas (d. 994), and Rhazes (860–932) made accurate descriptions of diseases such as smallpox and measles; made minimal improvements in surgery; and added many but-for-the-most-part ineffectual medicinal, botanical, and chemical substances to the medical armamentarium. But the teachings of Islam were similar to that of the Christian church in that autopsies or human dissections, which were absolutely necessary for the important study of anatomy, physiology, and pathology, were not performed. It is thus not surprising that the ideas of Galen continued to dominate the minds of the medical community.

It is certainly true that medical scholars were inspired by the new translations into Latin of the Hellenistic-Islamic works, but the emphasis was on books not on facts, such as are acquired by firsthand observations, and certainly not on experiments. Paracelsus (1493–1541), the fiery physician and alchemist, challenged the teachings of Galen in a dramatic manner that gave him great fame, but basically he substituted Galenic humors with equally unproven and untenable ones of his own. According to Garrison,[1] postmortem examinations began to be carried out on a limited basis toward the end of the thirteenth century, and a few more were performed in the cities of Venice, Florence, and Siena in the fourteenth century. Although it was inevitable that isolated pathological observations would have been made by these autopsies, it is unlikely that with their poor knowledge of normal anatomy the early dissectors would have been able to make significant findings. An exception was the work of Antonio Benivieni (1440–1502), a Florentine surgeon, which was entitled *On the Hidden and Wonderful Causes of Diseases*[2] and was based upon 100 autopsies. In this work he described the lesions associated with syphilis, which became almost epidemic during the last part of the fifteenth century. He also found gall bladder stones in a woman who had suffered from pain in that region, a "callus," which was undoubtedly a carcinoma, in the stomach of a man who could not longer eat, calculi in the urinary bladder, an erosion of the bones of the forehead, most likely a syphilitic lesion, and a perforation of the intestine. But for the most part dissections were primarily to demonstrate to medical students the validity of Galen's anatomy. Thus, whereas the Renaissance produced great works in art, architecture, philosophy, and literature, biology and medicine lagged greatly behind.

Before progress could be made in medicine, it was necessary to obtain the important knowledge about the structure of the human body which could only be gained by routine and systematic dissections carried out by learned men. This was a major problem. The church would only permit the occasional dissection on an executed criminal, which limited the routine and repetitive observations necessary for acquiring real knowledge of the structure of the human body, but the men who were supposedly qualified to teach anatomy for the most part came from a social class where manual and particularly odious tasks were performed by servants. Therefore for centuries, the anatomy professor, by traditional reading from the works of Galen, supervised the occasional dissection performed by a servant or barber while the cadaver was putrefying and the important structures were often disintegrating. If by chance there was a discrepancy between the findings of the servant and Galen, it was ignored because it was dangerous to contradict the Greek whose works were regarded as infallible by the church.

Andreas Vesalius

The change started with the career of Andreas Vesalius, a young Belgian born into an illustrious medical family in 1514 and who was fascinated with the anatomy of animals and dissected many rats, cats, and dogs. He studied first at Louvain but then went at age 17 to study in Paris under Jacobus Sylvius (1498–1555), a staunch and uncritical Galenist. He was not satisfied with the method of teaching anatomy in Paris, and returned to Louvain where he taught anatomy on the limited number of cadavers available to medical students. After a short time he went to Venice where independent ideas were tolerated and excellent opportunities were available for routine dissections without having to steal bodies from cemeteries and gallows. At the age of 22 he was awarded the medical degree and in recognition of his talent was appointed head of surgery and anatomy in nearby Padua. There he taught for five years and carried out dissections, noting errors in Galen's works, which finally resulted in his publication in 1543 of *On the Fabric of the Human Body*,[3] known historically as the *Fabrica*. He left Padua to monitor the printing of his books in Switzerland but was unprepared for the storm that occurred with its release. He was castigated, not only by his old mentor Sylvius, but by other prestigious anatomists in Europe. He offered to substantiate all of his findings that contradicted Galen but to no avail. In a fit of anger, he burned many of his manuscripts that had not been published, and retired from the field of anatomy. He became the court physician to Charles V and later to Philip II of Spain. Essentially he never performed dissections again, dying on the island of Zante on his way back from a pilgrimage to Jerusalem. But though he probably never realized it, his *Fabrica*, with its magnificent illustrations, would become the foundation of modern medicine until the time of William Harvey. There were other great anatomists [Bartolomeo Eustachi (1520-1570), Realdo Colombo (1516–1559), Gabriele Falloppio (1523-1562)] who were contemporaries of Vesalius and who added to the knowledge in the *Fabrica*. Some of them noted pathological findings in some of their cadavers. In 1554, Jean Fernel published his famous *Medicina*[4] in which he not only described appendicitis and endocarditis but suggested that syphilis could be responsible for aneurysms. He was the first to use the term *pathology* in the modern sense.

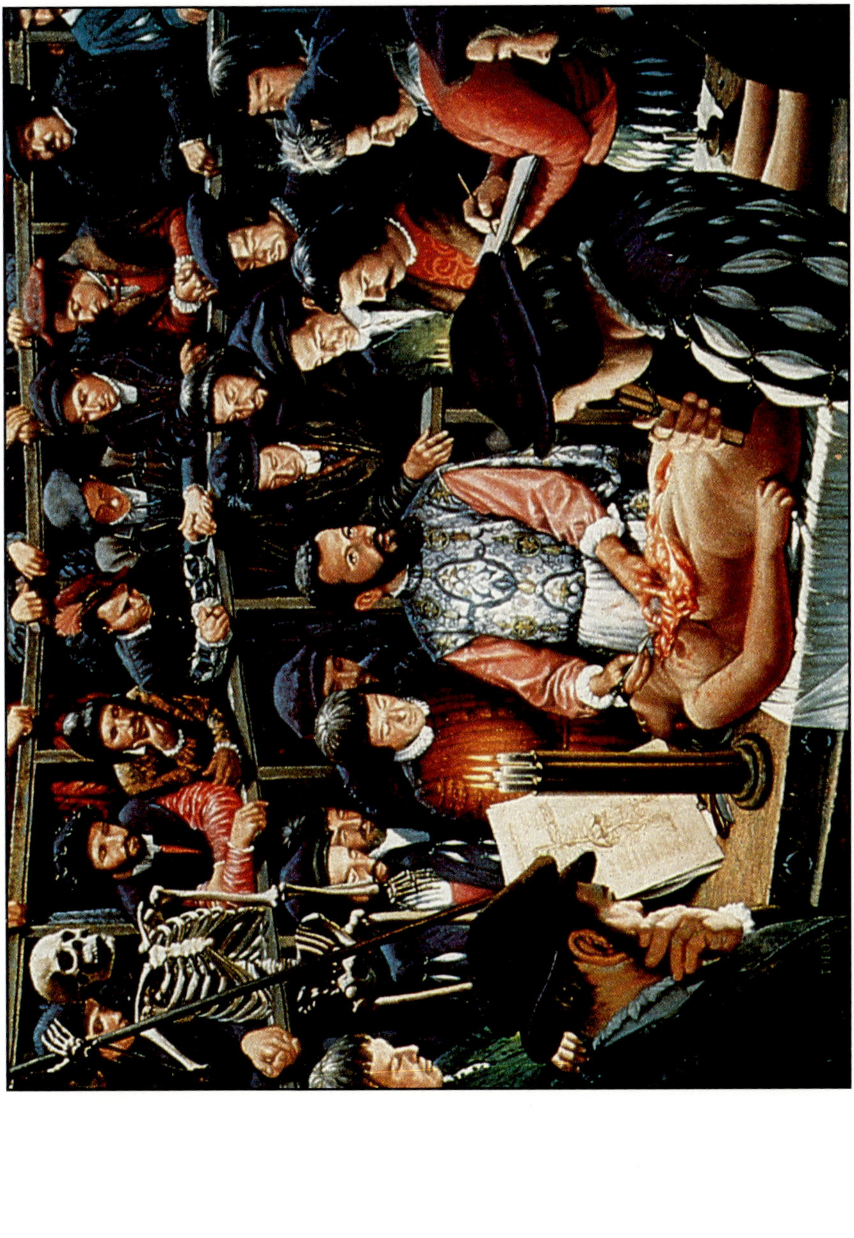

VESALIUS AND THE ANATOMY OF MAN

Science and Medicine during the Seventeenth Century — The Age of Reason

It was in the seventeenth century that the spirit of the Renaissance really showed its effects in science and philosophy. The intellectual climate of the Western World was never the same after this period. This was the time of Galileo (1564-1642), Newton (1642-1727), Kepler (1571–1630), Huygens (1629-1695), Pascal (1623-1662), Leibniz (1646-1716), and Boyle (1627–1691) in the physical sciences and mathematics; Locke (1642-1704), Bacon (1561-1626), Descartes (1596-1650) and Spinoza (1632-1677) in philosophy; and Harvey (1578-1657), Leeuwenhoek (1632-1723), Swammerdam (1637-1680), de Graaf (1641-1673), Malpighi (1628-1694), Sydenham (1628-1694), Willis (1621-1675), and Lower (1631-1691) in biology and medicine. And what was the essential ingredient of this new spirit? It was the recognition that true knowledge regarding nature could only be achieved by experimentation rather than by deductive reasoning. This was best expressed in Francis Bacon's publication *Novum Organum*, which first appeared in 1620. He wrote that:

> There are and can be only two ways of searching into and discovering truth. The one flies from the senses and particulars to the most general axioms, and from these principles, the truth of which it takes for settled and immovable, proceeds to judgment and to the discovery of middle axioms. And this way is now in fashion. The other derives axioms from the senses and particulars rising by a gradual and unbroken ascent, so that it arrives at the most general axioms last of all. This is the true way, but as yet untried. . . . Both ways set out from the senses and particulars, and rest in the highest generalities; but the difference between them is infinite. For the one just glances at experiment and particulars in passing, the other dwells duly and orderly among them. The one, again, begins at once by establishing certain abstract and useless generalities; the other rises by gradual steps to that which is prior and better known in the order of nature.[5]

It is difficult for a modern scientist, who has been taught the experimental method from his first dissection of a frog or his first experiment in the chemistry laboratory in high school, to realize that though this type of thought essentially started in the seventeenth century, it was only during the eighteenth and nineteenth century that it became widespread in use. In the most respected universities in Europe, such as Oxford and Cambridge, during the seventeenth century, the experimental method was non-existent, and the great scientists such as Newton and Boyle had to form the Royal Society to support their activities.

William Harvey

The English biologist William Harvey, like Vesalius before him, went to Padua where experimentation was encouraged. Just as Vesalius became the father of anatomy in Italy, William Harvey became the father of physiology there. He discovered the circulation of the blood, and his work was a classic in experimentation. By observing the contractions of the heart in many different species, and studying the valves in the heart and the veins, he came to the conclusion that the blood in the body flowed in one direction. Based on the size of the chambers, he calculated that each time the human heart contracted, at least two ounces of blood were driven into the large vessels leaving the heart, and that the weight of the blood pumped in one hour was greater than the weight of the entire body. He did not find any pores between the ventricles as stated by Galen, and the only logical conclusions from his findings was that the blood made a circle in the body. He published his findings in his classical 72-page *De Motus Cordis et Sanguinis in Animalibus* in 1628.[6] He did not work with the microscope, therefore the discovery of the capillary network to establish proof of the circulation of the blood had to await the observations of Malpighi in 1661.[7] Nevertheless, the work of Harvey was monumental, and more than two hundred years later William Osler stated with regard to the *De Motus Cordis et Sanguinis in Animalibus:*

> To the age of the hearer, in which men had heard and heard only, had succeeded the age of the eye in which men had seen and had been content only to see, but at last came the age of the hand — the thinking, devising, planning hand, the hand as an instrument of the mind, now reintroduced into the world in a modest little monograph from which we may date the beginning of experimental medicine. [8]

Osler was correct except that it would be more than a hundred years after Harvey's experiments that routine use of "the hand as an instrument of the mind" became commonplace, and would lead to an ex-

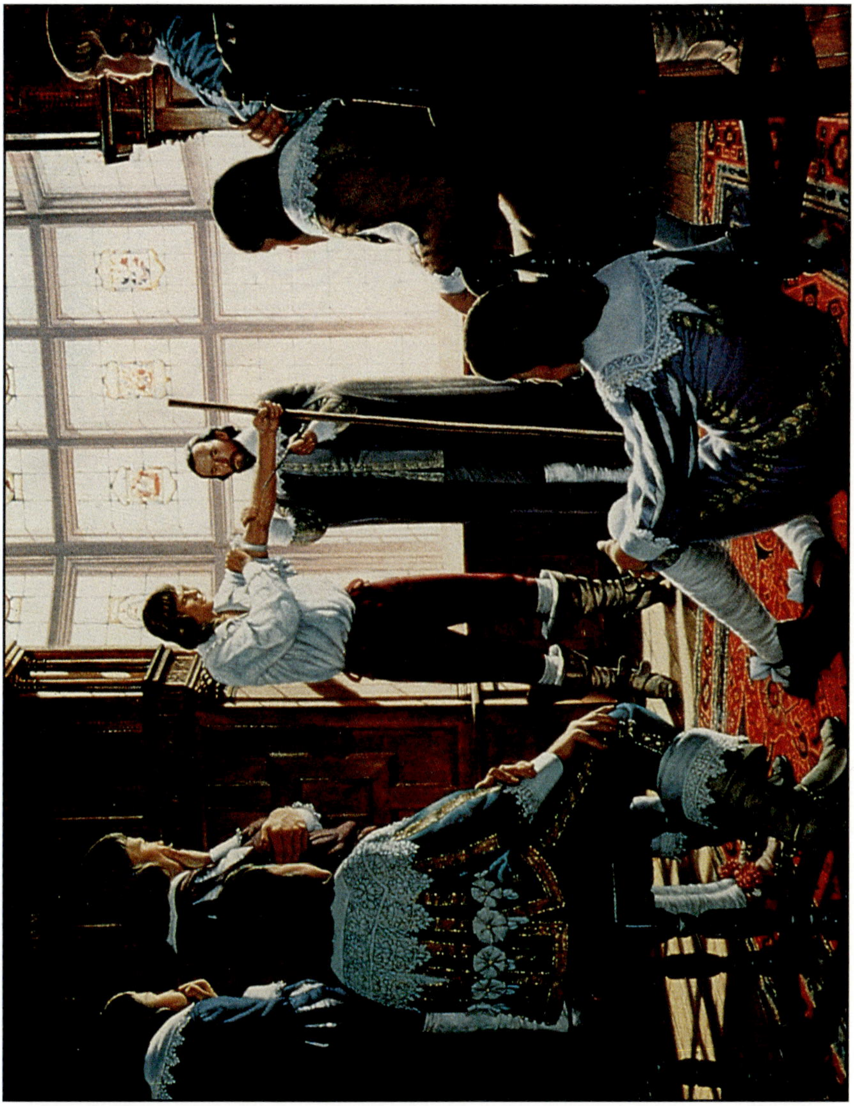

HARVEY AND THE CIRCULATION OF BLOOD

plosion in knowledge in biology and medicine. Other cultures, such as those in the Orient where dissection was prohibited or discouraged, made essentially no advancements in biology and medicine from ancient times.

The "Invisible Colleges"

It is interesting to note that because universities were not supportive of the experimental method, "invisible colleges" were organized outside of the institutions of higher learning.[9] The Royal Society was established in England in 1662, the Academie Royale de Sciences in France in 1666, and the Accademia de Cimento of Florence in 1657. They all encouraged experimental work and published the results of their members in their respective journals. The major individuals that these organizations supported during the seventeenth century were Issac Newton, who made monumental discoveries regarding gravitation, motion, and light; Robert Boyle, who carried out careful experiments in chemistry, and in his book *The Sceptical Chemist*[10] demolished the Aristotelian four elements of fire, earth, air, and water, which were believed for more than 2000 years; and finally Leeuwenhoek, who working at home in Holland and grinding his own microscope lenses made remarkable observations identifying blood cells, bacteria, and protozoa but made no speculations on their function.[11]

Minerva Medica Contemplates Moving from Italy to Holland

Although during the sixteenth and seventeenth centuries, northern Italy with its universities at Padua and Bologna were the sites of the great discoveries of Vesalius and Harvey, the anti-reformation influence of the Jesuits had an inhibiting effect on those institutions, and the seeking of new knowledge in science was discouraged. The result was that the more intellectually curious students no longer found those centers attractive. Fortunately one of the students of *Fabrica* at Padua, Jan Heurnius (1542–1601), returned to his home in Holland where he was appointed Professor of Medicine and Anatomy in Leyden in 1581. There in addition to his anatomical demonstrations, he had limited success in teaching medicine at the bedside using the method of Hippocrates. He was succeeded by his son, Otto (1577-1650), and after his son's death, by Francis de le Boë (1614-1672). The latter was a fine anatomist and had as his students, Willis, de Graaf, Stensen, and Swammerdam. He studied saliva, pancreatic juice, and bile, which he believed was important in converting food into blood. In pathology, he was the first to show that tubercles progress to cavities, but he seems to have taken the most pride in his teaching students at the bedside. He stated that:

> I led them by the very hand into the practice of medicine, that is, I took them daily into the public hospital for the purpose of seeing the sick to whose complaints and other notable symptoms I directed attention, asking immediately afterwards what they had observed in the disorders of their patients; their views as to the causes and proper treatment, and their reasons for the same. Whenever differences of opinion arose among them concerning these things, I, in a quiet way, pitted against each other those holding different opinions, in order that they might mutually satisfy themselves by as solid reasons as possible drawn from every source, finally giving my own judgment regarding the various views. With me they confirmed the happy results of the treatment, when God rewarded our labours by the return to health of the patients, or assisted in the examination of the cadavers when the patients finally paid the inevitable tribute to death.[12]

It is remarkable that in addition to medicine, other areas of human endeavors in Holland had their own special renaissance to the extent that it is fair to say that this small country became the intellectual and artistic center of the Western world. It illustrated one of the mysterious happenings when many creative geniuses in different fields appear in a small geographic area and in a comparatively short period of time. In addition to the medical scholars during this period of time, Spinoza, Leeuwenhoek, de Graaf, Huygens, Swammerdam in philosophy and science and Rembrandt (1606–1669), Vermeer (1632–1685), Hals (1580–1666), de Hooch (1629–1684), Ruysdael (1628–1682), and Hobbema (1638–1709) in art were active in Holland. It is possible that the economic success of the Dutch (their large merchant fleet, rich cities, a wealthy new middle class, freedom of speech and press, and toleration of various new ideas never before seen in Europe) encouraged these geniuses in art and science, but it is difficult to find a direct connection. In any case, it was under these influences that the medical school of Hermann Boerhaave arose at the end of the seventeenth century.

Science and Medicine during the Eighteenth Century — The Age of Enlightenment

Hermann Boerhaave

The Dutch physician Hermann Boerhaave (1668–1738) continued and expanded the pioneering work of Jan and Otto Heurnius and Francis de le Boë. Boerhaave was appointed Professor of Medicine in 1709 and taught there in Leyden to thousands of medical students until his death in 1738. The success of Boerhaave was based primarily on his personality; he was a sympathetic and kindhearted man with a genius for teaching and exposition using simple, practical, and graphic concepts in the manner of Hippocrates and Sydenham. He was also a tireless worker and wrote several books on medicine and chemistry, none of which ever showed him to be creative in a scientific sense. But, like William Osler, he must have been one of those true masters of the art of medicine, which enabled him to inspire medical students and patients alike. During his period of teaching, there were terrible epidemics of typhus and other diseases for which there was no therapy, but Boerhaave's popularity as a physician never diminished.

In 1718 the students found their days planned for them. Boerhaave lectured four or five hours each day, teaching physics, chemistry, physiology, and anatomy. Later in the day, he taught the students at the patient's bedside, all in systematic fashion. His students in the autumn of that year included several young men from Edinburgh, one being Alexander Monro (1697–1767). Monro, his son (1737–1817), and grandson (1773–1859), taught anatomy at the University of Edinburgh for a span of over a hundred years. John Rutherford (1695–1779) was another of Boerhaave's students and became Professor of Medicine at the same school, always using the Boerhaave approach to patients. It has been estimated that during Boerhaave's career as many as 1500 students from Scotland studied in Leyden, and several were instrumental in making Edinburgh a new Mecca for students during the eighteenth century. This important medical center will be discussed later because there were several very important English-speaking medical figures in the fields of pathology and medicine who studied there.

The Old Vienna School of Medicine

At the same time, while the Boerhaave school spawned the

Edinburgh Medical School in Scotland, it was also responsible for the establishment of the Old Vienna School of Medicine. Maria Theresa, the Empress of the Hapsburg Empire, recognizing the backwardness of medical practice in Austria, asked a disciple of Boerhaave, Gerhard van Sweiten (1700–1772), to come to Vienna in 1745 to rectify the stagnation of medical education there. To accomplish this task, the empress gave van Sweiten full authority as her Director of Health to make any changes he desired. Ruthlessly he discharged almost all of the professors of the old medical faculty and brought in new individuals that he thought could modernize the school. He hired Anton de Haën (1704–1776), also a student of Boerhaave, to be in charge of the Vienna City Hospital, where a new emphasis was placed upon careful observation and recording of data on each patient. There was a de-emphasis on medication, and reliance on the body to heal itself. It is noteworthy that de Haën used a thermometer to illustrate that a fever could occur during a severe chill and called attention to the sign of amenorrhea associated with a tumor of the pituitary. The newest knowledge in the fields of chemistry, botany, anatomy, physiology, surgery, and medicine was taught to the students, and van Sweiten gave special courses in anatomy to rural surgeons. The program was continued after the deaths of both van Sweiten and de Haën in 1776 under the leadership of such outstanding men as Anton Störck (1731–1803), Maximilian Stoll (1742–1788), and Johann Peter Frank (1745–1821). When the famous General Hospital was founded in 1784 and Frank was made director, he recognized that there were significant opportunities for developing anatomic pathology because there were as many as 14,000 patients passing through the hospital each year. Therefore he added a morgue, a postmortem room to the hospital, and appointed Alois Vetter (1765–1806) to be the first-full professor. Vetter dissected several thousand bodies and built a museum for interesting specimens, but he did not practice pathology in a systematic manner, and aside from the observation of gross oddities there was very little basic knowledge attained in pathology.

Giovanni Battista Morgagni

In spite of the fact that the center of medical excellence shifted to Northern Europe, Italy had its medical stars. The most illustrious figure in eighteenth century pathology was Giovanni Battista Morgagni (1682–1771), who when he died left to the world a magnificent work which he published in 1761 in five volumes called *De Sedibus et Causis Morborum.*[13] This work included the precise pathological and clinical observations and their correlation by both the author and his mentor A. Valsalva (1666–1723). The intent was to establish a methodology in which diagnoses and prognoses in various disease states could be made with better accuracy, by illustrating distortions of normal anatomy. Some of the more notable correlations were clearly related cerebral hemorrhage with apoplexy; brain lesions with paralysis of the opposite side; cardiac or aortic aneurysm ruptures with sudden death; vegetative endocarditis with urethral gonorrhea; and bone, liver, and brain disease in syphilis. He also described inflammatory consolidation of the lung associated with pneumonia, cirrhosis with acute yellow atrophy of the liver, intestinal ulcers, neoplasms of many different organs, and what, in retrospect, were most likely metastatic neoplastic lesions.

There was an essential difference in the work of Morgagni compared with the observations of other early autopsy studies made by such men as Jean Fernel (1497–1558), Felix Platter (1536–1614), Volcher Coiter (1534–1576), Marcello Donato (1538–1602), Pieter van Foreest (1522–1597), Johann Schenck von Grafenberg (1530–1598), Marco Aurelio Severino (1580–1656), Nicolas Tulp (1593–1674), Francis de le Boë (1614–1672), Johann Wepfer (1620–1685), Thomas Willis (1621–1675), Richard Morton (1637–1698), Marcello Malpighi (1628–1694), Theophile Bonet (1620–1689), Theodore Kerckring (1640–1693), Frederik Ruysch (1638–1731), Raymond de Vieussens (1641–1715), Jean Astruc (1684–1766), Jean Baptiste de Senac (1693–1770), Joseph Lieutaud (1703–1780), Giovanni Lancisi (1654–1720), and Eduard Sandifort (1742–1814). Morgagni's work was much more careful in the descriptions of lesions, and he was the first to make excellent correlations with many clinical signs and symptoms. Essentially, as an anatomist he was interested in finding the "seats of disease" in the form of lesions. However, there were other individuals, usually clinicians, who were not interested in anatomic pathology but thought that diseases could be classified like plants and animals on the basis of the various signs and symptoms. These were the "disease taxonomists" and theorists who developed elaborate systems to explain not only the cause of the disease but also attempted to explain the signs and symptoms of each malady. For the most part these ideas were throwbacks to the method of attempting to achieve new knowledge by deduction or superficial correlations of these signs and symptoms. Almost all of these ideas fell into disrepute by the end of the nineteenth century when experimentation negated their premises. But nevertheless some of their ideas had validity, and they will be discussed in the next chapter.

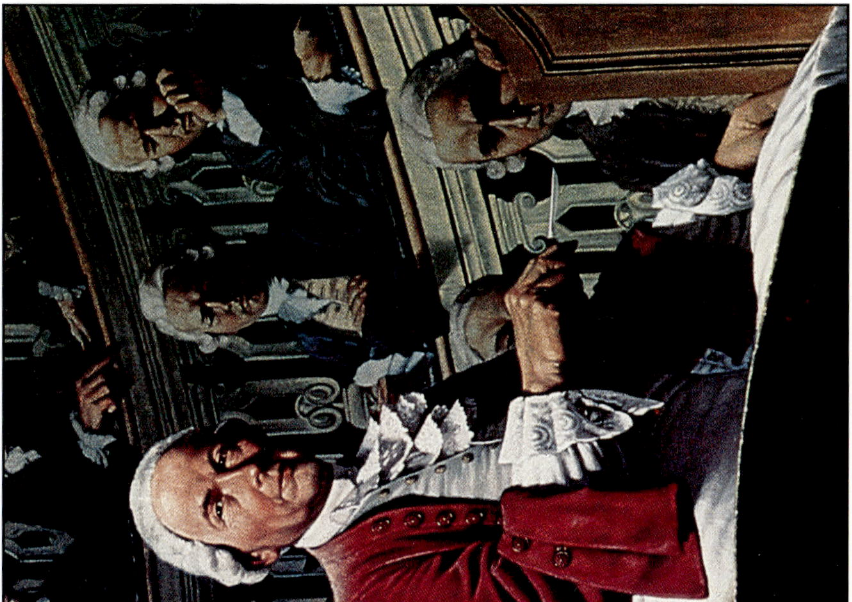

MORGAGNI AND PATHOLOGIC ANATOMY

Bibliography

1. Garrison, F.H., *An Introduction to the History of Medicine*, p. 228, 4th Edition. W.B. Saunders, Philadelphia, 1929.
2. Benivieni, A., *De abditis nonnulis ac mirandis morborum et sanationum causis*. P. Giuntae, Florence, 1507.
3. Vesalius, A., *De humani corporis fabrica libri septem*. Basel, 1543.
4. Fernel, J., *Medicina, Part 2 on Pathology*. Christian Wechel, Paris, 1548.
5. Bacon, F., First of Aphorisms, XIX, in *Works of Francis Bacon*, by J. Spaulding. Ellis and Heath, London, 1857.
6. Harvey, W., Exercitatio anatomica de motu cordis et sanguinis in animalibus. Fitzeri, Frankfurt, 1628. Translation in English in *Readings in History of Physiology*, J. Fulton, C. Thomas. Springfield, Ill., 1930.
7. Malpighi, M., De pulmonibus observationes anatomicae, B. Ferronius, Bonn, 1661. Translation in English in Readings in History of Physiology, C. Thomas, Springfield, Ill., 1930.
8. Osler, W., *An Alabama Student*. p. 329, Oxford Univ. Press, London, 1908.
9. Ornstein, M., *The Role of Scientific Societies in the Seventeenth Century*. Univ. of Chicago Press, Chicago, 1938.
10. Boyle, R., *The Sceptical Chemist*. Caldwell and Crooke, London, 1661.
11. Dobell, C., *Antony van Leeuwenhoek and His "Little Animals."* Dover, N.Y. 1960.
12. Newman, G., *Bicentenary of Faculty of Medicine of Univ. of Edinburgh, 1726-1926*. Univ. Edinburgh Press, 1926.
13. Morgagni, J.B., *De sedibus et causis morborum per anatomen indagatis libri quinque*. Remondiniana, Venice, 1761, English Translation by B. Alexander, London, 1769.

CHAPTER II

History is the essence of innumerable biographies.
— Carlyle

The Disease Taxonomists

With the advent of the Renaissance, other theories on the mechanisms of disease began to appear to take the place of or modify the theory of the four humors of Galen, although none had any experimental basis. Particularly in the sixteenth and seventeenth centuries, inroads were made into Galenism due to the advances in chemistry and physics, which led to the systems of iatrochemistry and iatrophysics.

Iatrochemistry was a point of view initiated by Paracelsus and promoted by Johann van Helmont (1577–1644), who emphasized the importance of ferments such as that in the stomach and intestine. Although he was not able to measure acid and base, he speculated that disease could be produced when these substances were out of balance. It would be a rather extreme extrapolation to believe van Helmont had any real understanding of our modern diagnoses of acidosis and alkalosis, any more than it is valid to consider Democritus the founder of the atomic theory of matter. Later Giovanni Borelli (1608–1679), a professor of mathematics influenced by his friend Marcello Malpighi when both were teaching at the University of Pisa, decided that physiology could best be explained by using mathematics and physics as tools rather than experimentation and was founder of the iatromathematical school.[1] He did study the movements of the musculoskeletal system with some interesting results, but he did not address the problem of disease in any more than a cursory manner. These ideas quickly lost their popularity as more medical and biological data became available. In the eighteenth century other medical systems developed, none of which had any lasting merit. Boerhaave had an eclectic system; Georg Stahl (1660–1734), a dynamico-organic system; William Cullen (1712–1790), a nervous pathology; Christoph Ludwig Hoffman (1721–1807), an irritation system; Johann Kampf (died 1753), the Doctrine of Infarctus, or fecal impaction with intoxication; Theophile de Bordeu (1722-1776), the "tripod of life" theory in which the heart, stomach, and brain are in balance and control health; Johann Christian Reil (1759-1813), the Doctrine of Vital Force where each organ has its own vital power, and disease is an aberration of these forces; Franz Mesmer (1734-1815), the theory of animal magnetism; J.B.T. Baumes (died 1815), the theory of generalized chyismus, which divided diseases into five classes, oxygenated, calorified, hydrogenized, nitrogenized, and phosphorized; John Brown (1735–1788), the Brunonian system based on external and internal irritations. Though the Brunonian system was popular for many years, it was based upon such nebulous ideas as excitement and irritation. The problem again was that these individuals essentially ignored the recommendations of Francis Bacon with regard to experimentation and continued to make speculative deductions.

Thomas Sydenham

Although Harvey had provided an experimental foundation for the study of physiology, there were still no comparable bases for the investigation of pathology. Nevertheless, there was still a need for careful observation in clinical medicine as a prelude to the further study of pathology and this was the message of Thomas Sydenham (1624–1689).[2] This practicing physician was an admirer of Francis Bacon, and took to heart his advice of collecting examples of diseases, making precise observations of the various signs and symptoms they presented, and then classifying them according to their similarities, which is the method used by botanists with various types of plants. Sydenham made careful notes regarding the time of year the disease appeared and that such general signs and symptoms such as malaise, fever, and headache should be discounted and only distinct ones were to be considered. With acute diseases such as smallpox, chickenpox, mumps, and measles, he did quite well and was able to differentiate measles from scarlet fever. With chronic diseases it was more difficult, but he was able to distinguish gout, syphilis, and chorea as distinct entities. Sydenham had no faith in any of the medical systems, but believed that, just as the Creator was responsible for creating each disease, He also prepared a specific therapy that remained for Man to find. He was led to this belief by his observation that quinine seemed to be specific for ague (malaria), and that he expected it would take centuries to prove this. However, Sydenham did not have any immediate followers after his death. Diseases such as those caused by ergot, mercury, and lead were described and appeared to be specific. Sciatica, trigeminal neuralgia, and possibly angina pectoris showed signs and symptoms of being discreet diseases, but the prominent medical minds appeared to be more fascinated with medical systems during the next two centuries. There were two major exceptions.

Francois Boissier de Sauvages and Carl von Linné (Linnaeus)

There appeared in 1731 a thesis written by Francois Boissier de Sauvages, a young graduate of the medical school at Montpellier, entitled *Nouvelles Classes de Maladies* in which he attempted to group diseases into classes, orders, and genera, just as the botanists and zoologists did with plants and animals. In this work, he attempted to identify for each disease an essential, constant, and, if possible, unique sign or symptom, which could be elicited by the physician. He stated that the etiologies, or the causes of disease, were hidden and that any classification of diseases on this basis was not possible. At that time, the approach of Sauvages was as scientific as possible, since he emphasized, as did Sydenham, the importance of making careful observations that could be documented and thereby would avoid unprovable hypotheses as to cause. It should be noted that he did not completely discount anatomical lesions, but regarded them as additional signs of each disease. Sauvages's book impressed Carl von Linné (1707–1778), the famous Swedish taxonomist of plants and animals, who was also a physician, and the two men corresponded for more than thirty years. Linnaeus produced his major classifications of diseases in 1763, which were also based completely on signs and symptoms. He proposed eleven major groups: (1) exanthemata, fever with skin eruptions; (2) critical fevers, fevers with a resulting red sediment in the urine; (3) inflammatory fever, fever with a hard pulse and local pain; (4) painful diseases; (5) mental illness; (6) loss of power of movement; (7) loss of control of movements; (8) impediments to external passages; (9) discharge of fluids; (10) physical deformities; and (11) palpable lesions.

From these groups Linnaeus had subcategories of 325 separate conditions. He was not able to distinguish the skin lesions of syphilis from that of smallpox. With regard to painful diseases, he listed as in the same class such diverse conditions as toothache, headache, arthritis, and sore throat. It is obvious to a modern physician that both Sauvages and Linnaeus were premature in their understanding of pathology and that the classifications of plants and animals were a much simpler task.[3]

Sauvages produced his main work in 1768, entitled *Nosologica Methodica Sistens Morborum Classes, Genera et Species,*[4] in which he lists 2,400 different diseases. He essentially used some of the categories of Linnaeus, but his problem was that in defining each disease species, he used signs and symptoms minutia that were not justified as unique to each disease. As a result he listed 18 different types of angina, 19 types of asthma, 20 types of lung infection, 12 species of nausea, and 29 species of vomiting.

William Cullen

One of the leaders of medicine during the Scottish Enlightenment, William Cullen (1712–1790) attempted to simplify the classifications of Sauvages and Linnaeus. In 1769 he published his *Synopsis Nosologiae Methodicae*[5] in which he reduced the eleven classes of Linnaeus and the ten of Sauvages to four. His motives in making a classification was primarily to teach young clinicians to organize their thoughts about their patients and to provide a starting point for further questions and observations. His first class was Pyrexias, and he subdivided it into (1) fevers without localized signs such as the intermittent and continuous forms; (2) localized inflammation as those in the throat or lungs; (3) the exanthemata; (4) fluxes such as the different forms of dysentery; and; (5) hemorrhagic, which were characterized by such conditions as nosebleeds, hemoptysis, and severe menstrual bleeding. His second class was the Neuroses, which were characterized by such signs as weakness, paralysis, seizures, syncope, and insanity. His third class was called Cachexias, which he subcategorized into three groups: (1) emaciations, (2) swellings, and (3) affections of the skin, which included such diverse entities as scrofula, syphilis, scurvy, and leprosy. His fourth class was the Locales, which could have been called Miscellaneous, because it included such symptoms, signs, or lesions as anorexia, speech loss, eneuresis, gonorrhea, aneurysms, buboes, various tumors, hernias, and even fractures. He eliminated the class of Dolores, which was prominent in the work of Sauvages and Linnaeus, since he recognized the great subjectivity of this symptom. It is interesting that Risse, in his study of the clinical records in the private practice of Cullen, found that this eminent physician did not use his published nosology in his diagnoses, which is a further indication that it was devised primarily for pedagogical purposes in the training of students at the Edinburgh Medical School.[6]

Philippe Pinel

The last famous taxonomist was Philippe Pinel (1745–1826). He told his medical colleagues "if you face a disease, determine its true character and its rank in a nosological table" and was extremely critical of physicians who "saw diseased people without seeing disease." He translated Cullen's work into French and then devised another complex classification of diseases based on signs and symptoms, which, as were the others, short-lived.[7] But he admired Morgagni and appreciated the work of Bichat, Laennec, and Corvisart. He was an outstanding and kindhearted clinician and did much to improve medicine and care in hospitals and insane asylums and thus was one of the leaders of the Paris School of Medicine during the first years of the nineteenth century.

The Taxonomists versus the Anatomical Pathologists

It should be pointed out that Thomas Sydenham, as one of the first disease taxonomists, or nosologists, did not think that postmortem examinations would throw much light on the study of disease. He wrote that:

> Others have more pompously and speciously prosecuted the promoting of this art (medicine) by searching into the bowels of the dead and living creatures, sound as well as diseased, to find out the seeds of (disease) destroying them, but with how little success such endeavors have been and are likely to be attended, I shall here in some measure make appear.[8]

And his friend, fellow physician and famous philosopher John Locke, agreed with him by writing that:

> That nature performs all her operations in the body so minute and insensible that I think nobody will ever hope or pretend even by the assistance of glasses or other inventions come to a sight of

> them. . . . Though we cut into the inside we see but the outside of things and make but a new superficies for ourselves to stare at.[9]

Morgagni took exception to this position almost one hundred years later and in part of his dedication of his book to Senac stated that:

> It is well known that there lived a physician at the end of the last century whom we would do an injustice if we denied that he was a careful observer of diseases. But he himself was biased against anatomy when he stooped to make assertions about it . . . which could not be defended even by his most ardent admirers. Indeed they easily could realize that the principle of his assertion could have led the inexperienced mind to the conclusion that the necropsy of victims of disease seem useless for the investigation of the causes of disease. . . . It was affirmed that the causes of health as well as of most maladies are inaccessible to our senses since they rest in hidden forms of invisible particles, in their connections and movements and in forces which control these movements and connections. From which, even if true, it does not follow that the effects of those causes necessarily also escape our senses; for they affect perceptible parts and the abnormal alterations, which we discern in them, are the manifest internal causes of very many diseases. (These critics) argue that the search for causes is useless because not all maladies can be cured when their cause is known. . . . Therefore they will consider it as worthless, even when anatomy will protect their reputation by demonstrating that a disease actually had been incurable . . . or when dissection will discredit common signs of maladies or throw doubt on them . . . or suggest certain new or less known signs for the diagnosis of a certain puzzling disease or finally pinpoint the correct seat and cause among many. . . . Autopsies promote our judgment in order that we do not accelerate the demise of patients by exhausting them with so many superfluous and possibly harmful remedies. . . . They also will check us from committing ourselves by hasty statements which the opening of the body will reveal as erroneous.[10]

Although Morgagni did not mention Sydenham by name, it is reasonable to believe that he was referring to the "English Hippocrates," and that his reputation, even one hundred years later, was significantly high that Morgagni hesitated to make a personal attack. At that time Morgagni was most likely a minority when he recommended routine and careful autopsies. However, it was not many years later, with the studies of Bichat, Laennec, and their followers in France, that the study of anatomic pathology superseded the taxonomic classifications, and placed the field of medicine on the road to scientific understanding.

Bibliography

1. Borelli, G., *De motu Animalium.* Bernabo, Rome, 1680.
2. Sydenham, T., *The Works of Thomas Sydenham.* The Sydenham Society, London 1848.
3. Linné, von, Carl, *Genera Morborum, in Audutorum Usum.* Upsala, 1763.
4. Sauvages de la Croix, F.B., *Nosologia methodica sistens morborum classes, genera et species.* Amsterdam, 1768.
5. Cullen, W., *Synopsis nosologiae methodicae.* Edinburgh, 1769.
6. Risse, G., *Hospital Life in Enlightenment Scotland.* Cambridge Univ. Press, 1986
7. Pinel, P., *Nosographie philosophique*, 3 vols., Paris, 1818.
8. Wolfe, D.E., *Bull. Hist. Med.*, **35**, p. 193, 1961.
9. Fox-Bourne, H.R., *The Life of John Locke, Vol. I.* p. 211, King, London, 1876
10. Morgagni, J.B., *De sedibus, et causis morborum per anatomen indagatis libri quinque, remondiniana.* Venice, 1761. English Translation by B. Alexander, London 1769.

CHAPTER III

What is the value of observation . . . if one does not know the seat of disease? You can take notes for twenty years from morning to evening at the sickbed on diseases of the heart, lungs and stomach, and you will reap nothing but confusion. The symptoms corresponding to nothing, will offer but incoherent phenomena. Open a few corpses, and immediately this obscurity which observation alone would never have removed, will disappear.

— M.F.X. Bichat

The Paris School of Anatomical Pathology

Medicine in France prior to 1800

At the beginning of the nineteenth century, the frontier of medicine moved to France. This was not capricious, but was part of the result of many factors that arose in France in the seventeenth and eighteenth centuries and were influential in producing the French Revolution. This, of course, was during the period of the Enlightenment in which Western thinkers, attempting to resolve the conceptions of God, reason, and the nature of Man, came to the tentative conclusion that with correct reasoning true knowledge could be found and lead Man to happiness.

Although the roots of the Enlightenment were in the works of Locke, Bacon, Spinoza, and Descartes, one of its major spokesmen in France was Jean Francois Marie Voltaire (1694–1778) This philosopher concluded that the purpose of life is not to reach heaven through penitence but to assure happiness to all men by progress in the sciences and the arts. Contemporaries Etienne de Condillac (1715–1780), who was a champion of Bacon's philosophy, and Julian La Mettrie (1709–1751), the materialist, led to the formation of a group, the ideologues, whose physician members George Cabanis (1757–1808) and Pinel (1745–1826) encouraged comprehensive observation of the patient, not the reading of books, as the way to further medical education. Of course, Hippocrates and Sydenham had stressed this earlier, but their teachings were isolated voices in medical history, while the ideologues were part of a large philosophical movement in pioneering the new scientific method in the last quarter of the eighteenth century. A little later Auguste Comté (1798–1857), in his philosophy of "positivism" noted that progress occurs in three stages which could be applied to that of pathology and medicine, (a) the theological stage that interprets the world in supernatural terms, (b) a philosophical stage that interprets the world in abstract ideas and forces, and (c) a positive stage that interprets the natural world by accumulating facts that lead to consolidation of phenomena into laws.

However, there were seeds of enlightenment of a more practical type that were sown during the rule of Louis XIV (1638–1715), although the final results of this planting [the execution of Louis XVI (1754–1793) following the Revolution of 1789] were not foreseen. The fact was that Louis XIV, the "sun king," in his attempt at self-glorification was attentive to anything that would enhance his regime. To accomplish this, he appointed brilliant men and encouraged competition among artists and writers. One of his advisors was the farsighted Jean Baptise Colbert (1619–1683), who, recognizing the possibility that men of a scientific bent could possibly advance France as a center of power and culture, persuaded Louis XIV to support a group of such people who were already meeting informally at various places in Paris. With the formation of the Académie des Sciences in 1666, Colbert selected eminent men in French life — physicians, mathematicians, astronomers, anatomists, botanists — and made them full-time workers for the crown, at a time when London's corresponding Royal Society was struggling for economic survival. Laboratories were designed in the Louvre, next to the king's library and by the end of the seventeenth century, there were senior scientists with paid associates and assigned students working in Paris. The academy continued into the eighteenth century, and as a result France was far in advance of other countries in all aspects of science. Technical schools were also established during the last half of the eighteenth century to train promising students in the physical sciences. But Louis XIV, in addition to taking the advice of Colbert, made a personal decision that was to result in a major advancement in medicine. In 1686 the king developed a severe anal fistula that was cured by the surgeon François Felix (died 1703) after the ointments and poultices of the royal physicians had failed. At that time surgery was considered a lowly trade that had traditionally been part of the barbering field, with its cutting of hair, shaving, and caring for wigs, whereas the physicians had a classical education in a university, spoke and wrote Latin, wore distinct robes, and for the most part had only a minimum knowledge of anatomy and did no surgery. The surgeons, on the other hand, learned how to treat lacerations and other types of wounds, such as those produced during wars or accidents, drained abscesses, performed amputations, and removed cancers and benign tumors on the surface of the body. Some of the more daring and skilled surgeons attempted to repair hernias, removed bladder stones, and trephined skulls. To show his appreciation to Felix, the king elevated him to a high court position, gave him a farm, and considerable money much to the chagrin of the royal physicians. His successor Georges Mareschal (1658–1736) was given even further power, and through the influence of the advisors of Louis XV (1710–1774) was able to obtain five professorships for surgical teaching at the College of St. Côme in 1724 in spite of the great public protests by members of the Paris Medical Faculty. Later Mareschal with the aid of Montpellier surgeon François de la Peyronie (1678–1747) established the Academy of Surgeons in 1731. The result was that surgery achieved professional parity with the Latin-speaking physicians. However, the groups continued to feud over privilege and power until after the French Revolution, when powerful new governments forced unification of the physicians and surgeons. A New Plan of the Society of Medicine, most likely written by Felix Vicq-d'Azyr (1748–1794) in 1790, stated that

> it is necessary, we shall not say merely to bring together but rather to reunite and fuse in the same habitation, in the same school, all the children of a family too long divided. All divisions must cease and the same status, prospects and rights must be extended to all. Has not surgery always been regarded as a part of medicine? . . . Why separate to the root the branches of a tree and then weaken it? Why two orders of Colleges? Why two academies? . . . Henceforth, medicine and surgery will be taught in the same schools. Those who have completed their studies will be subjected to the same examinations; they will enjoy the same rights, and all will be designated physicians (medecins). [1]

But the plan was not immediately implemented until Antoine Fourcroy (1755–1809), a chemist and physician with influence in the revolutionary government and exasperated with the continued bickering between the physicians and surgeons, wrote in a 1791 report:

> There will no longer be a ridiculous distinction between the two arts which are by nature inseparable. Henceforth citizens will find all knowledge united by the health officers. The scandalous quarrels will be ended forever.[2]

In 1794, Fourcroy, with the help of the anatomist Francois Chaussier (1746–1828), created the three Écoles de Santé — in Paris, Montpellier, and Strasbourg. The schools were equipped with the best facilities and equipment, and the students and professors were selected on the basis of merit. Twelve courses were given, dealing with both medical and surgical diseases. Pierre Joseph Desault (1744–1795), the most outstanding surgeon in Paris, was appointed Professor of Surgery, and Jean Nicolas Corvisart, the physician of Napoleon, was made the Professor of Medicine. The school in Paris was highly successful, and well-trained physicians and surgeons were soon working in the military, teaching, or working in private practice. It was soon recognized that the individual who wished to devote his career to surgery must spend a minimum of one extra year in a hospital carrying out various surgical techniques.

With regard to the study of pathology, two French physicians, were responsible for the beginnings of a movement in Paris that would come to fruition after the Revolution of 1789 and the reorganization of medicine under the new government, which eventually was headed by Napoleon Bonaparte. Jean Baptiste de Senac (1693–1770) and Joseph Lieutaud (1703–1780) attended Louis XV and were expert anatomists, members of the Académie des Sciences, and interested in pathological anatomy. Senac wrote a book,[3] published in 1749, in which he noted dilatation of the heart and hydrothorax during heart failure. He described pericarditis and warned that fluid could accumulate in the pericardial or pleural space independently, which was only possible to confirm at autopsy. He stressed the fact that palpatation was a common complaint, and usually no cardiac lesion accounted for this symptom. Lieutaud wrote books on medicine but is best known for his *Historia Anatomico-Medica* [4] which was published in 1767 and was a collection of more than 3500 autopsy reports culled from the literature and his own dissections. He included with each autopsy, a small amount of clinical information. He described neoplasms, and many abnormalities of the heart, but for the most part, the compilation of cases was made without any critical insight and was not as valuable a work as was Morgagni's published six years earlier.

Along with the new medical schools that combined medicine and surgery, there developed large hospitals that provided large numbers of patients for study. During the reign of Louis XVI, hospitals in France greatly expanded, especially in Paris; in 1788 there were 48 facilities with as many as 20,000 patients obtaining treatment at any one time. The conditions in most of the hospitals were appalling; as many as six patients were placed in one bed, and the contagious patients mixed with those with surgical problems. Often patients who had died were allowed to remain next to living patients for long periods of time. Surgery was performed in the middle of the ward with dirty instruments and blood present from previous operations. The screams during this pre-anesthetic period could be heard throughout the hospital. The mortality rate was higher than 20%.

Medicine in France during the First Half of the Nineteenth Century

Tremendous changes were made with the advent of the new revolutionary governments, especially following Napoleon's rise to power. New hospital facilities were built, one bed was assigned to each patient, wards were separated into medical and surgical cases, isolated operating rooms were constructed, and a central pharmacy and kitchen were established. Most importantly, the hospitals were integrated with the medical schools, and by 1801 competitive examinations were instituted for interns and staff members. Every type of medical condition was seen, and the hospitals of Paris were transformed from institutions of misery and hopelessness to cradles of learning and hope. The medical historian Erwin Ackerknecht called this period "hospital medicine" and stated "It was only in the hospital that the three pillars of the new medicine, the physical examination, the autopsy, and statistics, could be developed."[5] Wunderlich in his book *Wien und Paris* written in 1841 looked back on his training period in Paris, and wrote, "The hospital is the backdrop of all medical thinking; all is applied in the hospital; all can be confirmed only there or in the autopsy room."[6]

It was the surgeons who initially carried out the autopsies. By the nature of their work, they had long been forced into thinking about their cases in terms of Morgagni's "seats of disease," because they attempted to treat wounds, ulcers, abscesses, gangrene, stones, hernias, fistulas, and aneurysms. It was essential that they not only had to localize the lesion but also know, in detail, the anatomy surrounding it. Without this knowledge, the surgeon could not carry out his procedures with any chance of success. The autopsy was also important to him because it not only enabled him to evaluate the success or failure of his surgery but also allowed him the opportunity to think about improving his procedures.

The physicians, on the other hand, were dealing with internal and infectious diseases and traditionally thought about these maladies in terms of acrimonies, humors, crises, and irritabilities, and usually did not possess enough knowledge or interest in anatomy to even attempt to find these nebulous entities during an autopsy. Before the integration of medicine and surgery, the surgeons had no knowledge of or interest in internal diseases or the lesions that could be produced in these non-surgical conditions. However, with the combining of the two fields, three outstanding men who were skilled surgeons and anatomists became interested in internal diseases — Bichat, Corvisart, and Laennec. These individuals were responsible for more advancements in the fields of medicine and pathology in just twenty-five years (between 1800 and 1825) than in all the prior centuries.

Marie Francois Xavier Bichat (1771–1802)

Bichat was born in eastern France on November 14, 1771, and received his early education in Nantua. Later in Lyon he studied surgery under the direction of Marc Antoine Petit (1760–1840). In 1794 he went to Paris where Desault, the chief surgeon at the Hotel Dieu and Professor of Surgery at the new medical school, was teaching surgery to hundreds of young Frenchmen. Desault, quickly recognizing Bichat's great superiority over the other students, took him into his home and made him his first assistant and protege. Unfortunately Desault died the following year, but Bichat undertook to edit and publish all of his mentor's surgical works starting in 1798, even as he was losing interest in surgery as a career. He began to think about disease processes in terms of anatomy and physiology, and it was in these fields that he showed his genius. His capacity for work was prodigious; during the years 1795 until his death in 1802, he not only taught hundreds of medical students, cared for patients, performed hundreds of autopsies, and carried out experiments on animals, but he wrote several books. These are still classics,[7-10] especially those in which he showed for the first time that disease processes typically affect parts of organs rather than the whole organ itself. Thus, inflammation typically affects the outer layer or the serous or peritoneal tissue in the abdominal organs without necessarily affecting the underlying layers, and the same applies to the pleura and pericardium in the chest. The diseases resulting from this selective process later came to be known as peritonitis and pleuritis. When it occurs around the brain and spinal cord it is called meningitis. With this new knowledge, the field of pathology made a quantum jump, and Bichat became regarded as the father of histology even though he did not use the microscope, which did not become reliable for most individuals until the second quarter of the century. Bichat insisted that his student doctors know something about the status of the internal organs of their patients when they were making diagnoses and prognoses, and he knew that the only way they could achieve this knowledge was by routinely performing autopsies on their patients dead of their various diseases. He expressed his thoughts in this manner:

> It seems to me that we have entered an epoch where pathological anatomy must make a new effort. This science is not only that of the organic changes which arrive slowly or as consequences in chronic disease. It consists of the study of all possible alterations of our bodies whenever we examine their diseases. With the exception of certain fevers and nervous diseases, almost everything in pathology is in its domain. . . . Medicine was for a long time excluded from the exact sciences. She will have a right to belong to them, at least for diagnostics, when rigorous observation is everywhere combined with examination of organ changes.[11]

Bichat was also one of the first experimental physiologists, to perform experiments on animals. He investigated asphyxia by eliminating the function of the lungs by cutting the trachea and found that this affected not only the normal beating of the heart but also the brain in terms of alertness and motor function. By devising ingenious surgical techniques, he established that when dark (deoxygenated) blood was the only source of blood flowing to the brain from the heart, death quickly ensued. However if he connected the carotid artery of a normal dog to that of a dog whose lungs were not functioning, this blood that was bright red prevented death in the physiologically compromised animal. If he then cut the trachea of the donor dog, the blood in the carotids was soon dark, and both animals soon expired. During these experiments, Bichat also showed collateral circulation of the brain through the vertebral and basal arteries to maintain a temporary normal function of the brain when the internal carotids are compressed.

Discussion of these experiments and their historical significance to establish Bichat's contributions to experimental physiology are admirably discussed in a work by the science historians Lesch[12] and Albury.[13] Bichat was certainly a more modern figure in physiology than was Albrecht von Haller (1708–1777), who did his work in the prior century.[14] Bichat was also a transitional figure because he was a "vitalist," more speculative and certainly a tremendous contrast with the "mechanistic" François Magendie who succeeded him by only a few years as France's most eminent experimental physiologist. It is probably true, as Albury points out,[13] that in terms of their actual experiments, their vivisection approaches were quite similar. Thus, in spite of his "vitalism," this bias should not diminish his greatness, and it must be remembered that it was in pathology and medicine that Bichat did his most memorable work, particularly with regard to the practical aspect of his localizing inflammation to membranes. Bichat unfortunately died of infection, most likely contracted during his autopsy work, and the world was deprived of the discoveries this brilliant man would undoubtedly have accomplished in a long career. However, his astute disciple, Laennec, did build on his mentor's work and made major advances particularly in diagnoses of diseases of the chest.

Rene Theophile Hyacinthe Laennec (1781–1826)

Laennec was born in 1781 in Brittany. He received an excellent preliminary education at Nantes under the direction of his uncle, who was a senior physician in the local hospital. He then went to Paris to study under Bichat and Corvisart. His ability was quickly recognized and after the death of Bichat, he began a series of lectures in anatomic pathology which soon rivaled the course given by the famous Guillaume Dupuytren (1777–1835) who taught pathology from the standpoint of a surgeon. Laennec devised a classification[15] for abnormalities of organs produced by various illnesses, utilizing ideas he had received from both Bichat and Dupuytren. This classification was as follows: l. Alterations of nutrition with an increase producing a hypertrophy of an organ and a decrease producing atrophy. 2. Alterations in form or position such as

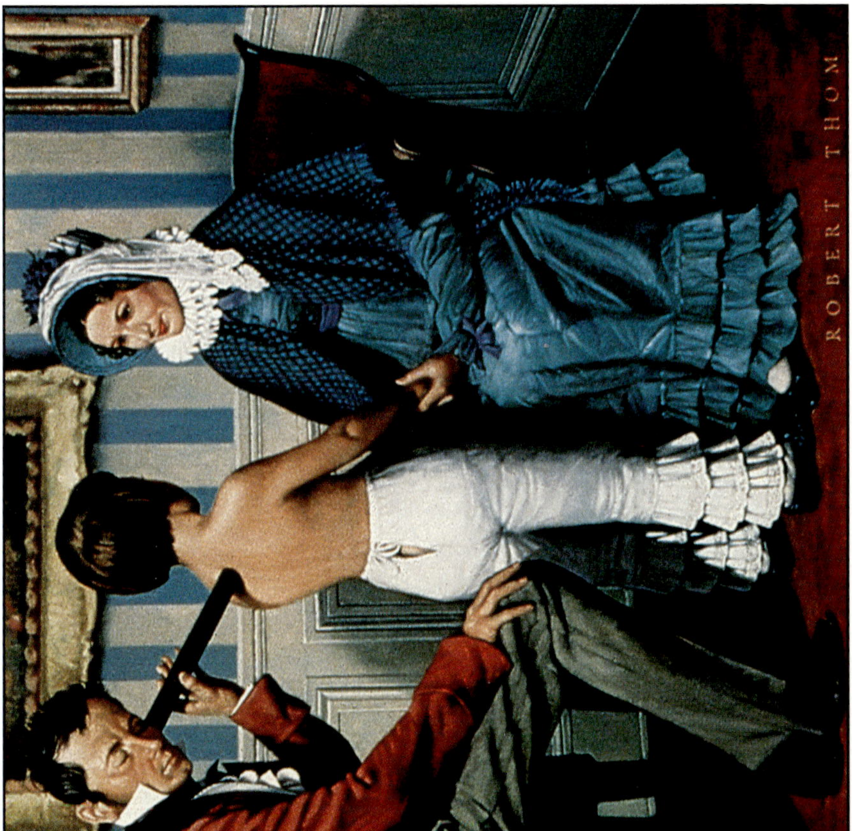

LAENNEC AND THE STETHOSCOPE

occurs in a hernia. 3. Alteration in the organ due to the presence of a foreign body or a parasite such as an insect or a worm. 4. Alteration in the texture of an organ. These he categorized as due to (a) a discontinuity in an organ because of a fracture or a wound; (b) inflammation or its consequences such as gangrene or suppuration; (c) the presence of fluid such as anasarca or hydrothorax; (d) the presence of an accidental tissue or one not normally present such as fibrous tissue, neoplasm, tubercle, or a cyst. This classification from a modern standpoint is not erroneous but simplistic in that there is very little insight into pathological processes themselves. Laennec always regarded pathology as his first interest, but, like other physicians at that time who were interested in doing research or teaching where there was no remuneration, he had to practice medicine. It was in 1816, while unsuccessfully attempting to examine the chest of an obese young woman with his ear to her chest, he decided to try the usefulness of listening through a cylinder made up of several sheets of paper. He was amazed at the amplification of the sounds that occurred, and that as he moved the cylinder to different parts of the chest, he heard entirely diverse sounds that not only correlated with the heart beats but also with respiration. Thus the first stethoscope was born and would soon replace forever the flask of urine as the symbol of the physician.

The acumen of Laennec manifested itself in how he utilized this finding. A lesser talent would probably have dismissed the finding as simply a curiosity, but for three years Laennec carefully recorded the sounds at different points on the chest, and correlated them, when possible, with postmortem findings. The results were published in his 1819 two-volume work,[16] which has become one of the classics of medicine. At this time Laennec was suffering from tuberculosis and retired to his home in Brittany, but two years later he was appointed Professor of Medicine at the College de France. He died in 1826 but not before he had been able to describe most of the pathological conditions of the lungs, including emphysema, acute and chronic pulmonary edema, bronchiectasis, pyemia, pneumothorax, pneumonia, bronchitis, pleuritis, and pulmonary infarction. Significantly, he was able to differentiate, during postmortems, tuberculosis and hydatid cysts from other types of chronic lung disease, all previously listed as phthisis. The problem had been that the lesions produced by the mycobacterium (not discovered until 1882 by Robert Koch) were easily confused with non-tubercular lesions such as those of carcinoma. However, Laennec was the first to recognize that certain lesions were simply stages in the various transformation of tuberculosis. He also showed that the lesions that occurred in the other organs and in the lymph nodes previously called scrofula were also related to the tubercular process. He described the transitions of the granulomas to cavities, and noted that the first major lesion was usually in the apex of the lung which he was often able to detect with the stethoscope. He devised descriptive terms for respiratory sounds such as bronchophony, egophony, pectoriloquy, metallic tinkling, cavernous respiration, and crepitus redux, some of which are still described in texts on physical diagnosis.[17] Laennec thought that many of these sounds were pathognomonic for certain lesions; this was later discredited by Josef Skoda in Vienna,[18] but there is no question that, before the invention of visualization techniques for diseases of the chest, Laennec's were the most useful techniques in the armamentarium of the physician. Before Laennec's time, essentially the only method of evaluating the thorax was the time-honored technique of succussion, even used by Hippocrates, which involved taking the patient by the shoulders and shaking him to hear if there was a splashing sound which would indicate hydrothorax, or measuring the distance on each side of the thorax from the sternum to the vertebra, with each respiration to determine whether there was asymmetry which could indicate pathological processes on a particular side. With regard to neoplasms Laennec called them "degeneration" and classified them as did his colleague Bayle in terms of their hardness.

Jean Nicolas Corvisart (1755–1821)

The other medical giant was Jean Nicolas Corvisart (1755–1821) who, like Bichat, was not only a pupil of Desault but was also primarily interested in internal diseases. As mentioned earlier, he was Professor of Medicine in 1794, and desiring to learn the best methods of diagnosis, he became aware of a little-read book by Leopold Auenbrugger (1722–1809) on percussion published in 1761.[19] He started to practice this technique, correlating his findings with autopsy findings of lesions of the heart, great vessels, and pericardium. In 1806, Corvisart published his work,[20] in which he also was the first to explain heart failure in mechanical terms. Then in 1808 he translated Auenbrugger's book and expanded on it with considerable discussion of his findings on this technique. He stated in his translation:

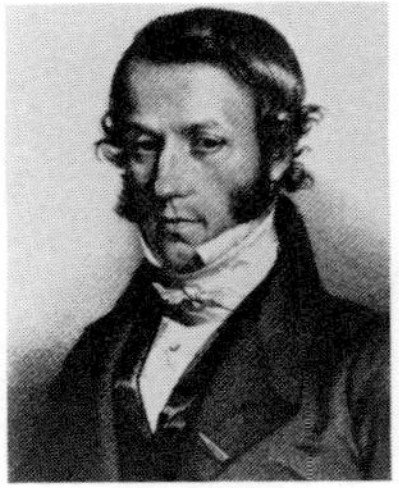
G. Andral

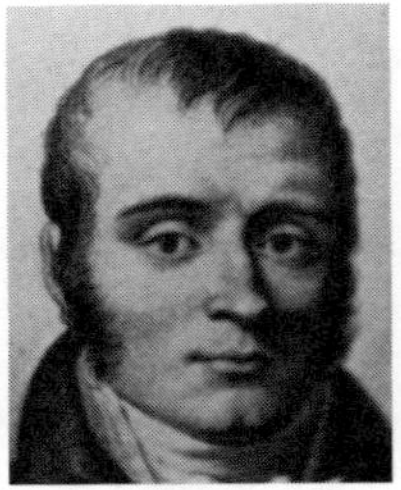
M. Bichat

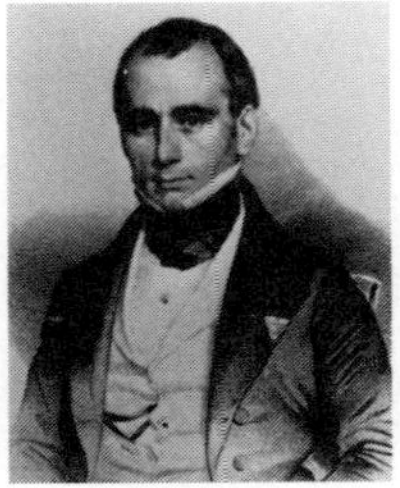
J. Bouillaud

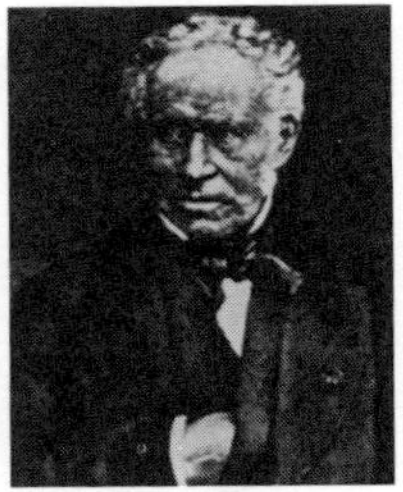
P. Bretonneau

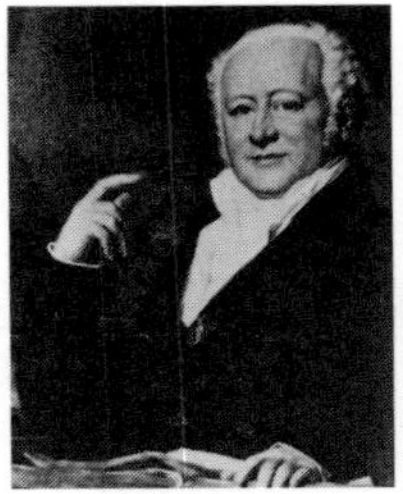
J. Corvisart

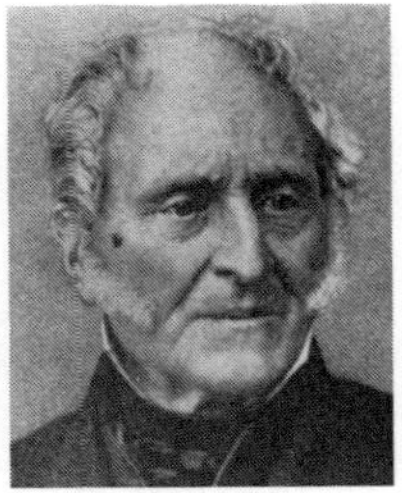
J. Cruveilhier

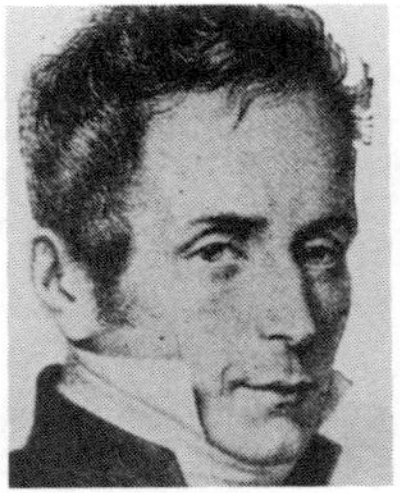
R. Laennec

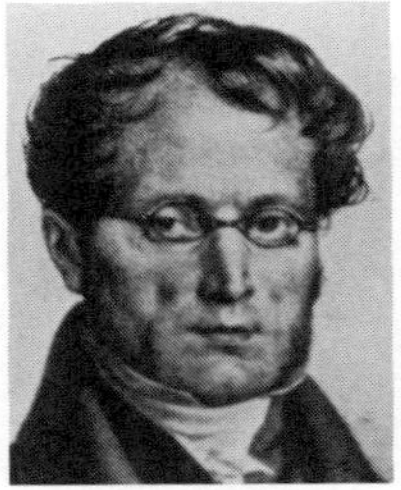
P. Louis

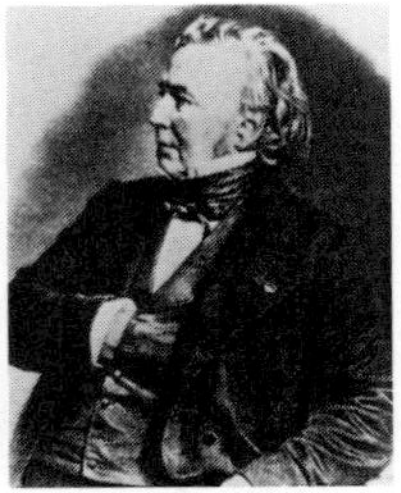
P. Rayer

THE EARLY NINETEENTH CENTURY PARISIANS

> Percussion made a strong impression upon me, and I think that since then I have practiced it unceasingly, whether in obscure diseases of the chest or in those that were simple and easily understood. It never led me astray if the condition of the patient was such as to allow me to make full use of it. On the other hand, I must frankly admit that I have known of many grave errors in diagnosis on the part of those who knew nothing of percussion or neglected it.[21]

With his considerable reputation, percussion quickly became popular among medical students. Before the time of Corvisart, physicians had difficulty evaluating heart disease. Although auscultation with the aid of a stethoscope had to wait a few more years, nevertheless Corvisart, by inspection, palpation, percussion, and immediate auscultation (ear directly against the chest), was able to make diagnoses of mitral valve disease, aneurysm when a thrill was present, hypertrophy or dilatation of the heart, and the evaluation of arterial pressure by feeling the pulse. He was also able to differentiate functional diseases of the heart from organic lesions and the significance of dyspnea in patients. Corvisart, the personal physician to Napoleon and in spite of his major contributions to medicine, retired into oblivion when the emperor was overthrown and exiled.

Other Eminent French Physicians during the Nineteenth Century

There were several other French medical men who contributed to pathology during this important period in France of "hospital medicine." Gaspard Laurent Bayle (1774–1816) was a colleague of Laennec and Corvisart and is best known for his work on tuberculosis and neoplasms. He performed hundreds of autopsies but emphasized that they often did not reveal gross lesions or the reasons for death. He summarized his conclusions on the value of autopsies in this manner[22]: 1. The necropsy is valuable in making classifications of disease. 2. The necropsy identifies organic lesions but sheds no light on their cause. 3. The necropsy almost never reveals the immediate cause of death. 4. The necropsy often reveals lesions of an organ that explains the failure in function of that organ. 5. The necropsy is often valuable in differentiating contagious diseases from certain non-contagious diseases with the same symptoms. 6. The necropsy is not of great help in studying diseases that are purely functional in nature, but it does exclude those with similar symptoms but organic lesions. 7. In contagious diseases the necropsy occasionally contributes information that is less specific in terms of organic lesions but may help in indicating that a given contagious disease is prevalent in the community. 8. The necropsy often serves to complete the history of a disease suspected from the clinical findings. Although these conclusions were made in 1813, they are for the most part still valid, but are often forgotten by clinicians today.

With regard to his work on tuberculosis, which he published as *Recherches sur la Phthisie Pulmonaire* in 1810,[23] Bayle concluded that this "longest and most dangerous of all chronic diseases" starts as with a minimum of symptoms, but at the end reduces the victim to a skeleton."[23] Bayle classified "phthis" into six categories on the basis of gross observations: tuberculous, granulous, melanotic, ulcerative, calcifying, and cancerous. Without the use of the microscope in the case of "cancerous" and without the knowledge of the mycobacterium, it was not possible to recognize that the other categories were most likely simply different stages of the same disease — tuberculosis. Bayle believed that these conditions were the result of a diathesis, or a constitutional predisposition to this disease, and was not contagious, but he recognized that similar lesions could appear in other organs such as the intestine, lymph glands, pleura, and larynx.

With his colleague J.B. Cayol, Bayle also wrote a long article on cancer[24] in which he attempted to categorize malignancies on the bases of their appearance and degree of hardness, which were the only means possible at the time. He described neoplasms in the breast, ovaries, testes, prostate, skin, kidney, bladder, liver, brain, thyroid, pharynx, esophagus, stomach, intestine, pancreas, and rectum. It is again clear that Bayle many times confused not only tuberculosis but other granulomatous lesions with malignancies. He also did not understand that ulceration, hemorrhage, gangrene, and suppuration were complications rather than specific characteristics of a particular tumor. However, he did recognize that some neoplasms were benign and that in the case of malignancy, the tumor could appear in adjacent organs, although the mechanism or use of the term metastases was not used. Bayle, like his teacher Bichat and his associate Laennec, died of tuberculosis, most likely contracted performing autopsies, at the age of only 42 years.

Gabriel Andral (1797–1876) was one of the next generation of French medical men who had a prodigious interest in pathology. He said he learned medicine three times, first as an anatomical pathologist, second as a physician learning percussion and auscultation, and third when he started in study of hematology. He wrote the pathology textbook[25] most-used during the second quarter of the nineteenth century, first published in 1829 in which he attempted to explain disease processes in terms of abnormalities of the capillaries, nutrition, secretion, blood composition, and nerve function. There was great speculation, and there is very little in his classification that in retrospect had any validity. A few years later he wrote the first major textbook on hematology.[26] He was the first to use the term "anemia" and "hyperemia," and while collaborating with the physician chemist Jules Gavarret (1809–1890), they analyzed the blood in normal and diseased states and found differences in fibrin content, particularly in maladies characterized by large amounts of inflammation. Andral was greatly influenced by François Magendie, who believed that the etiologies of many diseases would be found in disorders in the composition of the blood.[27] Andral's studies in turn influenced the Austrian pathologist Rokitansky, who extrapolated the Frenchman's findings into a theory of crases, which almost destroyed his reputation since the young Rudolf Virchow accused him publicly of attempting to return medicine to the old ideas of humors as a cause of disease. It is ironic that suggestions by Magendie, the greatest of sceptics and the debunker of unproven theories, could have so misled Rokitansky, the most renowned pathologist during the second quarter of the century. This dispute will be discussed in a later chapter.

Jean Cruveilhier (1791–1874) was the first recipient of a full-time chair in pathology in Paris in 1836, which was established by his wealthy surgeon pathologist and mentor Guillaume Dupuytren with whom he had collaborated over the years. Cruveilhier made significant studies on various diseases such as progressive muscular dystrophy, disseminated sclerosis, colon diverticula, hypertrophic pyloric stenosis, and gastric ulcers but he is best known as being responsible for the publication of one of the finest collections[28] of pathological drawings during the years 1829–42. He also had a predisposition to speculating on the causes of disease, stating that phlebitis was a primary factor in most organic maladies.

One individual who was a major voice in French medicine during the first half of the nineteenth century but whose accomplishments, retrospectively viewed, were almost nil was Francois Joseph Victor Broussais (1772–1838), a pugnacious, swashbuckling individual who served as an army physician in most of Napoleon's campaign during the years 1803–1814. Because of his military connections he became chief physician at the Val de Grâce, the military hospital and medical school, which he then used as a pulpit to promote his theories on disease. He was a spell-binding speaker and with the publication of his *Examen de la Doctrine Médicale Généralement Adoptée* in 1816, he expected to become the premier medical savant in France. He attracted hundreds of students to his lectures and called his ideas "physiological medicine."

He had as his patients many of the most eminent, non-medical individuals in Paris. His initial position was that diseases were not specific entities as proposed by Sydenham and Pinel, but abnormalities in function, an anti-ontology position that was continued in Germany for much of the remainder of the century by Virchow, Wunderlich, and Traube. The problem with Broussais was that as he became more powerful politically, his anti-ontological ideas became more and more another speculative system.[29] In 1822 he started his own journal to promote his ideas, and his books became simply polemics against anybody who contradicted him, much like his hero of the past in the political arena, Napoleon Bonaparte. His system finally resolved itself into the concept that diseases were due to irritations of organs and these irritations spread from one organ to another, especially if these organs had a special sympathy for each other.[30] He also speculated that most diseases started with irritation of the stomach. He regarded syphilis and smallpox as simply variations of inflammation produced by irritations, and tuberculosis and cancer were the aftermath of inflammation. He stated that malaria was the result of a periodic gastroenteritis. He later embraced the new phrenology of Gall, and by the time of his death in 1838, he had alienated his earlier followers, and students no longer found his lectures interesting. They were more fascinated by the work of Laennec and his followers who emphasized careful clinical observation correlated with postmortem findings together with the new statistical approach of Louis.

Also in contrast to Broussais was the work of Pierre Bretonneau (1778–1862), who had trained at the new École de Santé in Paris, but returned to his native Tours, where he practiced medicine and became the director of the local hospital. He achieved fame by his work on diphtheria and typhoid fever, which he early recognized as specific contagious diseases, characterized by specific types of inflammation, with the skin and mucous membranes being particularly susceptible. He noted the characteristic membrane with the inflammation of the throat which he called diphtheria and treated the condition with tracheotomy.[31] In cases of typhoid fever, he found at autopsy pustular inflammation of the intestine. He regarded these lesions of the mucous membranes in both diseases as specific for these conditions as the characteristic lesions of the skin in smallpox. However, he acknowledged that the etiologies of these specific diseases were still not known. Even though he was never part of a medical school, his reputation in Tours grew and he had as his disciples Armand Trousseau (1801–1867) and Alfred Velpeau (1795–1867). Bretonneau, by his ideas of specificity of diseases, certainly anticipated Pasteur's work with microorganisms.

Another important physician was Pierre Charles Alexandre Louis (1797–1872), who exerted a lasting influence, both in France and indirectly in the United States. He was responsible for the development of medical statistics, or the Numerical Method as it was called at the time. This involved carefully collating data on a large series of cases of a similar clinical condition with regard to the situations in which it is found, the various signs and symptoms, the pathological changes found at autopsy, and the effect, if given, of various drugs or therapy. In 1825, he published his work on tuberculosis,[32] in which he studied 960 clinical cases, correlating his findings by percussion and auscultation, with lesions observed in 358 autopsies. In 1829, there appeared his second great work on fevers. In 900 hospital patients, in which he performed autopsies on 133 fatal cases, he determined that in many cases, diagnosed as typhus fever, there were unique inflammatory lesions of the Peyer's patches in the intestine that did not appear in other cases of fatal fever cases. Louis called this condition typhoid,[33] although similar cases with the characteristic intestinal lesions were described by Bretonneau and called dothinenteritis a few years earlier. Then in 1835, Louis used his Numerical Method to determine the efficacy of Broussais's therapy of bleeding, using emetics, and blistering in the treatment of pneumonia patients and found them useless.[34] It is interesting that, while today statistics are an integral and required method in evaluating experiments and observations, the Numerical Method had its opponents when it was first introduced by Louis. Armand Trousseau told his students in 1867:

> I do not reproach the Numerical Method because it numerates, but I reproach it because it only numerates; in a word, because it depends, like the mathematician, upon an absolutely exact result. I reproach it for counting too much, for counting too long, for counting always, and declining to put any mind into the facts. This method is the scourge of the intellect: it transforms the physician into a calculating machine.[35]

Historically, Louis was important also for his influence on medicine in the United States, since even more than Andral, who had a greater reputation in France, Louis by his personality attracted an entire group of American students during the years 1830–1840. After a period of study with this Frenchman, many young American doctors returned to the two major medical schools, Harvard and Pennsylvania, as faculty members.[36]

There were other important French physicians at that time that contributed to the study of pathology, and there was for the first time the beginning of specialization in Paris. Pierre Rayer (1793–1867), who also started as an anatomical pathologist and wrote a thesis on the subject in 1818,[37] went on to become an expert on skin diseases, writing an excellent two-volume work[38] on the subject in 1826. However, his major accomplishment was his three-volume treatise[39] with an atlas on kidney disease published during the years 1839-41 in which he emphasized the importance of analyzing the urine. Rayer also was the first to recognize the contagious character of glanders[40] and worked with Davaine on anthrax[41] prior to Pasteur's and Koch's definitive studies.

Philippe Ricord (1800–1889) was a pioneer in the study of venereal diseases. He was the first to show that gonorrhea and syphilis were separate diseases and that the latter went through primary, secondary, and tertiary stages.[42] He was one of the first to recognize the complications of gonorrhea, including conjunctivitis and epididymitis.

Jean Bouillaud (1769–1881) was known as one of the outstanding diagnosticians during this period. He was the first to discover that aphasia is related to damage to the anterior lobes of the brain[43] and the first to note a correlation with certain inflammations of the heart with that of the articular joints. He later found the relationship between mitral valve disease and the same inflammation of the joints, but called this correlation a "law of coincidence."[44] His work was thus the beginning of the study of what later was known as "rheumatic fever" with its components of acute arthritis, acute carditis, and later scarring and damage of the mitral valve.

There were other outstanding physicians such as Leon Rostan (1790–1866), Pierre Piorry (1797–1879), Armand Trousseau (1801–1867), Jean Alibert (1768–1837), Guillaume Dupuytren (1777–1835), Joseph Malgaigne (1806–1865), Guillaume Duchenne (1806-1875), and August Chomel (1788–1856) However, as pointed out by Ackerknecht,[45] by the year 1848, the evolution of French medicine virtually came to a halt. The development of gross pathological anatomy and the physical examination had advanced medicine to a stage that could scarcely be envisioned fifty years earlier. In retrospect, the next major advances were to be made in the laboratory rather than in the hospital. Etiologies and physiological mechanisms in the elucidation of the pathogenesis of diseases required microscopic examination rather than simply gross visualization of lesions in addition to experimentation. Medical France was unable to rise to the challenge. Although François Magendie (1783–1855) was the outstanding physiologist at this time, he, as well as the experimentalists J. Legallois (1770–1840), J. Poiseville (1799–1869), M. Chevreul (1796-1889), R. Dutrochet (1776-1847), A. Donné (1801–1878) and later Claude Bernard (1813–1878), C. Brown-Sequard (1817–1894), E. Marey (1830–1904), P. Bert (1833-1886), C. Davaine (1812–1882), and Louis Pasteur (1822–1895), were outsiders with regard to the French medical establishment. They worked for the most part under the most adverse conditions with poorly equipped facilities, and none ever became professors of a French medical school. In addition, almost all of the students of these investigators, following graduation were without any opportunities for research and disappeared into the pool of medical practitioners. As an illustration of how the medical school professors felt about the relationship of the basic sciences to the practice of medicine, the following is a quotation of Armand Trousseu, the eminent French clinician, in his lectures to medical students in 1867:

> The successive admixture of physicochemical science with our art has produced so much evil and is calculated to lead astray disastrously young men commencing the study of medicine. The preparatory sciences bear the same relationship to the medical arts as the laws of light bear to painting, or stonecutting to architecture. . . . And moreover, gentlemen, it is undesirable that the increased means of investigation possessed in the present day, by multiplying elementary facts, or all events by rendering them more exact, does not fit the mind for producing more prolific, more practical or

> more reliable manifestations of art. . . . For Mercy's sake, gentlemen, let us have a little less science and a little more art.[46]

Even Louis Pasteur's studies on microorganisms were ignored by the medical community, and the French government appeared to be more interested in spending money on public buildings such as the Opera House instead of on laboratories. Pasteur, always outspoken when he was fighting for a just cause, sent an article to the Paris publication *Moniteur* in 1868 to attempt to shake the indifference of the public authorities. The following is a quotation from this memorable criticism:

> . . . The boldest conceptions and the most legitimate speculations can be embodied but from the day when they are consecrated by observation and experiment. Laboratories and discoveries are correlative terms; if you suppress laboratories, Physical Science will become stricken with barrenness and death; it will become mere powerless information instead of a science of progress and futurity; give it back its laboratories, and life, fecundity and power will reappear. Away from their laboratories, physicists and chemists are but disarmed soldiers on the battlefield. . . . The deduction from these principles is evident; if the conquests useful to humanity touch your heart — if you remain confounded before the marvels of electric telegraphy, of anesthesia, of the daguerreotype and many other admirable discoveries — if you are jealous of the share your country may boast in these wonders — then I implore you, take some interest in those sacred dwellings, meaningly described as laboratories. Ask that they be multiplied and completed. They are the temples of the future, of riches, and of comfort. There humanity grows greater, better, stronger; there she can learn to read the works of Nature, works of progress and those of barbarism, of fanaticism, and of destruction. Some nations have felt the wholesome breath of truth. Rich and large laboratories have been growing in Germany for the last thirty years, and many more are still be built; at Berlin, and at Bonn, two palaces, worth four million francs each, are being erected for chemical studies. . . . And France? France has not yet begun!"[47]

With Pasteur's influence, the king of France did start to take measures to build laboratories but it was too little and too late. The vigor and ambition of Bismarck and Germany that stimulated them to build scientific laboratories, including those in biology and medicine, also made it possible to make them militarily superior, and France, in its complacency, was crushed in the Franco-Prussian War of 1870 Thus, in spite of the work of a few great individuals such as Pasteur and Bernard, France was never again to achieve leadership in biology and medicine and Minerva Medica moved to Germany, where, as stated by Osler, the "temples" and "priests" of medicine reigned supreme.

Bibliography

1. Gelfand, T., *Professionalization of Modern Medicine*, p. 157. Greenwood Press, Westport, Connecticut, 1980.
2. Ibid, p. 166.
3. Senac, J.B., *Traité de la structure du coeur de son action et de ses maladies*. Chez Brosson, Paris, 1749.
4. Lieutaud, J., *Historia anatomico-medica*. Portal, Paris, 1767.
5. Ackerknecht, E. H., *Medicine at the Paris Hospital, 1794-1848*, p. 15. Johns Hopkins Press, Baltimore, 1967.
6. Wunderlich, K., *Wien und Paris*, p. 16. Ebner and Seubert, Stuttgart, 1841
7. Bichat, M. F. X., *Anatomie générale, appliquée à la physiologie et à la médicine*, 2 vols. Brosson, Gabon et Cie, 1801.
8. Bichat, M.F.X., *Traité d'anatomie descriptive*, 5 vols. Brosson, Gabon et Cie, 1801-03.
9. Bichat, M.F.X., *Recherches physiologique sur la vie et la mort*. Brosson, Gabon et Cie, 1800.
10. Bichat, M.F.X., *Traité des membranes en général et diverses membranes en particulier*. Richard, Caille et Ravier, Paris, 1800.
11. Ref. 7, Section XCIII
12. Lesch, J.E., *Science and Medicine in France*, page 70. Harvard Univ. Press, Cambridge, Mass., 1984.
13. Albury, W., *Experiment and Explanation in the Physiology of Bichat and Magendie, Studies in the History of Biology*, Vol. 1, p. 97, 1977.
14. Haller, von, A., *Elementa physiologiae corporis humani*, 8 vols. Lausanne, Berne, 1757-66.
15. Laennec, R.T.H., *Dictionaire des sciences médicales, anatomie pathologique*, Vol. 2, p. 46. Crapart, Paris, 1912.
16. Laennec, R.T.H., *L'auscultation médiate*, 2 vols. Brosson, Paris, 1819.
17. Adams, F.D., *Physical Diagnosis*, 14th Edition, Williams and Wilkins Co., Baltimore, 1958.
18. Skoda, J., *Abhandlung über Perkussion und Auskultation*. Vienna, 1839.
19. Auenbrugger, L. *Inventum novum ex percussione thoracis humani ut signo abstrusos interni pectoris morbos detegendi*. J. Trattner, 1761. See English translation in *Cardiac Classics*, p. 193, 1941.

20. Corvisart, J.N., *Essai sur les maladies et les lésions organiques du coeur et des gros vaisseaux*. Méquignon-Marvis, Paris, 1806.
21. Corvisart, J.N., *Nouvelle méthode pour reconnâitre les maladies Internes de la poitrine par la percussion de cette cavite.* Traduit d'Auenbrugger, avec des commentaires, Paris, 1808.
22. Bayle, G.L., *Dictionaire des sciences médicales*, Vol. 2, *Anatomie Pathologique*, p. 61. Crapart, Paris, 1812.
23. Bayle, G.L., *Recherches sur la phthisie pulmonaire*. Gabon, Paris, 1810.
24. Bayle, G.L., and Cayol, J.B., *Dictionaire des sciences médicales*, Vol. 3, *Cancer*, p. 537. Crapart, Paris, 1812.
25. Andral, G. *Traité de'anatomie pathologique*, 3 vols. Paris, 1829.
26. Andral, G., *Essai d'hématologie pathologique*. Fortin, Masson et Cie, Paris, 1843.
27. Magendie. F., *Lectures on the Blood.* Haswell and Barrington, Philadelphia, 1939.
28. Cruveilhier, J. *Anatomie pathologique du corps humain*, 2 vols. J.B. Baillière, Paris, 1829-42.
29. Broussais, F.J., *Examen des doctrines médicales et des systèms de nosologie*, 4 vols. Paris 1829-1834.
30. Broussais, F.J., *De l'irritation et de la folie*. Paris, 1828.
31. Bretonneau, P. F., *Des inflammations spéciales du tissue muqueux et en particulier de la diphthérite, ou inflammation pelliculaire*. Crevot, Paris, 1826.
32. Louis, P.C.A., *Recherches anatomico-pathologiques sur la phthisie*. Gabon et Cie, Paris, 1825.
33. Louis, P.C.A., *Recherches anatomiques, pathologiques et thérapeutiques sur la maladie connue sous les noms de gastro-entérite, fièvre putride, adynamique, ataxique, typhoide, etc.*, 2 vols. J.B. Baillière, Paris, 1829.
34. Louis, P.C.A., *Recherches sur les effets de la saignée dans quelques maladies inflammatoires, et sur l'action de l'émétique et des vésicatoires dans la pneumonie*. J.B. Baillière, Paris, 1835.
35. Trousseau, A., *Lectures in Clinical Medicine*, p. 34. The New Sydenham Society, London, 1869.
36. Osler, W., *Influence of Louis on American Medicine*. Johns Hopkins Hosp. Bull., Vol. viii, p. 161, 1897.
37. Rayer, P.F., *Sommaire d'une histoire abrégée de l'anatomie*

pathologique. Paris, 1818.

38. Rayer, P.F., *Traité théorique et practique des maladies de la peau*, 2 vols. and atlas. J.B. Baillière, Paris, 1826-1827.
39. Rayer, P.F., *Traité des maladies des reins*, 3 vols. and atlas. J.B. Baillière, Paris, 1839-41.
40. Rayer, P.F., De la morve et du farcin chez l'homme. *Mém. Acad. roy. Méd.* **6**, p. 625, 1837.
41. Rayer, P.F., Inoculation du sang de rate. *C.R. Soc. Biol. (Paris)*, **2**, p. 141, 1850.
42. Ricord, P., *Traité pratique des maladies vénériennes.* De Just Bouvier et Bouvier, 1838.
43. Bouillaud, J.B., Recherches expérimentales tendant à prouver que le cervelet preside aux actes de la station et de la progression, et non à l'instinct de la propagation. *Arch. Gen. Méd.* **15**, p. 64, p.225, 1827.
44. Bouillaud, J.B., *Traité clinique des maladies du coeur*, 2 vols. J.B. Baillière, Paris, 1835.
45. See Ref. 5, p. 121.
46. See Ref. 35, in Introduction.
47. Vallery-Radot, R., *The Life of Pasteur*, p. 152. Translated from the French by R.L. Devonshire, Doubleday, Page and Co., Garden City, NY. 1926.

CHAPTER IV

They tried to make an old woman of me; or that I should study Latin and Greek, . . . but these schemes I cracked (illustrating with his thumb on a table) like so many vermin as they came before me.

— John Hunter (describing his short period at Oxford in 1753 when his brother, William, attempted to make a "gentleman" of him.)

The Progress of Pathology and Medicine in Great Britain during the First Half of the Nineteenth Century

While France made significant advancements in medicine after the revolution of 1789 and for the first five decades of the nineteenth century, across the channel, the English-speaking medical community was struggling but succeeding, particularly during the years before 1820 when there were extremely difficult sociological conditions. The reasons were related to the organization of medical care, the unique characteristics of the general public and the manner in which the highest educational institutions, Oxford and Cambridge, looked at the practice of medicine and experimental science.

The Fragmentation of Medical Care

Medical care at the beginning of the nineteenth century was controlled by four different medical groups, each one protective and jealous of its rights under the law. The oldest group in England, the physicians, was made up primarily of those individuals who had received a classical, nonscientific education at Oxford or Cambridge and after graduation decided to become physicians. This was accomplished by spending perhaps a year with another physician, who charged the recent graduate or his parents a high fee for the privilege of being his assistant. Because medical knowledge at this time was very limited, the training was primarily learning how to take a medical history and then being able to make a very superficial examination of the patient by looking at the tongue, feeling the pulse, and then looking at the urine, almost in the manner of the ancients. After that prescriptions were written in Latin, most of which contained opiates or related substances from plants that gave the patient a better state of well being and relieved pain while his body either overcame or succumbed to the disease. There were other organic materials given that would produce diarrhea, sweating, or vomiting, all of which were thought to be of value in most internal diseases. There were also blistering agents, leeches, and poultices of varying types, none of which had any scientific basis but they were part of the art of medicine at that time. The only basic science on which there was any firm foundation was anatomy, but since the young, aspiring physician could see very little relationship of anatomy to the art of the physician, he gave only minimal attention to dissections. Following this non-structured training, it was possible for the young man to join the College of Physicians after a discussion in Latin with an examiner on some esoteric medical subject, which usually resulted in the medical degree. However, the number of members in the College of Physicians was never large, and they were a social elite, practiced in the major cities such as London, and had almost no contact with the general population.

The second group, the surgeons, had only recently separated themselves from the common barber by achieving Royal recognition with the establishment of the College of Surgeons. Their training was primarily through an apprentice program of several years with another surgeon without having to attend a university. They worked with their hands, took care of external lesions (broken limbs, wounds, abscesses), performed amputations, and were allowed to apply topical medications. However, they could not prescribe internal drugs, which was the province of the physicians. Most had a rudimentary knowledge of anatomy, either learned from their mentor or from attending one of the private schools of anatomy in the larger cities.

The third group was the apothecaries, which was made up of individuals with limited formal education but who had apprenticed under another apothecary for many years and worked out of a shop. He was considered a tradesman and could only receive remuneration for his drugs, not for his medical advice which was the prerogative of the physicians.

Eventually there evolved another type of practitioner who was essentially a product of the military campaigns. Due to a shortage of surgeons assigned to the army and navy, apothecaries and their apprentices found themselves by necessity performing surgery and learning on the battlefields. When they went back to civilian life, particularly after Waterloo, they naturally wanted to continue to use their new surgical skills. By a law passed in 1749, it had been established that medical personnel that had served in the military could practice after their discharge without having to belong to any of the other three groups. It was these individuals who served the needs of society because there were many small communities throughout Britain that could not support the services of both an apothecary and a surgeon. These apothecary-surgeons eventually became known as general practitioners, and as a group influenced the final consolidation of medicine and surgery late in the nineteenth century and provided most of the medical care in Britain until modern times.

The constant bickering between the various groups had economics as its basis, and each organization spent its time and energy attempting to increase its relative share of the medical marketplace rather than cooperating and attempting to bring better health care to the public. However, the influential members of British society had been imbued with the philosophy of Adam Smith that government should not undertake any actions or duties that were already or could be performed by individuals free of any restrictions. Lord Melbourne, who was prime minister twice in the 1830s, was famous for asking the question, "Why can't you let it alone?" which expressed his complete trust in individualism.[1] The basic values of the powers of British society at that time and to some degree many years later were contained in the ideas of self-help, volunteerism, individualism, and libertarianism. This philosophy was in great contrast to that existing in France and to an even greater extent in Germany, where enlightened despotism catapulted that country to supremacy in the sciences after 1850, a status maintained almost until the first World War. With the English government unwilling to take leadership in pressuring the physicians, surgeons, and apothecaries to work together for the good of society, several important problems related to medicine continued to inhibit progress in medical education. Essentially there was no national standard for medical education, and without the unification of medicine and surgery and the development of a structured curriculum including an objective examination system, the British medical men would show a complete spectrum of competence from excellent to atrocious.

Another problem was the antagonism of society toward the study of anatomy. There was a chronic shortage of bodies for dissection and perhaps more importantly for postmortem examinations. Prior to 1832, the only bodies that could be dissected were those of executed criminals, the idea being that this procedure was part of their punishment. With this philosophy it was natural that the general population would be disinclined to accept the idea that unclaimed bodies of innocent citizens would be made available for study or that their family members should be autopsied. The result was that with the diminishing number of executions, students and reputable anatomists or surgeons had either to rob graves themselves or work in collusion with thugs and murderers to obtain bodies for their studies. Many famous medical men in their memoirs relate how they carried out these activities. Dominic John Corrigan, the eminent Irish clinician wrote in 1789 about these earlier experiences in his career as follows:

> We employed our dissecting room porters to accompany funerals, and mark the recent graves which appeared to suit our purpose, and we had in our pay the old pensioner who kept the gatehouse, and used a lighted candle in the window as a signal. Night fell, and our operation commenced. We removed with our hands the clay and stones which covered the head and shoulders of the coffin — no more was uncovered; than a rope about three or four feet long was let down and the grapple, an iron hook with the end flattened out attached to the rope, was inserted under the lid of the coffin. The student then pulled on the rope until the lid of the coffin cracked across. The other end of the rope was now inserted around the neck of the dead, and the whole body was then drawn upwards and carried across the churchyard to some convenient situation, until four or six were gathered together awaiting the arrival of the car that was to convey them to some dissecting theatre. What added to the ghostly and ghastly character of the moonlight scene was that the bodies were stripped stark naked, for the possession of a shroud subjects us to prosecution.[2]

The results of these activities not only was demeaning to the medical men but infuriated the general public whose respect for the medical community was in general very poor. The use of sealed metal coffins were used to thwart the resurrectionists, and the cost of obtaining bodies increased. Eventually murders began to occur, and in 1827 two thugs, Burke and Hare, were convicted of killing innocent people to sell their bodies. As a result of this scandal, a parliamentary body was established, and hearings were held to rectify this problem. The Royal College of Surgeons was consulted and among others, the famous Astley Cooper made it clear that dissections were necessary in the education of a surgeon and that society had an obligation to provide a legitimate method for the obtaining of bodies. The result was that the Warburton Act, which was passed in 1832 after several years of controversy, abolished the dissection of executed criminals and provided for the obtaining of unclaimed bodies by licensed schools. This law helped in eliminating one factor, which had created the poor public image of the medical profession, but the internal milieu in the training of doctors was for the most part still disreputable. William Dale in his book *The Present State of the Medical Profession* published in 1860 states that in 1840:

> Drinking, smoking and brawling were the very rational occupations of the dissection room. In those days, it was no uncommon thing to see a regular battle among the students, parts of the human body forming their weapons.[3]

And Sir Henry Acland in his memoirs wrote the following of his experiences at St. George's Hospital during the same period of time:

> Everything wears the air of low men, of low habits, such as I have never hitherto come in contact with. . . . I was greatly horrified with the want of control and authority exercised among us students. The teachers truckle to us, joke; especially the evening lecturer, he will make any allusion for talk any folly to amuse the men. . . . At one o'clock on the first of October, the theatre of St George's Hospital was crowded to excess with medical gentlemen of all ages and grades; physicians, surgeons, accoucheurs, and pupils to all three, of all ages, sizes, appearances and station in life. In a few minutes a side door opened and Dr.—, the lecturer, appeared. He bowed repeatedly to his audience, and they in turn stamped and kicked uproariously. He began: "Gentlemen! (tremendous cheers) when I see before me so respectable an assemblage . . . my feelings are overpowered! You are about to begin your medical studies; the sole objects of such study are two; first, to get a name; secondly, to get money (violent applause)!"[4]

The cynicism and callousness that this reveals about the medical student during these Victorian times when many had been raised to be proper Christian English gentlemen is somewhat difficult to understand in comparison with the serious and disciplined demeanor of medical students at the present time. But considering that this was a time when ten-year-old boys were being sent into coal mines to work twelve hours a day, perhaps the gentility of the upper classes in Britain was simply a veneer, and that the starkness of the anatomy classes and the suffering and pain of hospital patients revealed the indifference and the callousness of people in general during that period of time.

Another factor that inhibited the reformation of medical training was the actuality that the teaching of science in the most elite institutions of learning, Oxford and Cambridge, was frowned upon by the deans and rectors that controlled the curriculum. Henry Acland describes his conversation with Edward Pusey, the famous theologian at Oxford when he asked why Oxford discouraged the teaching of natural science. The answer he received was "We notice that it engenders in those we know a temper of irreverence and often arrogance inconsistent with a truly Christian character."[5] But in spite of all these adverse factors, Great Britain produced some of the most brilliant and distinguished medical men of the nineteenth century.

Medicine in Scotland

It is remarkable that Scotland was more modern in outlook than England with regard to science. During the eighteenth century, Scotland underwent a period known as the Scottish Enlightenment, which was essentially independent of that occurring in France. It brought forth David Hume (1711–1776), Adam Smith (1723–1790), and Thomas Reid 1710–1796) in philosophy; Robert Burns (1759–1796), Allan Ramsay (1686–1758), Robert Fergusson (1750–1774), and others in literature; William Robertson (1721–1793) in history; and Joseph Black (1728–1799) and Daniel Rutherford (1749–1819) in chemistry. This was a period of freedom from warfare, and with the dominant church encouraging freer religious thought, the intellectual leaders created a positive climate for progress in both the humanities and science. Medicine was certainly the beneficiary of this liberalism, particularly in Edinburgh where a medical school that was modern in outlook arose. The University of Edinburgh had been established in 1592, but it was not until the eighteenth century that its medical school became its crowning glory. The seeds of this development occurred with the return of Alexander Monro (1697–1767), the anatomist, and John Rutherford, the physician, in 1719 after a period of study with Boerhaave in Holland. Caught up in the spirit of enlightenment and working together with the Edinburgh community, they were able to build a teaching hospital, the Royal Infirmary in 1738. This hospital, which was for the benefit of the poor, was built as a community project with the landowners contributing stones, merchants the timber, farmers the use of their carts, and masons and laborers donated one day of labor each month. The hospital was in close proximity to the medical school, which had an anatomical theater, a chemical laboratory, and a library and was part of the university complex. The medical school was the most modern in its time with a premedical program of four years in the classics and the medical curriculum including chemistry, botany, materia medica, anatomy, surgery, and midwifery. The better students were then appointed as "physician assistants" and were given further training at the Royal Infirmary. So by the middle of the eighteenth century, there was created in Edinburgh a new mecca to which eager young men would flock, remain awhile, and then return to their respective communities and hospitals where by practicing and teaching they would give forth the new knowledge they gained. Essentially the medical philosophy was that of Boerhaave and his student John Rutherford. The professor of medicine always started his lecture series with this comment:

> The method I propose to pursue is to examine every patient before you, I shall conduct this by a plan which will be the most useful. . . . I shall give you the history of his disease in general; second, enquire into the cause of it; third, give you my opinion how the disease is likely to terminate; lay down the indication of cure which will arise; or when any contrary symptom arises, you shall have notice of it; that you may see the reason for altering my prescriptions. . . . If you find me mistaken, I hope you will excuse me, for the Art of Physic is not infallible, nor do I myself by any means set up for infallible. I shall make as accurate observations and as just conclusions from them as I can. I hope this will produce a good result and help to make you real Physicians.[6]

When William Cullen (1711–1790) became professor of medicine in 1766, he stated that Boerhaave's system was still entirely in force except that it had incorporated new ideas and discarded the obsolete ones.

A survey of the backgrounds of the outstanding English-speaking medical men of the eighteenth and first half of the nineteenth centuries reveals that almost all of them spent some time in Edinburgh. In the 1700s it was the anatomy taught by Alexander Monro and his students, so necessary in surgery, that brought many of them to Scotland. Medicine however was still primarily an art and was to remain so until the development in France of the new physical examination by Corvisart and Laennec and based upon anatomic pathology. The following eminent medical men from Great Britain, either had received their medical degree at Edinburgh or had spent some time studying there: Thomas Addison (1793–1860), Thomas Bateman (1778–1821), Charles Bell (1774–1842), John Bell (1763–1831), Benjamin Bell (1749–1806), Richard Bright (1789–1858), Robert Christison (1797–1882), James Clark (1788–1870), Astley Cooper (1768–1841), Abraham Colles (1773–1843), David Craigie (1793–1856), William Cruikshank (1745–1800), John Cheyne (1777–1836), John Forbes (1787–1861), Robert Graves (1796–1853), Marshall Hall (1790–1857), Francis Home (1719–1813), James Hope (1801–1841), Thomas Hodgkin (1798–1866), Herbert Mayo (1796–1852), Charles Scudamore (1779–1849), William Stokes (1804–1878), and John Thomson (1765–1846).

Most of the well-trained American medical men during the 1700s had trained in Edinburgh, some with the encouragement of Benjamin Franklin who knew William Cullen there. Before 1765, there were 15 Americans who graduated from Edinburgh, but from 1765 to 1799, in spite of the American Revolution, there were at least 113 who had trained there. Some of the prominent ones were John Morgan (1735–1789), William Shippen, Jr. (1736–1808), Benjamin Rush (1745–1813), Adam Kuhn (1743–1817), Caspar Wistar (1760–1818), and Alexander Garden (1728–1791). The significant factor about most of these men was that they knew anatomy, which was necessary for the understanding of anatomic pathology. Eighteenth-century surgeons certainly had more opportunities than physicians for studying morbid anatomy, not only because they were the teachers of normal anatomy, but because they were called upon by physicians when a postmortem was necessary. For example, when George II (1683–1760) died, he had been attended by physicians but was autopsied by the surgeon Caesar Hawkins (1798–1884). This association of necropsies with surgeons continued well into the nineteenth century in England, because unlike France, the physicians simply did not have enough surgical and anatomical training. And as long as the surgeons did the postmortem examinations, the understanding of internal disease could not develop significantly. However, there were a few more conscientious physicians who were Edinburgh graduates, such as Hodgkin, Bright, Addison, Graves, and Stokes, who recognized the importance of autopsies and were able to perform them on their own patients. As a result they were able to make discoveries related to internal diseases.

The Edinburgh Influence

There were three major schools spawned from the Edinburgh mecca that influenced the study of pathology in Great Britain; those of William and John Hunter, Guy's Hospital, and the Dublin School.

The School of William and John Hunter

The first was that of William Hunter who had studied anatomy under Alexander Monro and William Cullen. Hunter was first an anatomist, then a surgeon, later an obstetrician, and finally considered himself a physician. He was fined by the College of Surgeons when he elected to become a member of the College of Physicians. However, it has been said that William Hunter's greatest discovery was the talent of his brother John (1728–1793), who had rebelled so much as a youth that he essentially had no formal education and resulted in his being apprenticed out to a cabinet maker. When this was unsuccessful, the educated William offered him a last opportunity to become his assistant dissector at the Great Windmill Street School of Anatomy, which had been established by William in 1748.

John quickly developed into an expert dissector, and William then obtained a position for him as a surgeon apprentice to the well-known surgeon William Cheselden (1688–1752). Thus, John Hunter became a skilled surgeon, but he had no ambitions to be either a famous anatomist or practicing surgeon. He was essentially a curious man and his interest was the entire domain of biology, and he asked questions about nature that his colleagues found boring or irrelevant. He was a scientist rather than a practitioner, and, though he hated to see patients, there were great demands for his services. He used the huge funds he earned from fees to buy a country estate where he kept all types of animals, including zebras, leopards, snakes, and a large pond for freshwater life. He was fascinated with comparative anatomy and dissected more than 500 animals. He created a huge museum for all types of animal specimens, including human ones, both normal and abnormal. He did the first definitive study on teeth on various animals; noted the descent of the testes in some animals; studied the air sacs in birds, the pregnant uterus, venereal disease; and made the original description of the olfactory nerve. He was interested in pathology, particularly inflammation, and studied it in great detail. However, because of his lack of formal education, he found it very difficult to write and publish his findings. His major work was his *A Treatise on the Blood, Inflammation and Gunshot Wounds*, published a year after his death although many of his ideas on inflammation were also in his *Principles of Surgery*, a series of lectures given in 1786. He was the first person to attempt to explain the Celsus cardinal signs and symptoms of inflammation, which were tumor (swelling), rubor (redness), calor (heat), and dolor (pain), in terms of the anatomy and physiology of his time. John Hunter's ideas regarding inflammation were as follows:

> The operation in the body called inflammation is one of the most common and most extensive in its effects, and requires our greatest attention. It is the cause of many effects, both salutary and diseased, producing abscesses, fistulas, diseased bones, etc, and in many diseases is the first step toward a cure; so that it becomes a first principle of surgery. Inflammation would appear to be produced by an increased action of the vessels, but it is most probably in the smallest vessels, for it may be confined almost to a point where none but the smallest vessels exist. 1. Swelling of the parts (tumor) in inflammation is greatest in the middle, and gradually lessens from that till it is lost in the surrounding parts. It is owing to the extravasation of coagulable lymph and some serum being squeezed out as the coagulable lymph thickens . . . causing edema. 2. Color of the inflamed parts (rubor) . . . is visibly changed from the natural hue, whatever it was, to red. This red is of various hues, according to the nature of the inflammation; if healthy, of a pure scarlet red; if less healthy the color is more of a purple. . . . This increase of red would appear to arise from two causes; first, dilatation of the vessels, by which a greater quantity of blood is sent into those vessels . . . and second, the formation of new vessels. . . . 3. Heat of the inflamed part (calor). . . . The inflamed part

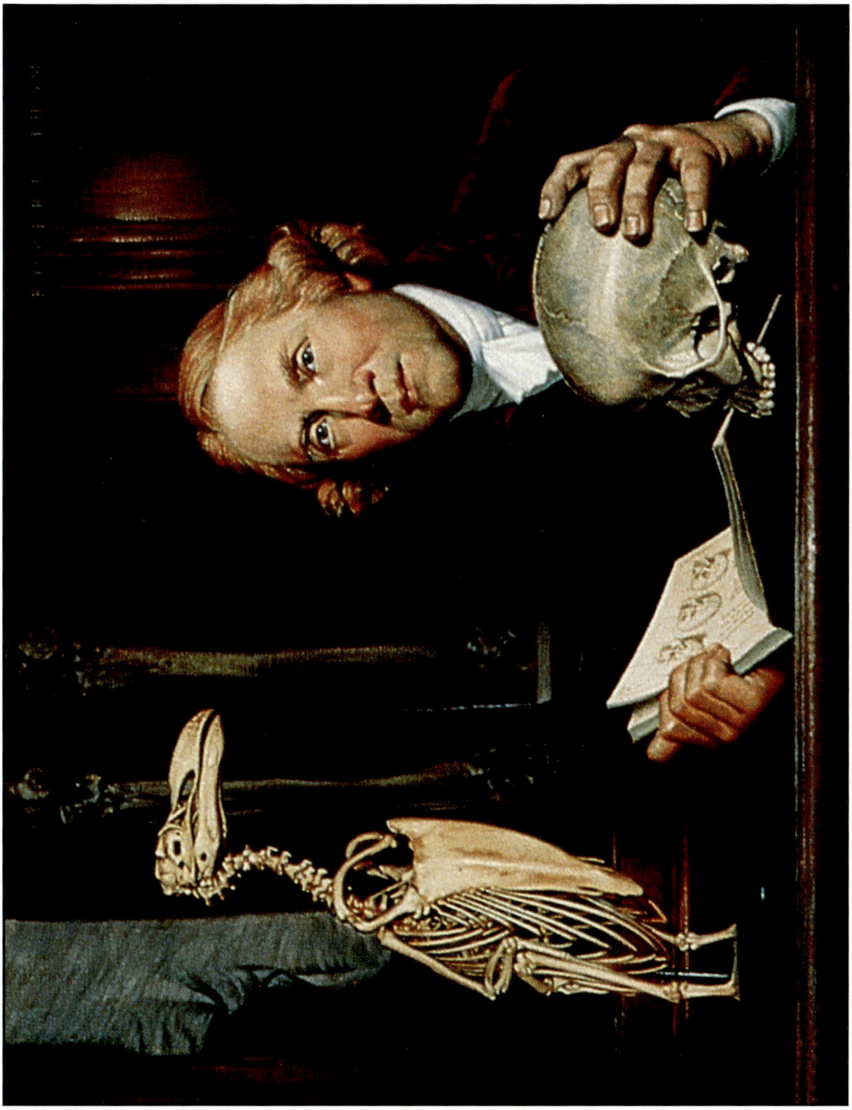

HUNTER: FOUNDER OF SCIENTIFIC SURGERY

> is hotter than common. . . . From all the observations I have made, I do not find that a local inflammation can produce local heat above what is natural to the animal. 4. Pain (dolor). . . . As inflammation is passing from the adhesive to the suppurative, the parts then undergo a greater change than before, and the pain grows more and more. . . . The nerves also acquire at that time a degree of sensibility which renders them more susceptible of impression than when they are in their natural state; thus an inflamed part is not only painful in itself, but it communicates impressions to the mind independent of pain, which do not arise from a natural sound part.[7]

It was by his astuteness that Hunter was the first to realize that inflammation was a defensive response of the body and that it was the first step in healing. And even though he did not use a microscope, he was able to understand what was occurring at a lower level of such activity. It should be remembered that in 1794, thc electrical nature of the nerve impulse, the sensory cells that respond as pain, the nature of heat, and the exudation of white blood cells from the blood was completely unknown. Virchow in 1895 in his essay *One Hundred Years of General Pathology* said this about John Hunter:

> In England it was especially John Hunter, a highly regarded surgeon, who recognized the significance of pathological anatomy. To him we owe the founding of the first great museum of pathological preparations, one which has become the prototype of the many continental institutions of the same kind. He introduced the experimental method into pathology, and henceforth observations on living animals were used for the correction and extension of anatomical investigations. On the basis of such experience it was possible for the investigator named to set up general doctrines of proven significance. These soon became the standards of general pathology in England, and maintained their rank into modern times.[8]

Hunter had many students, Edward Jenner, Astley Cooper, John Abernethy, William Clift, James Parkinson, William Blizard, and Philip Syng Physick from Philadelphia, and, because of his interest in pathological processes such as inflammation, he is given credit for bringing the practice of surgery from a craft to a science.

After Hunter's death, his nephew and pupil Mathew Baillie (1761–1823) continued as one of the proprietors of the Great Windmill

Street Anatomical School and was instrumental in publishing in 1793 the first textbook in the English language dedicated to the new field of anatomical pathology.[9] This text was followed by an atlas that was issued in ten parts over the years 1799–1802, which consisted of specimens beautifully drawn by William Clift that were mostly from John Hunter's collection.[10] These were accompanied by clear and concise descriptions of the lesions with little discussion about pathogenesis, although Baillie stressed this was the goal of pathology. The texts and atlas went through several editions and were the best available until Jean Cruveilhier published his two-volume work during the years 1829–1842. James Hope published an excellent pathology atlas in 1834,[11] but it was not the equal of Robert Carswell who released his *Illustrations of the Elementary Forms of Disease* [12] in 1838. This was followed by the books of Herman Lebert, who published in 1845 a two-volume text with an accompanying atlas entitled *Physiologie Pathologique* composed primarily of illustrations of lesions as seen under the microscope.[13] This work was followed by his most definitive work, the four volume *Traité d'Anatomie Pathologique*, published in 1857, which incorporated the most advanced knowledge about pathology and contained magnificent color illustrations of disease processes, both gross and microscopic,[14] and was the envy of Rudolf Virchow, a friend of Lebert.

Guy's Hospital School

The second school spawned from the Edinburgh mecca was that of Guy's Hospital, which flourished during the first half of the nineteenth century. There were four men who were primarily responsible.

Astley Cooper

Astley Cooper not only studied in Edinburgh but was a pupil of John Hunter and was to become the most famous surgeon in England at Guy's Hospital during the first quarter of the century. From his experience with Hunter, he became a pioneer in vascular surgery and was the first to ligate a common carotid and external iliac artery for repairing aneurysms, and in 1817 made a daring ligation of the abdominal aorta. But because of his stimulation by Hunter, he was also a constant dissector and anatomist. When he was not performing surgery on both royalty and the poor in London, he was either teaching, doing experimental surgery on animals, or dissecting cadavers. He had a dissection room both at his home in London and at his country estate, and, just as did Hunter, he would arise at 5:00-6:00 A.M. and dissect the entire day if possible. It is said that he was unhappy if a day went by when he was unable to perform a postmortem examination or some type of dissection. His usual day was to see outpatients until 1:00 in the afternoon after his dissections, visit hospital patients until 2:00, lecture on anatomy until 3:00 when he would help at the student dissection rooms or perform surgery until 7:00, after which he would have dinner, take a nap, and then lecture or visit patients until midnight. He was the shining light at Guy's Hospital during the early years of the nineteenth century, and trained many outstanding surgeons, such as Aston Key (1793–1849) and Benjamin Travers (1783–1858). However, when three young physicians, Richard Bright, Thomas Addison, and Thomas Hodgkin, came down from Edinburgh after 1810, already having been stimulated by the Scottish faculty and perhaps by visiting in France, the stage was set for outstanding progress in pathology and internal medicine.

Richard Bright

The first of the young men was Richard Bright, a cheerful, courteous, and even-tempered man, who was loved by both his students and his patients. He was an excellent anatomic pathologist, spending hours in the postmortem room, examining every organ with extreme care and correlating his findings with each clinical detail. His discoveries were monumental:

1. He found that "dropsy" could most often be correlated with lesions of the kidneys with protein in the urine and with a semi-quantitative increase in urea in the blood. In his two volume work, *Reports of Medical Cases Selected with a View of Illustrating the Symptoms and Cure of Diseases by a Reference to Morbid Anatomy* in 1827 he said that:

> There are other appearances to which I think too little attention has hitherto been paid. They are those evidences of organic disease, which occasionally present themselves in the structure of the kidney, and which, whether they are to be considered the cause of the dropsical effusion or as the consequence of some other disease, cannot be unimportant. Where these conditions of the kidney to which I allude have occurred, I have often found the dropsy connected with the secretion of albuminous urine, more or less coagulable on heat. . . . I have never yet examined the body of a patient

> dying of dropsy attended with coagulable urine, in whom some obvious derangement was not discovered in the kidneys.[15]

In 1836 Bright wrote his final thoughts on his discoveries in Guy's Reports. Because they were of such significance for both internal medicine and pathology his conclusions are given here:

> The importance and extensive prevalence of that form of disease, which after it has continued for some time, is attended by the peculiar changes in the structure of the kidney, now pretty generally known by the names of 'mottling', 'white degeneration', 'contraction' or 'granulation' impresses itself every year more and more deeply on my mind. . . . It is indeed, a humiliating confession, that, although much attention has been directed to this disease for nearly ten years, and during that time there has probably been no period in which at least twenty cases might not have been pointed out in each of the large hospitals of the metropolis . . . yet little or nothing has been done towards devising a method of permanent relief, when the disease has been confirmed. . . . I am most anxious . . . to impress upon the members of our profession the insidious nature of this malady, that they may be led to watch its first approaches, with all the solicitude which they would feel on discovering the first suspicious symptoms of phthisis, or of epilepsy. . . . The first indications of the tendency to this disease is often hematuria, of a more or less decided character; this may originate from various causes. . . . Scarlatina has apparently laid the foundation for future mischief . . . or without having made any such observation, he awakes in the morning with his face swollen, or his ankles puffy, or his hands edematous. If he happens, in this condition, to fall under the care of a practitioner who suspects the nature of his disease, it is found that already his urine contains a notable quantity of albumen; his pulse is full and hard*, his skin dry, he has often headache, and sometimes a sense of weight or pain across his loins. . . . Sometimes without any treatment, the more obvious and distressing of these symptoms disappear; the swelling is no longer observed and the urine ceases to evince any admixture of red particles . . . and the symptoms are gradually lost sight of or are absolutely forgotten. Nevertheless, from time to time the countenance becomes bloated, the skin is dry, headaches occur with unusual frequency, or the call to micturition disturbs the night's repose. After a time . . . weakness or pain in the loins increase, and headaches, often accompanied by vomiting add greatly to the general want of comfort and a sense of lassitude, and of depression

* This was an indication of hypertension, but an instrument for routine measuring of blood pressure would not be available for another 70 years.

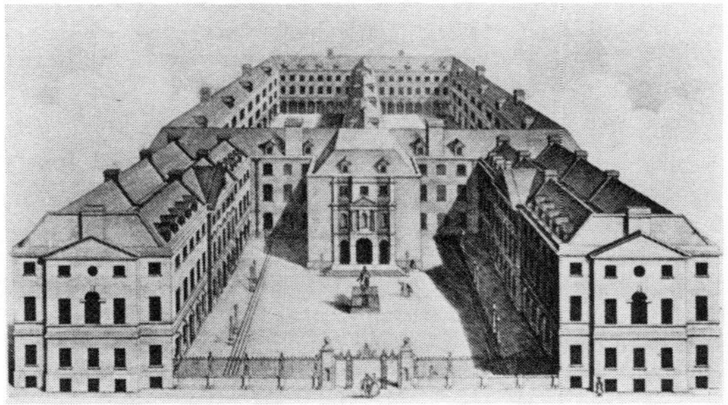

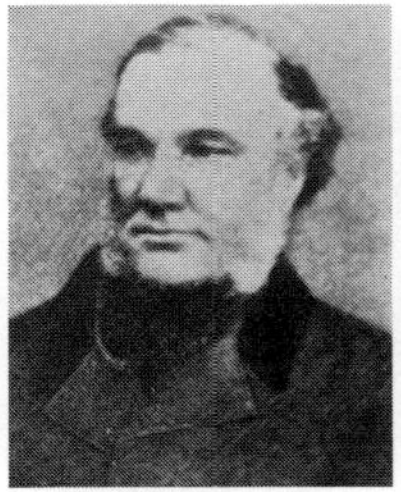

T. Addison

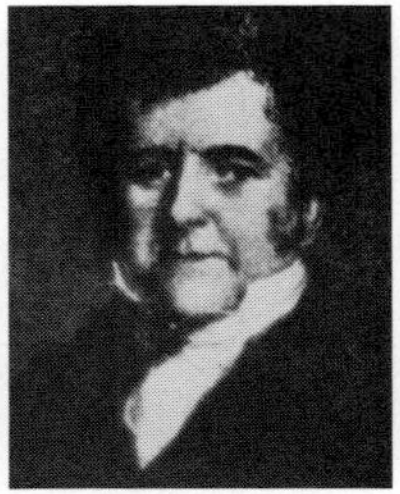

R. Bright

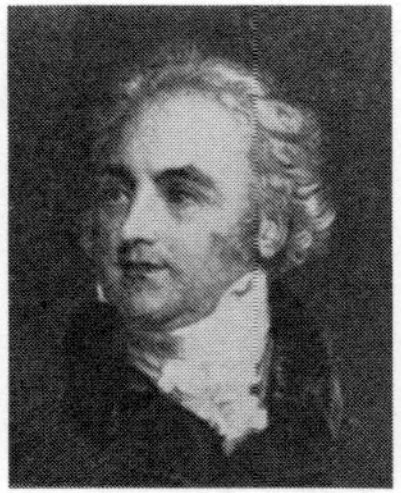

A. Cooper

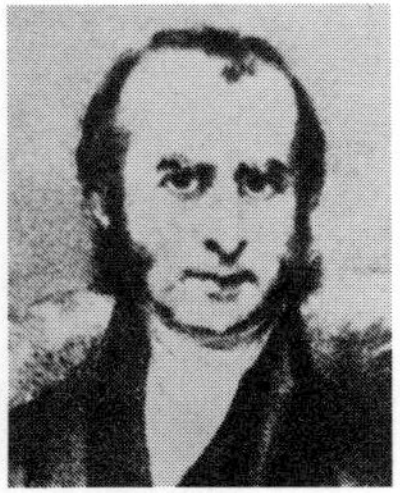

T. Hodgkin

THE MEN OF GUY'S HOSPITAL

> gradually steals over the bodily and mental frame. If blood is drawn, it is often buffed, or the serum is milky and analysis will frequently detect a great deficiency of albumen, and sometimes manifest indications of the presence of urea. . . . (Sometimes) the patient is restored to tolerable health, or if he is, perhaps less fortunate — the swelling increases, the urine becomes scanty, the powers of life seem to yield, the lungs become edematous, and in a state of asphyxia or coma, he sinks into the grave. He may be suddenly seized with an attack of pericarditis, or peritonitis, which without any renewed warning, deprive him, in 48 hours of his life. His hearing may be depraved, his vision indistinct and he may have a convulsive fit and become blind. Of the appearance after death . . . do we always see the lesion in the kidney? After ten years . . . I am ready to answer this question in the affirmative and yet I confess that I have occasionally met with anomalies which have been somewhat difficult to explain. . . . [16]

Thus, in spite of the vast numbers of cases that Bright studied, it was several years before the medical world accepted the disease of glomerulonephritis as a distinct entity.

2. Bright was the first to correlate jaundice and fatty stools with lesions of the pancreas or its duct leading into the intestine.[17]

3. Bright was one of the first to describe acute yellow atrophy of the liver which he described in 1836 with two cases in which he found intense jaundice without any mechanical obstruction of the ducts.[18] He came to the conclusion that the disease was due to an inflammatory action in the substance of the liver and noted that the condition was accompanied by mental confusion and multiple hemorrhages. He described the liver in both cases as being small, soft, and yellow. The reader should be aware that at the time of Bright's work, microscopic work and the study of histology was just getting started due to the improvement in the compound microscope by Joseph Lister, and therefore Bright was only able to make gross descriptions.

Thomas Addison

Thomas Addison was the second of the bright young men. He was described by a contemporary in this manner:

> The personal power which he possessed was the secret of his position, much superior to what Bright could ever claim, and equal, if

> not greater than that of Sir Astley Cooper. For many years he was the leading light of Guy's, so that every Guy's man during his thirty or forty years of his teaching was a disciple of Addison, holding his name in the greatest reverence, and regarding his authority as the best guide in the practice of the profession. . . . He was dogmatic in his teaching, and thus the pupils accepted as pure gospel every word which flowed from his lips. The force of his words was enhanced by his mode of delivery and by the presence of the man himself. Addison was of good height and well made, stood erect, with coat buttoned up very high, over which hung his guard and eyeglass. He wore a black stock with scarcely visible shirt-collar, and this further elevated his head. He had . . . dark hair and side whiskers, large bushy eyebrows and smallish dark eyes, nose thick, as were also his lips, which enclosed his firmly knit mouth. His features were not refined, but belonged to a powerful mind and showed no trace of any kind of sentiment. His penetrating glance seemed to look through you, and his whole demeanor was that of a leader of men, enhanced by his somewhat martial attitude.[19]

Addison made four significant contributions. These were as follows:

1. The first clinical discussion of appendicitis and its complications was published in the book *Elements of Practical Medicine* that he wrote with Richard Bright in 1839. This was the description that was entitled "Inflammation of the Caecum and Appendix Veriformis," and expanded on the work of Hodgkin in 1836:

> The patient is suddenly seized with severe pain, sometimes with chills and vomiting. A hardness and tumefaction are soon very evident to the hand in the part first affected; this continuing general symptoms of peritonitis often takes place, and terminates fatally; but under careful treatment the inflammation remains circumscribed and becomes even less extensive, assuming the form of a local deep-seated abscess. The threatening symptoms of peritonitis subside; the tumefaction just above the iliac crest is more and more obvious to the touch, and gradually shows a tendency to point; in process of time it either opens of its own accord, or is assisted by the lancet, and a discharge of ill-conditioned pus follows, which from its peculiar fetid smell, is soon discovered to be mingled with feculent matter. The discharge continues for many weeks and the

> patient often sinks at length from exhaustion. In other cases, when the powers of the system are previously unbroken, the abscess closes and permanent recovery is obtained. The morbid appearance shows a fecal abscess in the right iliac region that has arisen from disease set up in the appendix caeci. It is found that this organ is very subject to inflammation, to ulceration, and even to gangrene . . . this little wormlike body is often detected in the midst of the abscess, with a perforation at its extremity; of by ulceration higher up in its parietes.[20]

2. At a time when lobar pneumonia was exceedingly common, Addison, by careful microscopic examination stated correctly in 1839:

> Pneumonia may be defined to be an inflammation of the air cells of the lungs, speedily producing an effusion into them of a serous looking fluid commonly mixed with blood; causing, if unchecked, such a degree of thickening of their parietes as apparently to fill them up for a time; or leading to the deposition of an albuminous matter, which is either solid or of a puriform character; and seldom, if ever, terminating in the formation of a genuine abscess.[21]

3. Addison made the first clinical description of pernicious anemia (shortly to be called Addisonian anemia) in 1849:

> For a long time I had from time to time met with a very remarkable form of general anemia, occurring without any discoverable cause, whatever, cases in which there had been no previous loss of blood, no chlorosis, no purpura, no renal, splenic, or miasmic or malignant disease. It makes its approach in so slow and insidious a manner that the patient can hardly fix a date . . . of that earliest feeling of that languor which is shortly to become so extreme. The countenance gets pale, the whites of the eyes pearly, the frame flabby rather than wasted . . . there is an indisposition to exertion, with a feeling of breathlessness on attempting it; the heart palpitates, the lips, gums and tongue seem bloodless and the appetite fails and edema appears above the ankles. The patient eventually cannot rise from his bed, his mind wanders, and he falls into a half torpid state and at length expires. Nevertheless, to the very last, and after a sickness lasting perhaps several months, the bulkiness of the frame and the obesity often present a most striking contrast to the failure and exhaustion observable in every other respect. . . . After death I have failed to discover any organic lesion that could prop-

> erly or reasonably be assigned as an adequate cause of such serious consequences.[22]

4. In 1855 Addison published a small book entitled *On the Constitutional and Local Effects of Disease of the Suprarenal Capsules* in which he describes hypoadrenalism, which is still known as Addison's disease, while he was over the years still trying to find the lesions that could produce his pernicious anemia. He wrote the following:

> The leading and characteristic features of the morbid state to which I would direct attention are anemia, general languor and debility, remarkable feebleness of the heart's action, irritability of the stomach, and a peculiar change of color in the skin, occurring in connection with a diseased condition of the suprarenal capsules. . . . This discoloration is sufficiently marked, indeed, as generally to have attracted the attention of the patient himself or of the patient's friends. This discoloration pervades the whole surface of the body, but is commonly most strongly manifested on the face, neck, superior extremities, penis, and scrotum and in the flexures of the axillae and around the navel. We may suspect some malignant or strumous disease — we may be led to inquire into the condition of the so called blood making organs but we discover no proof of organic change anywhere — no enlargement of the spleen, thyroid, thymus or lymphatic gland. . . . I believe that the anemic prostration and peculiar condition of the skin will present a corresponding character, and that whether acute or chronic, provided the lesions involve the entire structure of both organs, death will inevitably be the consequence.[23]

Although it is obvious to the modern reader that Addison was having difficulty differentiating pernicious anemia from hypoadrenalism, the reason was that the understanding and definition of anemia had not been established. The word was loosely used to describe the clinical features of pallor, feeble pulse, palpitation, faintness, and lack of energy, all of which can be found in both clinical entities, although it is not clear how Addison, who was such an astute clinician, did not note on occasion the often characteristic inflamed tongue, the slight icterus, premature graying hair, and the tingling of the fingers and toes of patients with pernicious anemia. However, the basic problem was that the diagnostic and simple methods for determining the number of erythrocytes or hemoglobin per unit of volume of blood had not been accomplished in 1855, and microscopic examination of the blood and bone marrow were not performed until Ehrlich developed the staining methodology. Thus Addison could not have known that hypoadrenalism does not usually produce anemia. Nevertheless, Addison's work was monumental, particularly the correlation of the pigmentation of the skin with lesions of the adrenal glands, and although he did not realize it, his discovery was important in the later understanding of the still undiscovered endocrine system.

Thomas Hodgkin

The third great man of that period at Guy's Hospital was from a personality standpoint the strangest — Thomas Hodgkin. He was a devout Quaker, dressed in their quaint clothes of that time, used *Thee* and *Thou* in his speech, and championed all the down-trodden people on the earth, including the American Indians, the black slaves, the insane, and the poor people of London. He was very outspokenly critical of any institution that encouraged injustices. But in common with Bright, Addison, and Cooper, his first love was anatomical pathology. However, his perspective in that field was more French than British, because he had gone to Paris in 1821 to study under Laennec, who took a liking to the Quaker. Although he obtained his medical degree at Edinburgh, he eventually returned to Guy's Hospital where he was determined to interject into British pathology the anatomic pathology of Bichat and Laennec with its emphasis on tissues and membranes. But his efforts were not very successful, and he states about his lectures to the English medical student:

> For the three years that I have filled the unprofitable thankless post of lecturer on Pathological Anatomy I have been cut short not by the termination of the subject but by the desertion of my audience. I am painfully sensible how strongly this bespeakes the want of talent in the lecturer. But . . . by the recent acts of an important body, you are recommended not to neglect this study and what is more it is rendered incumbent upon you to become acquainted with legal medicine. Now morbid anatomy is to legal medicine what mineralogy is to Geology — I might almost say what letters are to language.[24]

Poor man! Considering the fact that the typical medical student was so crude and mercenary as described earlier in the chapter by Acland, it is surprising that with his idealism, Hodgkin even stayed in the field of medicine, let alone trying to imbue academic pathological anatomy into most of the medical students at the time. Hodgkin wrote a book in 1837 entitled *Pathology of Membranes* in which he summarized his thoughts on the value of pathological anatomy and perhaps his opinions of the medical students he tried to teach:

> To those who may place the summum bonum of medical practice in converting the largest quantity of physic into gold, morbid anatomy must, I am aware, be an object of disgust, rather than attraction; but those who are aspiring to become worthy members of a profession which has for its object the restoration of health to our suffering fellow-creatures, must see that morbid anatomy or the investigation of those physical derangements which as the consequences of disease or accident, it is their business to avert or remove, constitutes a study the most essential to their art. We can only become properly initiated into our profession by personal acquaintance with disease, founded on our own patient investigation at the bedside of the sick, and by a diligent examination of the effects of disease, as brought to light by cadaveric inspection. The practice of examining the dead for the purpose of ascertaining the seat and effect of disease, is absolutely necessary to complete those ideas which it is impossible for the best verbal descriptions perfectly to convey; and it is also necessary, as the means of detecting that which yet remains to be either wholly discovered or more fully elucidated.[25]

Hodgkin's medical knowledge was highly respected by his colleagues, but politically he was such a maverick that he was eventually maneuvered out of Guy's Hospital. He went to St. Thomas' Hospital but with little more success and eventually left the field of medicine, went to Palestine to help the "poor Jews" and died there in 1866.

But he made significant discoveries and is remembered for four of them.

1. The most important was his description of a particular disease of the lymphatic system that he described in 1832 in a paper *On Some Morbid Appearances of the Absorbent Glands and Spleen* [26] which was a classic description of what Wilks in 1865 referred to as "Hodgkin's disease." Perhaps since this was one year before his death, he might have known about the honor bestowed upon him by Wilks while he was in Palestine.

2. In his *Lectures on the Morbid Anatomy of the Serous and Mucous Membranes* published in 1836, he was one of the first to describe "appendicitis" as an inflammation in the iliac fossa produced by ulceration and perforation of the appendix with fecal contamination of the fossa, which sometimes remains localized but other times becomes diffused over the entire abdomen, which proves fatal.

3. In 1827, he wrote a paper *On Retroversion of the Valves of the Aorta* [27] in which he describes damage to the valves of the aorta allowing blood on systole to flow back into the left ventricle, or what is now known as aortic insufficiency. Hodgkin was the first to describe this condition, although Corrigan four years later gave a much more extensive clinical and pathological description of this condition.

4. In 1827 he published with his fellow Quaker Joseph Lister a paper, *Notice of Some Microscopical Observation of Blood and Animal Tissues,*[28] which contains the first clear description of muscle cells and erythrocytes. This paper could be considered the beginning of the discipline of histology.

The Dublin School

The third school that was spawned by the Edinburgh Medical School was that of Dublin, which also had a triad of internists, William Stokes (1804–1878), Robert James Graves (1796–1853), and Dominic John Corrigan (1802–1880), who all received training in Scotland. The creativity of these men rivaled that of Bright, Addison, and Hodgkin at Guy's Hospital. During the last quarter of the eighteenth century there were a great number of Irish students who enrolled at Edinburgh because Ireland did not offer any comparable training. Other pioneers of this Dublin school were John Cheyne (1777–1843), who first described hydrocephalus and then the Cheyne Stokes respiration; Abraham Colles (1773–1843), who wrote the classic description of fracture of the carpal end of the radius; Robert Adams (1791–1895), who gave the classic description of gout; and James Macartney, the great Irish surgeon and anatomist. Perhaps the most famous clinician was Robert Graves, who was the first to bring the German method of assigning medical students to make the initial examination of hospital patients as part of their training. Before that time the students were only observers at the bedside. Graves also recognized the importance of postmortem examinations in the teaching about disease. One of his students, Andrew Young, wrote of Grave's opinions about the value of autopsies when he was asked by this physician

> to make post-mortem examinations of some bodies which had been living the night before but died of fever a few hours previous to my taking up the task, at his desire. There were few of us who like to be inhaling the emanations from a body recently dead from fever, or other such ailments, on empty stomachs, and often I have been busy for hours, until the afternoon, and alone when he would return to the dead room where I had been making careful dissections of the diseased parts. He would scrutinize these carefully, and make his remarks aloud for my instruction, and finally say "Young, this is the true way to study pathology. Here we see the changes which caused the symptoms we watched at the bedside with so much anxiety, and which are still fresh in our memory. . . . Now run home and take your breakfast."[29]

The major discovery by Graves was his first accurate account of exophthalmic goiter accompanied by palpitation of the heart, written in 1835. The description is as follows:

> A lady, aged twenty, became affected with some symptoms which were supposed to be hysterical. This occurred more than two years ago; After she had been in this nervous state about three months it was observed that her pulse had become singularly rapid . . . and was constant, never being under 120, and often much higher. She next complained of weakness on exertion, and began to look pale and thin. Thus she continued for a year, but during this time she manifestly lost ground. It was now observed that the eyes assumed a singular appearance, for the eyeballs were apparently enlarged, so that when she slept or tried to shut her eyes, the lids were incapable of closing. When the eyes were open, the white sclerotic could be seen to a breadth of several lines around the cornea. In a few months, the action of the heart continuing with increasing violence, a tumor, of a horseshoe shape, appeared on the front of the throat and exactly in the situation of the thyroid gland. This was at first soft but soon became harder . . . and is now thrice the natural bulk of the gland in a female. From an early period of the disease, a remarkable disproportion was found to exist between the beats of the radial and of the carotid arteries, the former feeble and the latter violent causing a most evident throbbing of the neck and accompanied by a loud rustling sound.[30]

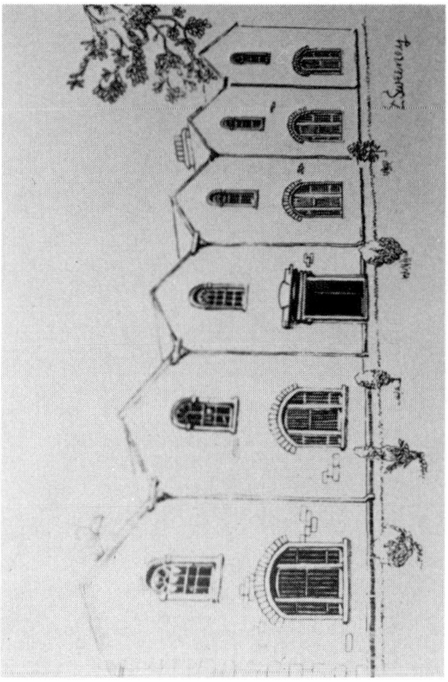

Trinity Medical School

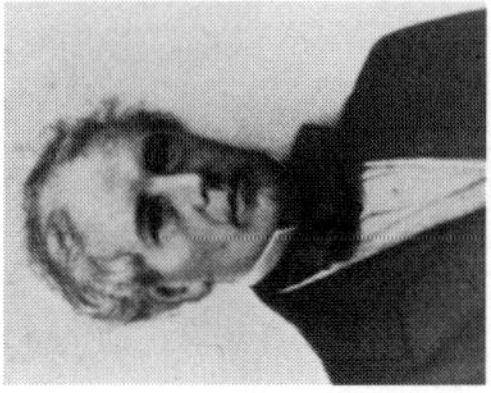

D. J. Corrigan

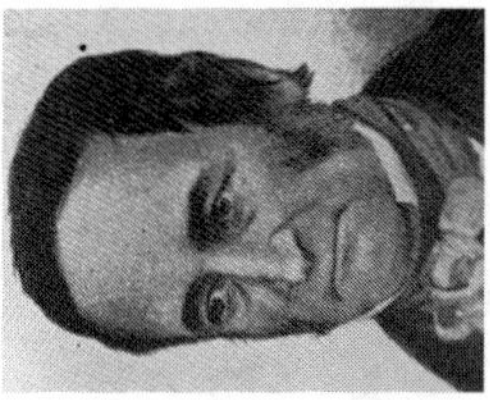

R. Graves

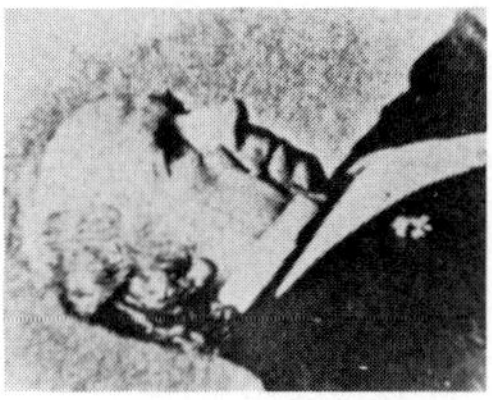

W. Stokes

THE DUBLIN TRIAD

William Stokes was first a pupil and then a colleague of Graves. He is best known for detecting the phenomena of heart block with syncopal attacks and a slow pulse which became known as the Stokes-Adams syndrome (with Robert Adams).[31] In his book *The Diseases of the Heart and Aorta*, published in 1854, he gave an account of fatty degeneration of the heart in a case in which there was the characteristic periodic breathing which became known as Cheyne Stokes breathing. He also gave the first description of paroxysmal tachycardia.[32]

The other member of the Dublin triad, Dominic John Corrigan was very much interested in pathology and is most known for his characterizing the typical pulse of aortic insufficiency, the "water hammer pulse," which became known as the Corrigan pulse. He logically concluded that the hypertrophy of the left ventricle in aortic insufficiency is a compensatory mechanism and not a primary disease.[33]

Later Developments in Scotland

Back in Edinburgh itself, anatomic pathology was making progress, although the postmortem examination of patients was not routine and was often cursory and unsystematic. This was due primarily to the public attitude before the Warburton Act of 1832. John Thomson had been chosen for the first chair of pathology, and the long tradition of excellent anatomy resulted in excellent surgeons who always used dissections for improving their techniques and correcting their errors.

Experimental pathology also made progress. John Bell regarded as the founder of surgical anatomy, was the first to ligate the gluteal artery, the common carotid, and internal iliac in his treatment of vascular injuries.[34] Charles Bell, the brother of John, was the first to show that the ventral spinal nerve root had a motor function and showed that the fifth cranial nerve had both motor and sensory functions. He also was responsible for showing that injury to the seventh cranial nerve results in "Bell's palsy."[35] James Syme (1799–1870) was the first to treat a case of iliac aneurysm by ligating the common iliac and the internal and external iliac arteries,[36] and also wrote a book on pathology related to the practice of surgery, emphasizing the new antiseptic techniques originated by his son-in-law, Joseph Lister.[37] Robert Lister (1794–1847) was the first surgeon in Great Britain to use ether anesthetic and he originated the idea of observing the larynx using a mirror.[38]

Edinburgh had one of the most famous and original gynecologists in the nineteenth century in James Young Simpson (1811–1870), who was the first to use chloroform instead of ether as an anesthetic[39] and devised new instruments for obstetrics and surgery. Simpson also invented new surgical techniques for ovariotomy and made pathological studies of female diseases.[40]

In medicine, Edinburgh had several famous physicians, among them John Hughes Bennett (1812–1875), who following his graduation in 1837, spent two years in clinical medicine in Paris, and then two years doing research in Germany where he learned to become an expert microscopist. When he returned to Edinburgh in 1841, he commenced a series of lectures in histology and microscopic pathology, which was the first of its kind in Great Britain. He was later pathologist to the Royal Infirmary and lectured on both medicine and pathology. All of his pathological cases were carefully annotated and illustrated with microscopic drawings by his own hand. Bennett also gave in 1845 the first description of death by leukemia with abnormalities of the spleen and liver, but was interpreted as "suppuration of the blood."[41] However, Virchow, only six weeks after Bennett's publication, also published a report on the necropsy of a patient with the same symptoms. He gave the condition the name of "leucemia,"[42] and is usually given credit for the discovery. It is true that Bennett described the condition as pyemia of the blood, and Virchow called it "white blood." In Bennett's case, there appeared to be enlarged lymph nodes, and it is likely that this was a lymphatic leukemia, whereas Virchow's case does not appear to have enlarged nodes, and he describes some of the white cells as having horseshoe shaped nuclei, which indicates he was dealing with a myelogenous leukemia. In either case, the situation indicates that anatomic pathology was being actively pursued at that time and priorities for discoveries of new diseases would become problems for the medical world until the present time. John Goodsir (1814–1867) was an anatomist at Edinburgh who also used the microscope and recognized the importance of the cell in his research,[43] and Virchow recognized his research and dedicated his famous book *Cellular Pathology* to Goodsir. David Craigie (1793–1865) also contributed to the field of pathology and wrote a text that was an attempt to summarize the latest concepts in pathology, the best part being a description of lesions of the pancreas.[44] Robert Christison, a professor of medicine and toxicology, was most famous for his work on poisons and various drugs,[45] and he also wrote a major paper *On Granular De-*

generation of the Kidneys[46] in 1839 confirming and extending the work of Bright.

Two other Scottsmen went to France in the 1820s to study pathology. The first was James Hope (1801–1841), who taught pathology at St. George's Hospital and did an excellent correlation of auscultation with lesions of the heart, which was published in 1832 and underwent several editions and translations.[47] The second was Robert Carswell (1793–1857), who, like Hodgkin, was more idealistic on how to bring pathological anatomy to Great Britain, and, like the Quaker, was doomed to failure because there was no financial support for such an endeavor. But Carswell was a superb artist and as mentioned earlier drew approximately a thousand illustrations of pathological specimens, which he published in 1838. He finally left the field of pathology to become the physician to the king of Belgium.

Thus in Great Britain in the first half of the nineteenth century, as in France, there were individuals such as the forerunner John Hunter (who was a naturalist, surgeon, and pathologist), then Astley Cooper, and finally Bright, Addison, and Hodgkin, who, building on the techniques of their predecessors and the Frenchmen Laennec and Corvisart, brought internal medicine into the modern age. For the remainder of the century, the elicitation of the physical signs at the bedside was the prime activity of almost every physician, and on the basis of his skills in these techniques which were evaluated by the postmortem examinations, he was measured by his peers and the public. But as he tapped and listened to the internal mechanisms of his patient, after having taken a careful history of the illness, the thoughts of the conscientious physician would soon reflect the explosion of knowledge about the nature of disease, which during the last half of the century would surpass all the cumulative knowledge of the thousands of years before. Although Louis Pasteur in France made the greatest contribution with his discovery of microorganisms as etiological factors in infectious diseases, most of the discoveries were made in Germany, the subject for the next chapter.

Bibliography

1. Morrell, J.B., *Individualism and the Structure of British Science in 1830. Historical Studies in the Physical Sciences*, **3**, p. 183, 1971.
2. Widdess, J.D., *A History of the Royal College of Physicians of Ireland, 1654-1963*, p. 184. E. and S. Livingston Ltd., Edinburgh, 1963.
3. Dale, W., *The Present State of the Medical Profession*, p.38, 1860.
4. Atlay, J.B., *Sir Henry Acland Memoirs*, p. 82. Smith, Elder Co., London 1903.
5. Ibid, p. 140.
6. Newman, G., *Bicentenary of the Faculty of Medicine of Edinburgh, 1726-1926*, p. 42. J. Thin, Edinburgh, 1926.
7. Hunter, J., *Lectures on the Principles of Surgery*. Harwell, Barrington and Harwell, Philadelphia, 1839.
8. Virchow, R., One Hundred Years of General Pathology, (1895) in *Disease, Life and Man*, and translated by L. Rather. Stanford Univ. Press, Stanford, California, 1958.
9. Baillie, M., *The Morbid Anatomy of Some of the Most Important Parts of the Human Body*. J. Johnson and G. Nicol, London, 1793.
10. Baillie, M., *A series of engravings accompanied with explanations which are intended to illustrate the morbid anatomy of some of the most important parts of the human body*. W. Bulmer and Co. London, 1799-1802.
11. Hope, J., *Principles and Illustrations of Morbid Anatomy*. Whittaker and Co., London, 1834.
12. Carswell, R., *Illustrations of the Elementary Forms of Disease*. Longman, London 1838.
13. Lebert, H., *Physiologie pathologique*, 2 vols. and atlas. J.B. Baillière, Paris 1845.
14. Lebert, H., *Traité d'anatomie pathologique, generale et speciale*, 4 vols. Baillière, Paris, 1857.
15. Bright, R., *Reports of medical cases selected with a view of illustrating the symptoms and cure of diseases by a reference to morbid anatomy*, Vol. I. Longmans, London 1827.
16. Bright, R., Cases and Observations Illustrative of Renal Disease, Accompanied with the Secretion of Albuminous Urine. *Guy's Hospital Reports*, No. 1, p. 338, 1836.

17. Bright, R., Cases and Observations Connected with Disease of the Pancreas and Duodenum. *Med. -chir.* Trans. **18**, p. 1, 1832.
18. Bright, R., Observations on Jaundice. *Guy's Hosp. Reports*, **1**, p. 604, 1836.
19. Hale-White, W., *Great Doctors of the 19th Century*, p. 110. Edward Amold and Co., London, 1935.
20. Bright, R., and Addison, T., *Elements of Practical Medicine*, p. 498, 1839.
21. Addison, T., Pneumonia, *Guy's Phys. Soc.* 1837 and 1843.
22. Addison, T., Anemia: Disease of the Suprarenal Capsules. *Lond. Med. Gaz.*, **43**, p. 517, 1849.
23. Addison, T., On the Constitutional and Local Effects of Disease of the Suprarenal Capsules. In *A Collection of the Published Writings of the Late Thomas Addison, M.D.*, p.211. New Sydenham Society, London, 1868.
24. Maulitz, R.C., *Morbid Appearances*, p. 205. Cambridge Univ. Press, N.Y., 1987.
25. Hodgkin, T., *Lectures on the Morbid Anatomy of the Serous and Mucous Membranes*. Sherwood, Gilbert and Piper, London, 1836-1840.
26. Hodgkin, T., On some morbid appearances of the absorbent glands and spleen. *Med. -chir. Trans.*, **17**, p. 68, 1832.
27. Hodgkin, T., On the retroversion of the valves of the aorta. *Lond. Med. Gaz.* **3**, p. 43, 1828-29.
28. Hodgkin, T., and Lister, J., Notice of some microscopical observations of blood and animal tissue. *Philos. Mag.* **2**, p. 130, 1827.
29. See Ref. 2, p. 162.
30. Graves, R. J., Newly Observed Affection of the Thyroid Gland in Females. *Lond. Med. Surg.* J., Vol. VII, pt.2, p. 516, 1835.
31. Stokes, W., Observations on some cases of permanently slow pulse, *Dublin Quart. J. Med. Sci.*, **2**, p. 73, 1846.
32. Stokes, W., *The Diseases of the Heart and Aorta.* Hodges and Smith, Dublin, 1854.
33. Corrigan, D.J., On permanent patency of the mouth of the aorta, or inadequacy of the aortic valves. *Edinburgh Med. Surg. J.*, **37**, 225, 1832.
34. Bell, J., *The Principles of Surgery*, 3 vols. T. Cadell and W. Davies, Edinburgh, 1801-1808.

35. Bell, C., *The Nervous System of the Human Body*. Longmans, London, 1830.
36. Syme, J., Case of Iliac Aneurysm., *Med. -chir. Trans.* **45**, p. 381, 1862.
37. Syme, J., *Contributions to the Pathology and Practice of Surgery.* Sutherland and Knox, Edinburgh, 1848.
38. Lister, R., *Practical Surgery*. J. Churchill, London, 1837.
39. Simpson, J., Discovery of a new anesthetic agent. *Lancet*, **2**, p. 549, 1847.
40. Simpson, J., Contributions to the Pathology and Treatment of Disease of the Uterus. *Lond. Edinb. Month. J. Med. Sci.* **3**, p. 547,1843.
41. Bennett, J.H., Case of hypertrophy of the spleen and liver in which death took place from suppuration of the blood. *Edinburgh Med. Surg*. J. **64**, p. 413, 1845.
42. Virchow, R., Weisses Blut. *Froriep's Notizem a.d. Geb. d. Natur. u Heilk.* **36**, p. 155, 1845.
43. Goodsir, J. and Goodsir, H., *Anatomical and Pathological Observations*. Edinburgh, 1845.
44. Craigie, D., *Elements of General and Pathological Anatomy.* Edinburgh, 1828.
45. Christison, R., *A Treatise on Poisons.* A. Black, Edinburgh, 1829.
46. Christison, R., *On Granular Degeneration of the Kidneys.* Waldie, Philadelphia, 1839.
47. Hope, J., *A Treatise on the Diseases of the Heart and Great Vessels.* W. Kidd, London, 1831.

CHAPTER V

The Progress of Pathology and the Organization of Science in the Germanic Countries during the Nineteenth Century

While progress was being made in medicine and pathology in France and Great Britain during the years 1800–1850, the situation in the Germanic countries was entirely different. Following the French Revolution and the invasion and humiliation of the Germanic aristocracy by Napoleon's armies, two movements occurred in Germany and Austria, which were in many ways at cross-purposes to each other.

The first movement was the development and embracement by Germanic intellectuals of the Natural Philosophy of Friedrich Wilhelm Joseph von Schelling (1775–1854), which essentially rejected the realism, materialism, and egalitarianism identified with the new France. The theme of Natural Philosophy, which influenced all fields of scholarly endeavors, was that true knowledge could only be achieved by aspiring to the German concept of Wissenschaft, which was the "unity of all learning." von Schelling believed that Nature is not to be understood simply from the perspective of empirical observation and scientific theory; it is rather "a reality of its own which speculative or intellectual intuition has to interpret."[1] This regressive "romantic" period in German philosophy led to elaborate theories whereby the foremost physicians and biologists used nebulous concepts such as polarities, irritabilities, and sensitivities. The emphasis was on synthesis, and admired research was primarily cerebral and deductive. Analytical experimental studies were ridiculed by the intellectual community as "bread study" (brotstudius).[2] And utilitarianism of any type was considered unworthy as a university objective. This, of course, was somewhat the same point of view at Oxford and Cambridge during the same years, except that the English institutions had essentially no interest in science of any type and did not adopt the Natural Philosophy of the German scholars. To give an idea of how pervasive Natural Philosophy affected the thoughts of outstanding biologists, the following is taken from Rudolf Virchow's eulogy of Johannes Müller (1801–1858), his teacher and a great pioneering physiologist:

> The natural philosophy of von Schelling had taught men to deduce all phenomena from the idea of the absolute. Such was the epoch in which Müller became a doctor of medicine . . . he had diligently consulted nature; and he had early learned to know and imitate Humboldt and Goethe. But he was arrested by the antithesis of Natural Philosophy which seemed so ingenious; and he believed that he had discovered something of great importance, when, resting on the experiments of Ritter, he demonstrated expansion and bending of muscles as the pole of the organic column, from which all of these, each in a straight line, diverged in the form of a circle. His descriptions revelled in all manner of half-intelligible comparisons, whose distinctness was not increased by the Latin tongue. How very easily might the whole of his great development have been injured at this point! But salvation was nigh at hand. Müller was obliged to go to Berlin to pass the state-examination for a physician's license, and was absent from the atmosphere at Bonn for almost one and one half years. When in Berlin he had the good fortune to come into close contact with Rudolphi, who was then engaged with the publication of his Elements of Physiology; and whose tendencies in this science, as Müller himself says, were overpoweringly anatomical and skeptical. At least it did not fail in taking effect on Müller, who henceforward betook himself zealously to the province of careful anatomical investigation.[3]

Fortunately those scientists such as Müller recognized that Natural Philosophy was an invalid method of furthering knowledge and by 1830 it was losing its popularity. However, as we shall see, it still showed its influence in the writings of Karl Rokitansky and Jacob Henle, although these individuals were also outstanding observers and experimentalists. It was only toward the end of the century that it completely lost its influence.

The second movement in the Germanic countries was one which had a positive influence. This movement was major change in German education from kindergarten to the university. Following the defeat by Napoleon, it was recognized by some of the German rulers that to achieve political, economic, and military superiority over its neighbors, it was necessary to attempt to take the leadership in the Industrial Revolution, which at that time belonged to England. Wisely, they understood that this could only occur through massive improvement in education and the development of scientific laboratories and institutions. The seeds of this growth were planted by the Prussian King Frederich William III

(1770–1840), who following his defeat by Napoleon at Jena in 1806, appointed Wilhelm von Humboldt to overhaul the Prussian schools. von Humboldt mandated that school would be compulsory for all children, and took measures to modernize the entire primary and secondary schools. More importantly, he took measures, during the first quarter of the century, to instill modern thought and organization into the earlier medieval German universities, activities which did not occur in other European countries until much later in the century. The result was that the duties of the faculties changed from primarily teaching to emphasis on original work and publications. This was in keeping with von Humboldt's idea that such activities were the fundamental duties of true scholars. In the sciences, the various German states in the Confederation of the Rhine and Prussia ensured that science professorships were well endowed, and great research institutes with equipment and staff were established, particularly after the failed Revolution of 1848. Because of these benefits, the competition for the professorships was very keen and only the most brilliant individuals were chosen. By the middle of the century, the scientists in Germany and Austria were career professors. It is important to point out that next to the aristocracy and the army officer corps, the university professor was at the top of the social hierarchy. He was usually a high-ranking civil service officer and was entitled to retirement with full salary, which was usually more than adequate. Additionally, he was permitted to receive fees from students for the courses he gave, and if he was well known in his field, a fine lecturer, or if the course he gave was a requirement for the curriculum and therefore had hundreds of students in his class, he accumulated income that allowed him to live in grand style. The more advanced courses, which only attracted specialized students, were often left to the junior members of the faculty, the private docents, who not only received fewer student fees, but received no salaries except perhaps small ones, and only if they acted as assistants to the professor. It was difficult to become a docent, since this title was awarded two to five years after having received a doctorate, and required not only performing additional research, but also, finally, an oral examination. The individual could then remain a docent for the remainder of his life without a salary, but if his research was outstanding he could sometimes receive the title of "extraordinary professor." The only way the docent could improve himself financially was to be appointed professor in his department, or in another university if the prior professor died, took another position, or retired. It is interesting that in spite of the security that the professors had in their positions, most of them seldom stayed at one university. They often secured new positions in which they were promised new facilities and new challenges. One feature of this system was that it provided maximum mobility for the student. The curriculum of the medical student was very flexible with regard to faculty control, class attendance, and routine examinations. Usually the student attended two or more universities depending upon his interest in studying under different professors. In this manner, he became acquainted with many distinguished names in his own special field of interest, but also had the opportunity to be exposed to the ideas of eminent individuals in other sciences. This wandering from one university to another prevented him from becoming one-sided. The professors, because their fame and fortune was partially related to the number of fee-paying students in their classes, made a special effort to keep their courses interesting and current and to justify the adulation they sometimes received. The surgeon Theodor Billroth (1829–1894) wrote in his book:

> There are professors who affect their students as the piper of Hamelin affected children. Now, if the student makes his choice with enthusiasm, he will study with enthusiasm also. It furthers study more than most people think — more than all study programs and all curricula. In my own experience, I have found men who were wasting their time in a stupid and blasé manner at one university, and who migrating to another, were suddenly seized by such an admiration for some teacher that they became the most industrious of students.[4]

After two years of study and attending classes at different universities, the medical student took a so-called "tentamen physicum," which was a comprehensive examination in zoology, botany, embryology, anatomy, physiology, chemistry, and physics. When he passed, he continued for approximately three years taking courses in the fields of medicine, surgery, obstetrics, pathology, and materia medica. He again took a written, oral, and practical examination in which he could be asked to perform an autopsy or demonstrate a surgical procedure on a cadaver. If he passed, he received the certificate of physician, but if he wanted the title of doctor, he was required to write a thesis. With regard to the study of pathology, in the medical schools and the affiliated hospitals, the morgue became a well-equipped institute for pathology and the professor of pathology, the director. In addition, these institutes were equipped with laboratories where experimental work was being done in the areas of histology, physiology, chemistry, and pharmacology.[5] With organization such as this in many universities, the German-speaking countries raced far ahead of their neighbors, particularly in the basic sciences.

Bibliography

1. Kroner, R., J. von Schelling, in *Encylopedia Brittanica*, Vol. 19, p. 1149. Benton, Chicago, 1973.
2. Turner, R.S., The Growth of Professional Research in Prussia, 1818-1848, Causes and Context. *Historical Studies in the Physical Sciences*, **3**, p. 137, 1971.
3. Virchow, R., Johannes Müller, the Physiologist, a Eulogy Pronounced in the Hall of the University of Berlin, translated by A.M. Adam. *Edin. Med. J.*, **4**, p. 452, p. 527, 1858.
4. Billroth, T, *Uber das lehren und lernen der medizinischen wissenschaften an den universitäten der Deutschen Nation nebst Allgemeinen Bermerkungen über Universitäten*. 1876. English Translation, MacMillan Co., 1924.
5. Flexner, *A. Medical Education in Europe*. Boston, 1912.

CHAPTER VI

No generalization is wholly true, not even this one.

— Oliver Wendell Holmes, Jr.

Vienna, Karl Rokitansky, and Neohumoralism

It will be remembered that in Vienna in 1745, Empress Maria Theresa appointed Gerhard van Sweiten to reorganize medicine in Austria. As a result of his modernization, one of his later successors, Johann Peter Frank (1745–1821) appointed Alois Rudolph Vetter (1765–1806) in 1796 as the first pathologist in the new Allgemeines Krankenhaus (Vienna General Hospital). He performed thousands of autopsies during the years 1796–1803, and wrote *Aphorisms from Pathological Anatomy* giving his experience over those years. His book was not a success and he left his unpaid position to go to Cracow to be professor of anatomy and physiology. However, he soon returned to Vienna where he died of tuberculosis in 1806, a martyr to anatomic pathology like Bichat, Bayle, and Laennec because the infectiousness of the disease was not recognized. In 1812 Lorenz Biermayer was appointed pathologist, and during the years 1812–1825 he performed as many as 600 autopsies per year. In 1829 he was replaced by Johann Wagner and on the latter's death, Karl Rokitansky took his place.

Karl Rokitansky – The Early Years

Karl Rokitansky was born in Bohemia in 1804, studied at the University of Prague under Purkinje, but went to Vienna because he found the curriculum at Prague narrow and harsh with required memorization in Latin from antiquated textbooks. He became Wagner's unpaid assistant and remained in this position for two years after receiving his medical degree. He learned dissection from Wagner, but he read constantly the works of Bichat, Andral, and Hunter. When he took over the position of Wagner in 1832 he quickly established himself as a first-class investigator with his expressed goal of

> First . . . sorting the facts scientifically on a purely anatomical basis and thereby creating the subject of general pathological anatomy which would justify its separate existence as such second, demonstrating the applicability of the facts and their utilization for diagnosis in live patients. [1]

He insisted that case histories be given together with the cadavers. In 1834, he was appointed extraordinary professor, legal anatomist, and custodian of the museum at Vienna General Hospital which was a combined civil and military hospital and where every patient who died was automatically subject to be autopsied. As a consequence, over the years 1832–1866, Rokitansky either performed or supervised approximately 30,000 necropsies, and he was able to record innumerable details and identify pathological changes in organs that were characteristic of different diseases. Most importantly, he was able to compare these alterations with variations in normal organs and postmortem changes that traditionally led to wrong conclusions. He worked closely with the superb diagnostician Josef Skoda (1805–1881), who aided him in correlating postmortem findings with the clinical symptoms. Of course, the French clinician pathologists, such as Laennec, Corvisart, and Louis, had done this, but there was a significant difference in that the Frenchmen were not only specializing in certain regions of the body, but did both the clinical and pathological studies themselves. On the other hand, Rokitansky was a full-time pathologist, not a clinician, and not only brought more objectivity to the postmortem findings, but was much more comprehensive than the French workers. As a result, the new specialties such as orthopedics, dermatology, ophthalmology, obstetrics, gynecology, general surgery, and neurology also greatly profited. Rokitansky was essentially the first in the Germanic countries to employ an anatomic basis for the idea of a "disease process," which over a period of time changed physicians from thinking about disease in terms of signs and symptoms — fevers were often erroneously called diseases, such as "catarrhal fever" when there were secretions from the upper respiratory tract, "catarrhal-rheumatic fever" when there was aching in the muscles, and "gastro-catarrhal fever" if vomiting occurred during respiratory inflammations. Both Rokitansky and Skoda emphasized that the most var-

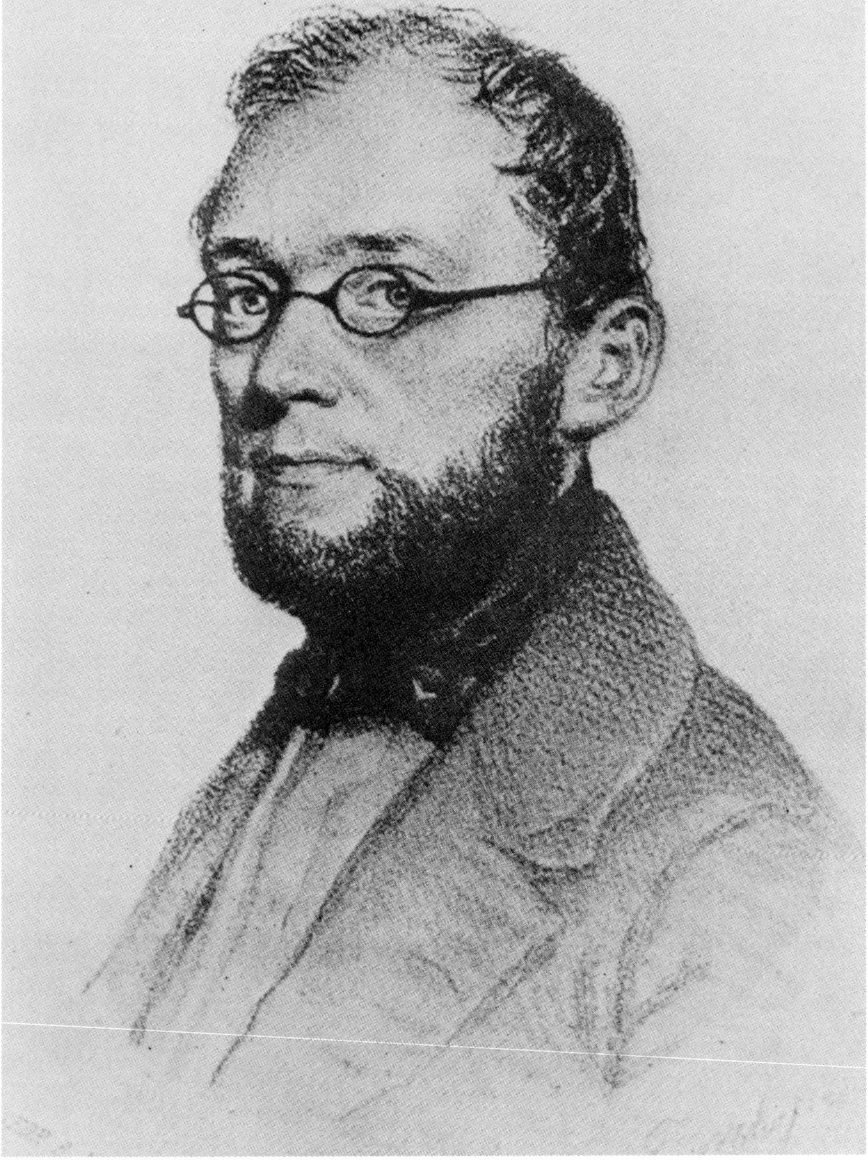

KARL ROKITANSKY

ied signs and symptoms can be found with similar anatomical changes, and, conversely, similar signs and symptoms could often be correlated with diverse anatomical changes. After ten years of monumental labor, Rokitansky started work on his distinguished manuscript *Handbook of Pathological Anatomy,*[2] which today is considered a classic and which Rudolph Virchow described in 1895 as follows:

> (Rokitansky's) famous textbook of pathological anatomy appeared piecemeal from 1842 on, immediately proving itself the best of all available textbooks in this discipline and the real basis of practical medicine. Without any reservation, one may designate it the finest flower of organicism. For it went far beyond Cruveilhier's textbook in the masterful vividness and precision — equal to the classics of the descriptive natural sciences — of its depiction of particular organ diseases, as well as the richness and trustworthiness of its author's personal observations. Even today it remains unequaled.[3]

Reading through Rokitansky's four volumes of observations today, one is impressed with its comprehensiveness. For every organ system, the author has organized pathological changes under the headings of variations in: (1) developmental abnormalities; (2) size; (3) deviations of position; (4) continuity as in injuries such as fractures; (5) tissues such as neoplasms, infarction, and inflammation; and (6) foreign bodies and abnormal contents such as shrapnel or calculi. There are clinical correlations with such pathological phenomena as intussusception and volvulus, perforation of ulcers, lesions and tumors of the gallbladder and its ducts, defects of the heart or its valves or septa. The fact is that Rokitansky was the Linnaeus of anatomical pathology, and although his discoveries were not as dramatic as those of Pasteur, Virchow, Bright, Addison, Laennec, Koch, or Ehrlich, his observations are embodied in the common knowledge of every modern pathologist. Rokitansky was by nature a very undramatic person and in his autobiography relates how he was plagued by mental depression and had a pessimistic view on life. Adolf Kussmaul who studied with him in 1847 relates an incident that somewhat reveals the personality of Rokitansky:

> Everybody worshipped him. He was astonishingly silent. In the mortuary, he opened his mouth only to dictate the proto-

> col. After four months of regular use, the scalpels happened to be resting one fair autumn morning, and I used to pause to step outside for a breath of fresh air. Soon after, Rokitansky came out and stood near me in the sun; the warm air in the yard visibly comforted him. Suddenly, he turned to me, nodded in a friendly way and observed; "Nice weather today!" I was startled. I could not have been more astonished. Still, I pulled myself together and replied; "Yes, it is indeed a beautiful day!" With that, the conversation came to an end; it was the first and only time I heard from him. (However) Rokitansky would suddenly be transformed from his usual impersonal and dry appearance as soon as something unusual came to light during the autopsies. Then he caught fire; one could see it by his shining eyes. He would immediately transfix the strange finding, grasp the scalpel and scissors, sit himself down at a little table, and become entirely absorbed by the anatomical problem before him, preparing and reflecting at the same time. Rokitansky was a great anatomist, but a mediocre teacher.[4]

This was confirmed by Osler in 1874 when he visited Vienna and Rokitansky and said that:

> Medicine and pathology is infinitely below that of Berlin. After having seen Virchow, it is absolutely painful to attend postmortems here — they are performed in so slovenly a manner and so little use is made of the material.[5]

The Attack by Rudolf Virchow

Perhaps it was because of his introverted and retiring manner that as the most renowned pathologist in the world at the time he accepted, without defending his position or retaliation, the severe castigation given to him by the young Rudolph Virchow, regarding his speculative ideas about diseases in which no significant pathological lesions could be found. Virchow's audacity was astonishing because at that time the young pathologist, by his own admission, had contributed almost nothing to the field of pathology. Since this was one of the events that propelled Virchow into prominence in the medical world, and was one of the major controversies during the nineteenth century, it is of interest to investigate its background. In Volume I of his handbook, Rokitansky expressed the following ideas:

> Humoral pathology is simply a requirement of common practical sense; and it has always held a place in medical science, although the limits of its domain have, no doubt, been variously circumscribed or interpreted at different times. Of late years it has met with a new basis and support in morbid anatomy, which, in the inadequacy of its discoveries in the solids to account for disease and death, has been compelled to seek for an extension of its boundary through a direct examination of the blood itself. Not alone has pathological anatomy demonstrated the existence of blood diseases in unlooked for detail; it has at the same time solved a problem of the weightiest import. It has, we think, decided in favor of a humoral pathology, by demonstrating a primitive anomaly of blastemata; by demonstrating the endogenous impairment of the blood within the vascular system, in inflammatory process, as the basis of the variations in exudates; lastly by demonstrating the dependence of local morbid action upon pre-existent impairment of the general circulation. Our attention will be directed to the diseases of the blood in its totality, and to local dyscrasial processes, with inflammation at their head, only in so far as these offer the basis and starting point for consecutive disease of the entire blood mass. It is remarkable, however, and no less important for practice than for science, perhaps, that the essential forms of these local dyscrasial processes occur, likewise, as primitive affections of the entire blood mass. Thus, primitive pyemia, fibrincrases, sepsis of the blood, severally occur independently of all local beginning, and of all infection.[6]

In as much as Natural Philosophy (with its emphasis on synthesis and theories) still had its residual influence on many of the German scientists at the time, it is very likely that considering his respected reputation his speculations in his monumental handbook would have been ignored or at most perhaps cause a raising of the eyebrows of other men versed in pathology. But this was not to be because the brilliant, pugnacious, and above all ambitious Virchow wrote a review of Rokitansky's book in which he excoriated him for his speculations. The review read as follows:

> This is no longer the simple pathological anatomist whom we have learned to know in the earlier parts (of the book); it is the recognized master for whom his inherited territory has become too small. We know indeed from where this mania for enlargement takes its origin. We wish to say this openly; it comes from the indolence of the pathologist, the clinician, and therapist. Finally, when we summarize our judgment of the book we must confess that we have rarely seen one more dangerous for medicine, and that we have rarely read one with sadder feelings. Great powers have natural tendency toward arbitrariness, toward despotism, yet is it not sad when one after another we see them follow the same path and again destroy with their own hands, the blessing that they had only just revealed to the human race?[7]

The result was that, without a rebuttal, Rokitansky simply removed the entire speculation section from the next edition of his handbook. Fifty years later, Virchow justified his castigation of Rokitansky by writing:

> Rokitansky's Handbook of Pathological Anatomy, proclaiming the new humoral pathology of the Viennese school, appeared in 1846. It was necessary to protect science from this false pathology of humors. This I did in a critical review . . . in December 1846. To my great pleasure, Johannes Müller expressed his appreciation in warm terms to me, and it soon appeared that my brief essay had also an effect in Vienna. The "crases" have not since appeared in the scientific marketplace. The last "system" of general pathology was buried with them.[8]

It is ironic that what Virchow called "indolence" on the part of Rokitansky was really an over-enthusiastic reaction to the work and comments of Magendie and Andral. Just as Bayle earlier realized that all diseases, even fatal ones, did not always produce gross lesions, Rokitansky must have been frustrated in his efforts to be comprehensive in his handbook, and he therefore proposed that in those cases without visible seats of disease, it was logical to assume the answer was to be found in the blood. This, of course, was a throwback to the humoralist ideas of the past, but to a certain extent this was suggested by both

Magendie and later Andral. François Magendie, the supreme skeptic, had cast doubt on the anatomical approach to studying disease which led him to state in his lectures on blood:

> I set but little value on the minute examination of the traces left by disease on our organs though that pursuit has been pompously styled pathological anatomy. The lesions found at our autopsies are frequently produced after death, and consequently the plan hitherto followed in such inquiries is fallacious, and can only lead to vague information and error. The effects of disease have long been studied; let us search for their causes . . . my persuasion . . . is that we shall find in the blood the cause of a host of diseases.[9]

Then Andral, impressed with the ideas of Magendie, set about the analysis of blood in different diseases and in his resulting publication stated that:

> I design to make known the alterations that the blood has presented me in different diseases, under the triple view of its physical properties, and of its chemical and microscopical constitution. I have exhibited the results that I have obtained, in seeking to appreciate the variations in proportion that some of the principles of the blood, to wit, the fibrine, the globules, the solid elements of the serum, and the water may confer, whether in disease, or in different states of the physiological conditions.[10]

Rokitansky in his enthusiasm about the possibilities of finding the causes of diseases in the blood, not only accepted Andral's work uncritically, but encouraged the German chemists to undertake the studies of blood. He said in his book:

> Upon the chemical pathologist we would strongly urge an unremitting prosecution of his researches. We would recommend him to direct his labors more particularly towards ascertaining the precise character of the impairment suffered by the proximate ingredients of the blood, and of the anomalies impressed upon its elementary composition. The interests of hematopathology would, after all, perhaps, be best served by the examination, in the above sense, of blood taken from the

> dead subject, the diagnosis of the case having previously received the light of a general post-mortem examination.[11]

This encouragement had mixed reactions from the physiological chemists, who were already aware of Virchow's criticism of Rokitansky. Carl Lehmann, in his well-known textbook *Physiological Chemistry* published in 1849 wrote the following:

> We are convinced that the principal object had in view by Rokitansky, in writing the first volume of his celebrated work, which has been so severely criticized, was simply to indicate to pathologists the points of view he had himself established, might be most fully comprehended. But it has unfortunately happened that his followers have frequently borrowed, from physics and chemistry, phrases and modes of representation, without seizing the spirit of these sciences, or even comprehending their methods of operation. Hence there has emanated from this school a multitude of the most unsubstantial medical fictions which, for shallowness, yield to none of the earlier schools. There has been an over estimate of the value of chemical auxiliaries, and a complete ignorance of the present condition of organic chemistry. Have the numerous analyses of morbid blood instituted during the last few years fulfilled the expectations of physicians? It must be admitted that when we seriously inquire into the recompense for all of the labors and sacrifices (of investigators), we find that the result, although too dearly bought, was altogether inadequate to satisfy the requirements of pathology. Animal chemistry is still wholly unable to afford us a precise, and at the same time a practically useful method of investigating blood; and how should it be otherwise while we continue to be in doubt regarding the chemical nature of its ordinary constituents. The mineral substances of the normal blood are not yet determined — we scarcely know the names of the fatty matters it contains. We are also ignorant of the excrementitious substances in the blood. How then, amidst these and a thousand other uncertainties and doubts, can an investigation of the blood be scientifically and trustworthily conducted?[12]

However the warnings of Lehman did not inhibit Justus Liebig, who dominated the field of analytical and organic chemistry during his lifetime, from an incursion into the study of living phenomena. Like

Rudolph Virchow, who was soon to monitor all ideas about pathology, Liebig used his international reputation to allow him to pontificate on biological subjects about which he had little understanding, but gave him confidence to criticize and ridicule others such as Louis Pasteur who disagreed with him. As a result, he published one of the first books on biochemistry *Animal Chemistry* or *Organic Chemistry in Its Application to Physiology and Pathology,* which was very popular and widely quoted for many years, but in retrospect was a monumental work of speculation and oversimplification. It is likely that Liebig's ideas also influenced Rokitansky since their publications appeared almost at the same time. These are statements in Liebig's book that illustrate his unjustified conclusions:

> The organs are formed from the blood, and contain the elements of the blood; they become transformed into new compounds, with the addition only of oxygen and water. Hence the relative proportion of carbon and nitrogen must be the same as in the blood. If then we subtract from the composition of blood, the elements of the urine, then the remainder, deducting the oxygen and water, which have been added, must give the composition of the bile. Or if from the elements of the blood, we subtract the elements of the bile, the remainder must give the composition of urate of ammonia or of urea and carbonic acid. The analyses of Playfair and Boeckmann gave for flesh, (fibrine, albumen, cellular tissue, and nerves) and for blood, as the most exact expression of their numerical results, one and the same formula, namely $C_{48}N_6H_{39}0_{15}$. This may be called the empirical formula of blood. The urine of herbivora contains no uric acid, but ammonia, urea, and hippuric or benzoic acid. By the addition of 9 atoms of oxygen to the empirical formula of their blood multiplied by 5 we obtain the elements of 6 atoms of hippuric acid, 9 atoms of urea, 3 atoms of choleic acid, 3 atoms of water, and 3 atoms of ammonia.[13]

The obvious fact that impressed Liebig was that the primary analyses of beef muscle and blood gave essentially the same percentages of carbon, hydrogen, oxygen, and nitrogen as did egg albumen, pus, gelatinous material, and arteries. Then on the basis of his knowledge of inorganic and organic compounds of low molecular weight which had such diverse percentages of the elements, it must have seemed logical that all protein molecules were similar in their structure and that only a few modifications could change them one into the other. Although the amino acids glycine and leucine had been discovered in 1820 by Braconnot and Liebig himself had discovered tyrosine in casein,[14] the possibility of the existence of an infinite number of proteins with similar primary compositions produced by 20 different amino acids connected by peptide bonds with additional covalent and hydrogen bonding to give various shapes to the molecules that can also have a molecular weight as high as a million was not remotely conceivable by Liebig and his contemporaries. Only a few brave souls criticized and contradicted Liebig, since he was able to use his journal to demolish his adversaries, as Louis Pasteur found when he proposed that it was the living activities of yeast that converted glucose to alcohol. However, Berzelius in Sweden correctly accused Liebig of carrying out "writing table" chemistry with regard to living organisms and stated that this type of activities simply encumbered physiology with erroneous ideas.[15] Kohlraush in 1844 pointed out that using Liebig's methods, it was possible that beginning with any complex formula containing carbon, hydrogen, and oxygen and then adding or subtracting enough water, ammonia, or oxygen in a arbitrary manner, it was possible to arrive at any other preconceived substance using the same elements. He illustrated this fact by using Liebig's logic to show that an oxidation of protein could produce the compound hydrogen cyanide and the explosive compound fulminic acid.[16] The fact that it would take another 150 years to show that there were thousands of reactions occurring at the same time in every living cell, each promoted by individual enzymes which in turn were controlled and produced by the action of DNA and RNA, would have been completely incomprehensible in 1842.

The results of these premature studies and conclusions based upon crude gravimetric methods of analyzing blood discouraged extensive studies during the second half of the century. The chemists were making major progress in both inorganic and synthetic organic chemistry and didn't want to be involved in what they called "slime chemistry" as they called analysis of living organisms.[17] However, the pathologists and anatomists using the microscope after 1835 were also making lasting discoveries in pathology and they also lost interest in looking for disease processes in blood.

This digression was made to illustrate how scientists in their desire to explain biological phenomena before the discovery of innumerable but necessary facts that seemed insignificant at the time, devise theories that within a few years seem simplistic and incredibly naive to their successors.

The Declining Years of Rokitansky

Rokitansky, in spite of his "crases" theory that got him into trouble with Virchow and the chemists, was appreciated in Vienna and was honored more than any contemporary Nobel Prize winner. The following is Osler's description of the celebration in Vienna for Rokitansky on his 70th birthday in 1874:

> The city, university and students all combined to celebrate the event in a manner worthy of themselves and of the distinguished man who has so long shed lustre on their school. Not only, however, here but throughout the medical world great interest was shown in it, as the long string of delegates from the various universities and societies attested. The proceedings began in the fest salon of the Academy of Science at 11 AM when the deputations were received and the addresses read. By the appointed hour not an available seat was free in the spacious hall, and it was indeed a stirring sight to see such a goodly assembly gathered together to do honor to the "pioneer of modern pathology". At the conclusion of the opening oration by the Dean of the medical faculty, a beautiful bust, hidden by curtains, was unveiled with great effect, amid the cheers of the students. Then followed a jubilee song by the members of the University Musical Society after which the work of the morning began — the receiving of the deputations. These, to the number of thirty-four, coming from all quarters of Europe, presented their congratulatory addresses. Of more general interest was the grand torch-light procession of the students, which took place in the evening. The weather had been most unpropitious, and towards evening the snow, which had been falling, changed to rain, but, nothing daunted, the procession formed and marched around the Ring, the fine wide street surrounding the inner town to the Cour-Salon, where a university dinner was going on. About fifteen hundred students, all provided with torches, and many wearing the fantastic uniforms of their societies, composed the procession. Thousands of people turned out to see the sight, and every

> window of the tall houses on each side of the street possessed its occupants. Inside the City Park, in front of the Cour-Salon, they halted, and Professor Rokitansky surrounded by his family, appeared in one of the lower galleries. Here there was an address, followed by a reply and the evening was spent in true German fashion.[18]

It would be surprising if ever again any society would ever honor its great intellectual achievers in this manner.

Bibliography

1. Rokitansky, K., *Selbstbiographie und Antrittsrede*. ed. Erma Lesky, p. 64, Hermann Bohlaus, Vienna,1960.
2. Rokitansky, K., *A Handbook of Pathological Anatomy*, 4 vols. English Translation by W.E. Swaine. The Sydenham Society, London, 1854.
3. Virchow, R., *One Hundred Years of General Pathology*, (1895) in *Disease, Life, and Man*, and translated by L. Rather. Stanford Univ. Press. Stanford, 1958.
4. Kussmaul, A., *Memoirs of an Old Physician, 1899*, p. 249. Translated in 1981, Amerind, Pub. Co, New Delhi, 1981
5. Osler, W., Allgemeines Krankenhaus, *Canada Medical and Surgical Journal*, **Vol. II**, p. 451, 1873-74.
6. Ref. 2, Vol. I, p. 362.
7. Rather, L., Virchow's review of Rokitansky's Handbook in the Preussische Medizinal-Zeitung, Dec. 1846, *Clio Med.* **4**, p. 127, 1969.
8. Virchow, R., *One Hundred Years of General Pathology* (1895), in *Disease, Life, and Man*, and translated by L. Rather. Stanford Univ. Press, Stanford, 1958.
9. Magendie, F., *Lectures on the Blood*, p. 9. Haswell and Barrington, Philadelphia, 1839.
10. Andral, G., *Essai d'hématologie pathologique*. Fortin, Masson et Cie., Paris, 1843.
11. Ref. 2. p. 363.
12. Lehmann, C.G., *Physiological Chemistry*, Translated by G.Day, p. 7. Harrison and Son. London, 1851.
13. Liebig, J., *Animal Chemistry,* Translated by W. Gregory, p. 132. Taylor and Walton, London, 1842.
14. Schmidt, C., *Chemistry of the Amino Acids and Proteins*. Charles Thomas, Springfield, Ill. 1945.
15. Fruton, J.S., *Molecules and Life*, p. 97. Wiley Interscience, NY, 1972.
16. Florkin, M., A History of Biochemistry, in *Comprehensive Biochemistry*, Vol. 30, p. 181, Elsevier Publ. Co. Amsterdam, 1972
17. Ibid, p. 1.
18. Ref. 5.

CHAPTER VII

Medicine has reached a point, of which Microscopical Anatomy appears to constitute its foundation . . . and when a profound study of Physiology and Pathological Anatomy is impossible, without an accurate acquaintance also, with the most minute structural conditions.

— A. Kölliker (1852)

The Advancement of Normal and Pathological Histology

The Evolution of the Microscope

During the years 1830–1850, with the decline in the number of discoveries in pathology made by the gross postmortem examinations of organs and the recognition that pursuit of the causes of disease in the neohumoralistic analysis of blood (as proposed by Rokitansky, Andral, and Magendie) was premature, an important series of events occurred that made possible a quantum jump in pathology. This was the development of the achromatic compound microscope in 1830, which allowed investigators to observe lesions, pathological processes, cells, and microorganisms for hours at a time without undue fatigue at three hundred magnification and moderately good resolution. Although Zacharias Jensen is credited with the invention of the compound microscope in 1590, as greater magnifications were possible, the image formed by the two or more lenses in the objective had such severe spherical and chromatic aberrations that the object being viewed was so distorted that no definitive conclusions could ever be made. On the other hand, the single lens, or magnifying glass had less distortion and allowed more light at comparable magnification. But at higher magnifications the single lens had to be extremely small, limiting the visual field and shortening the focal length so that any slight movement of the lens or the eye of the observer would lose the image. Only Antony van Leeuwenhoek (1632–

1728), who was a man of infinite patience and was able to grind lenses as small as a grain of sand, was successful in making major observations. Starting in 1673 and continuing for the next fifty years, Leeuwenhoek described such living material as bacteria, protozoa, spermatozoa, and blood cells. It appears that his best microscopes, out of the hundreds he designed, consisted of a tiny biconvex lens mounted in a metal plate with the object mounted on a thin piece of glass or in a capillary tube and glued on the end of a needle. The distance of the object from the lens was adjusted by screws attached to the metal plate. The maximum magnification he achieved was probably about three hundred, which would have made unstained and living bacteria in a capillary tube very difficult to describe. Leeuwenhoek's biographer Clifford Dobell believes that the microscopist found a secret means of achieving a dark-field illumination that enabled him to observe the shape and motion of bacteria.[1]

In the meantime, opticians and mathematicians throughout Europe continued to strive to improve the compound microscope, but with little success. During the eighteenth century, they created beautiful instruments in terms of metal and mechanical work, but the spherical and chromatic aberrations prevented the microscope from becoming a useful scientific tool, and thus it was simply a toy of the rich and curious. The comments of various investigators illustrates the poor reputation of the microscope at the beginning of the nineteenth century. John Hunter said "I am led to believe that we may be deceived by the appearances viewed through the magnifying glass"[2] and a few years later John Bostock offered that:

> An historical detail of the errors into which this instrument has led even those who have been most skillful in its application would have the effect of inducing us to place little confidence in hypotheses and speculations which are derived from objects which can only be detected by the use of high magnification.[3]

However, in 1829, the culmination of many years of work on combinations of lenses by Joseph Jackson Lister (1786 –1869), the father of the famous surgeon, resulted in a solution to the aberrations. He did a study with this new microscope with Thomas Hodgkin and they published the work in 1827, in which they correctly noted the difference between smooth and striated muscle fibers and the fact that there was no

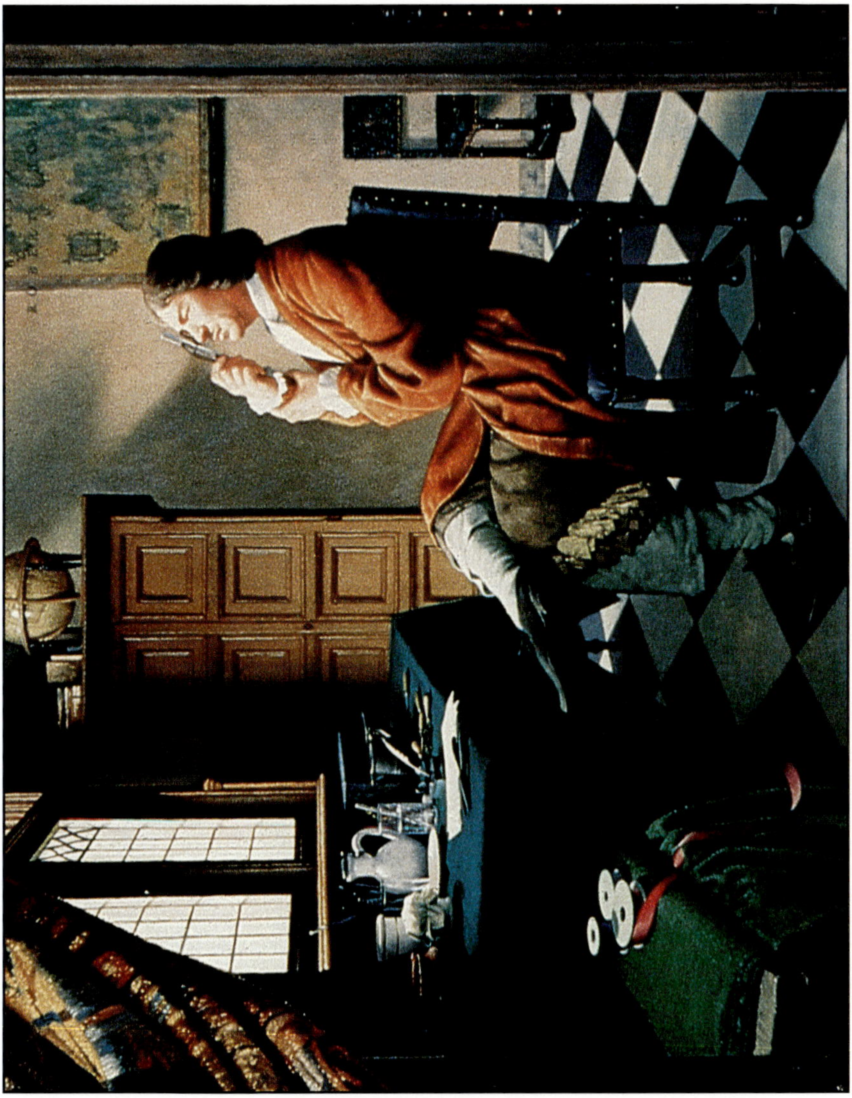

LEEUWENHOEK AND THE "LITTLE ANIMALS"

nucleus in the human erythrocyte.[4] Following this paper, three English opticians, Powell, Ross, and Smith, started the commercial production of the new microscope design. Then soon after, Oberhauser in France, Plossel and Schiek in Germany, and Amici in Italy implemented the optical improvement and began to compete with those in England. The resolution of these microscopes could separate points only one micron apart, but by 1870, with the development of the oil immersion lens of Ernst Abbe at the Zeiss factory, the resolution was such that lines only one-quarter of a micron could be separated.[5] This, of course, was fortuitous since the study of bacteria necessitated this degree of resolution. But in 1840, for the study of tissue, the Lister design was sufficient for good work, and as the microscopes poured out of the various factories of Europe, thousands of eyes started to explore the microscopic world, animal and plant, both normal and abnormal and the race was on in the scientific institutions for discoveries and fame. This period was described by Hughes Bennett in this way:

> Achromatic microscopes now could not be manufactured with sufficient rapidity; crowds of investigators besieged the workshops of Schiek and Piston in Berlin, Ploesch in Vienna, and Frauenkofer in Munich. Animated with the hope of being the first to explore the untrodden region, and by means of the new instrument to clear away the obscurity in which the ultimate structure of organs was involved, the young anatomist soon was enabled, not only to rival, but to surpass his teachers. A new race of observers was thus created, who at present fill all the chairs of anatomy and physiology in Germany, and their labors, combined with the more tardy cooperation of some investigators in Britain and France, have now so far advanced the study of histology, as to render an acquaintance with it absolutely imperative on the anatomist, physiologist and pathologist. It must be acknowledged that the Germans have taken the lead in histological studies, and the names of Ehrenberg, Müller, Schwann, Schultze, Wagner, Weber and Valentin, whose reputations principally depend on the discoveries they have made by means of the microscope, must be well known to you. The activity, also, the Germans now display, in the examination of healthy and morbid structures, is extraordinary, and can only be appreciated by an actual observer. Many individuals in the present day have become good microscopists by their own perseverance but the years they have devoted to this, the difficulties they have over-

> come, and the mistakes they have made are only known to themselves. Things are infinitely changed when a teacher stands by the student, and points out and explains the difficulties which fall in his way. A phenomenon which may have puzzled a solitary observer for months and been led astray for years, when explained by a teacher is at once easily understood. Hence it is that this study has made such progress in Germany and in consequence, the young anatomist commences a career with a knowledge that would have astonished the older observers.[6]

Although the English had developed microscopy as a hobby, and there were microscopical societies, the emphasis was on preparation of materials for their beauty and wonder rather than as a tool for obtaining new knowledge about the structure of living organisms. Private courses in microscopy were given by museum curator John Quekett in London and Hughes Bennett in Scotland. The surgeons R.B. Todd and W. Bowman had also published a book on anatomy and physiology that included material on histology.[7] However, there was no systematic full-time academics that would have considered themselves histologists or pathologists. Lionel Beale was a professor of physiology at King's College and wrote a popular book on the use of the microscope.[8] He gave an interesting table on the microscopic differences between benign and malignant tumors as follows:

Cancerous.	*Epithelial Growths.*
Cells not connected with the matrix in a regular manner, or forming laminae.	*Cells connected with the matrix, often forming distinct laminae.*
Cells differing much from each other in size and form.	*Cells resembling each other in size and general outline.*
Cells readily separable from each other.	
Cells not connected together at their margins; their edges seldom forming straight lines.	*Cells often cohering by their edges, which generally form straight lines; three or four cells being frequently found united together.*
Cells containing several smaller cells in their interior often met with.	*Cells usually containing one nucleus.*
Nuclei varying much in size and number in different cells.	*Nuclei not varying much in size in different cells.*
Juice scraped from the cut surface containing many cells floating freely in the fluid, and not connected with each other.	*Juice scraped from the cut surface, containing small collections of cells, which are often connected with each other.*

The situation in France was no better. Private courses in microscopy were given in Paris during the 1840s by three Germans, Louis Mandl, David Grüby, and Hermann Lebert, and two Frenchmen, Alfred Donné and F.V. Raspail. But as in Great Britain, the application of the microscope was primarily as an aid to the clinician when possible, and a great dispute arose when Herman Lebert and his pupil came to the conclusion that the microscope could be used to differentiate malignant from benign tumors.[9] Lebert took the position that cancer cells could be morphologically identified in the juice of squeezed tumors. He noted the large size of the nucleus, which was often lobulated or irregular compared to normal cells. Lebert was, of course correct that cancer cells actually exist, but, without stains at the time, his work could not have been definitive, and the Parisian surgeons thought they could more definitively differentiate benign from malignant tumors by gross examinations and that Lebert's criteria were subject to great error. This was most likely the true situation since pathologists were unhappy with cytological criteria of cancer cells even after the monumental work of G.N. Papanicolaou almost one hundred years later.

The School of Johannes Müller in Berlin

The Germans, on the other hand, in the universities and new institutes worked together to bring about significant advances in histology. It was under Johannes Müller in Berlin that the distinguished school of microscopic anatomy and biology originated and was to have such an exceptional effect on the fields of anatomy, physiology, and pathology from 1830 until 1858 when Müller died. This stimulating teacher had as his disciples Rudolf Virchow, Jacob Henle, Theodore Schwann, Emil DuBois-Reymond, Ernst Brücke, Robert Remak, Gabriel Valentin, Karl Reichert, Rudolf Kölliker, Herman Helmholtz, Benno Reinhardt, Karl Kupffer, Max Schultze, Johanne Miescher, Joseph Gerlach, Eduard Pflueger, and Hermann Stannius, who together with their respective students almost completely dominated all the fields of biology up to the period before the first World War. Most were expert microscopists and used this instrument to produce a body of knowledge that filled many books and journals, particularly in the fields of histology, embryology, physiology, and pathology. Who was Johannes Müller, the man whose personal research has almost been forgotten, but who stimulated so many young men to make important achievements during their own lives? Virchow said of Müller:

> We have to inquire what it was that raised Müller to so high a place in the estimation of his contemporaries; by what magic it was that envy became dumb before him; and by what mysterious means he contrived to enchain to himself the hearts of beginners, and so to keep them captive through many long years? Some have said — and not without reason — that there was something supernatural about Müller, for his whole appearance bore the stamp of the uncommon; and that his commanding influence did not wholly depend on his extraordinary original endowments, is certain from what we know of the history of his mental greatness.[10]

The years 1830–1850 were those of prodigious microscopic activity in Müller's laboratories. By the end of this period, textbooks such as those of Rudolf Kölliker[11] were available that described in infinite detail all of the organs of the body, including such complex structures as the retina, the cochlea, the various nerve cells of the brain and spinal cord, the taste buds, and the blood vessels. This was at a time when microscopical techniques were still comparatively crude.[12] Fixing, hardening, softening, and clearing was accomplished with such solutions as alcohol, acetic acid, chromic oxide, mercuric chloride, and turpentine. The tissue was cut into sections with a scalpel and mounted on glass slides with canada balsam or glycerin after removal of water by alcohol. Slides were in existence but thin glass for coverslips became available only in 1840.

Later Developments in Microtechniques

Embedding and infiltrating the tissue with paraffin before sectioning was not done before the 1880s. Stains were not available until the 1850s when carmine started to be used. However, in the study of tissues, the importance of stains was certainly helpful but was not essential, because the major studies of the various tissues were done without them. Nevertheless, the discovery of new stains became a fascinating area for research in histology, perhaps for their aesthetic qualities but certainly there were diminishing returns for the efforts involved in terms of new knowledge about tissues gained from the new assortment of colors. Haematoxylin (extracted from logwood) was used as early as carmine and was an excellent nuclear stain when it was realized that a mordant, such as alum, must be used with it. When William Perkin discovered the aniline dyes in 1856, an assortment of colors became available that were soon used in histology. In 1862 Beneke used Perkin's mauve; in 1863 Waldeyer used Paris blue and rosaniline, and Waldeyer, Frey, and Roberts all tried using basic fuchsin; in 1864 Chrzonszczewsky used indigocarmine; in 1874 Ranvier used cyanine, and Lieberkuhn alizarin; in 1875 Cornil used methyl violet and Fischer eosin. Then Paul Ehrlich, as a student of Waldeyer in Strasbourg, and later of Julius Cohnheim, Carl Weigert (Ehlich's cousin), and Rudolf Heidenhain in Breslau (who were among the best histologists and pathologists at that time), did his thesis on the use of aniline dyes in histology, which he studied from the standpoint of organic chemistry. In this treatise[13] published in 1878, and several other papers over the next few years,[14, 15] Ehrlich not only introduced several aniline dyes to histology — methyl blue, nigrosin, aurantia, tropaeolin, acid fuchsin, orange G, and bordeaux — but developed a theory of action of these dyes on the bases of their chemical structures and reactions toward certain cell components. During the years 1880–1888, Ehrlich made pioneering studies on blood, which allowed the field of hematology to develop.[16] Specifically, he was able to differentiate the various white blood cells with his stains, but he essentially left the field to morphologists to trace and study the normal and abnormal blood cells and their precursors — these individuals would eventually be called hematologists. Ehrlich then helped the bacteriologists such as Koch with stains of microorganisms,[17] and then went on to pioneer the fields of immunology[18] and finally chemotherapy.[19]

The cytologists during the period 1875–1895, Flemming, Oscar and Richard Hertwig, and Boveri, went on to improve the staining techniques in their study of mitosis and chromosomes, which eventually formed the basis of genetics.[20] However, in pathology, aside from the development of exfoliative cytology, such intracellular studies did not show their importance until late in the twentieth century when chromosomal abnormalities were found to be etiological factors in certain human developmental abnormalities and the production of specific diseases. The anatomical pathologists had sufficient problems to undertake with their microscopical study of such processes as inflammation, necrosis, degeneration, repair, and neoplasms to keep them busy for the last part of the nineteenth century and the early part of the twentieth century.[21, 22] During this period the nature of these processes were redefined in terms of activity of the various cells that were migrating from different areas, undergoing multiplication or hyperplasia, or showing effects of injury with cloudy swelling. The tissues that can regenerate, such as most types of epithelium or liver, were compared with tissues that cannot, such as muscle cells and nerves. Virchow, and later Cohnheim showed the effects of abnormal clotting in blood vessels with the formation of thrombi and emboli. And most importantly, the nature of neoplasms and their differentiation from other growths, such as tuberculosis, and other granulomatous lesions was accomplished by microscopic examination. Later in the century, the improvement of staining techniques made possible the better visualization of histological structures and patterns, and the result was that progress was made in differentiating malignant from benign growths.

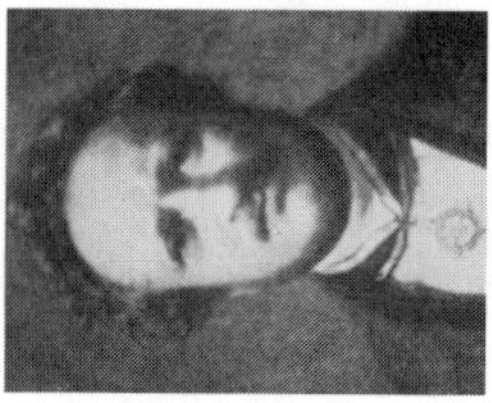
J. Müller

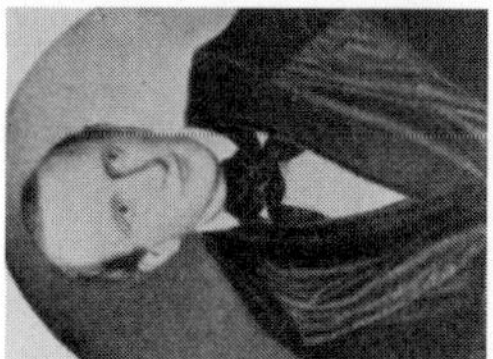
E. Brücke

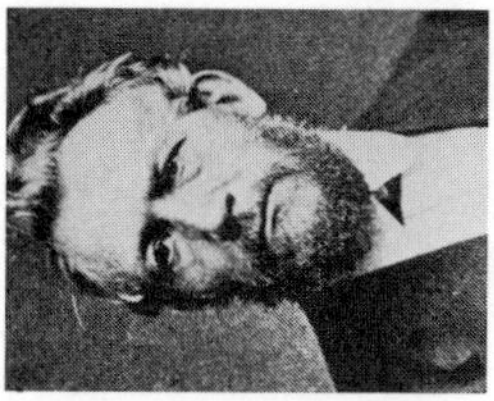
E. Dubois-Reymond

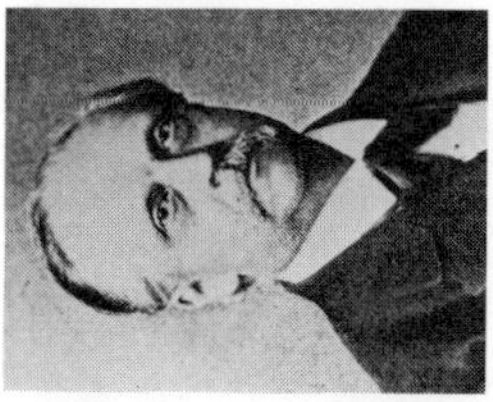
H. Helmholz

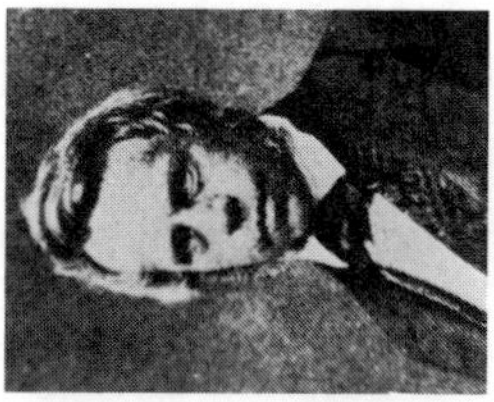
J. Henle

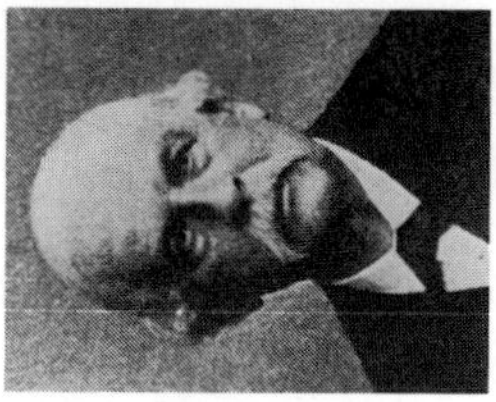
R. Kölliker

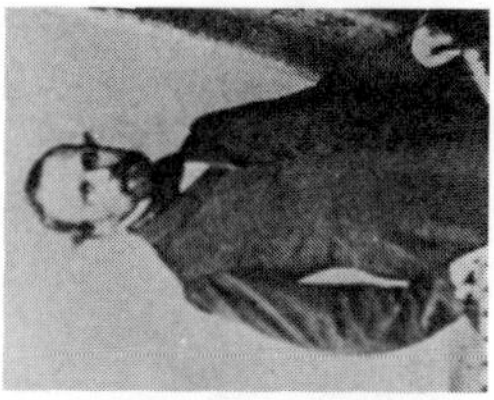
R. Remak

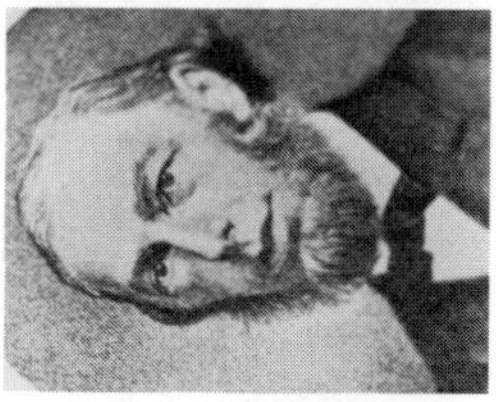
M. Schultze

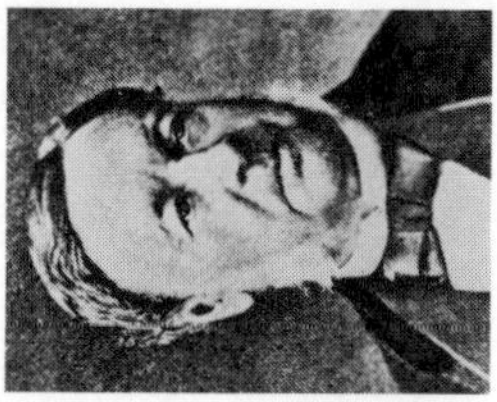
T. Schwann

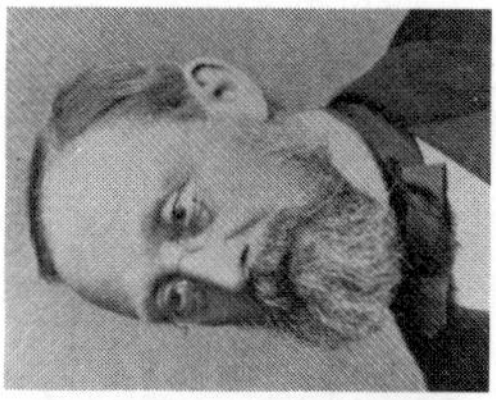
R. Virchow

JOHANNES MÜLLER AND HIS STUDENTS

Bibliography

1. Dobell, C., *Antony van Leeuwenhoek and his "Little Animals."* New York, Dover , 1960.
2. Foster, W.D., *A Short History of Clinical Pathology*, p. 11. E.S. Livingston, Edinburgh, 1961
3. Ibid., p. 11.
4. Hodgkin, T., and Lister, J., Notice of some microscopic observation of blood and animal tissues. *Philos. Mag.*, **2**, p. 130, 1827.
5. Turner, G., The Microscope as a Technical Frontier in Science, In *Historical Aspects of Microscopy*. Edited by S. Bradbury and G. Turner, Heller, Cambridge, 1967.
6. Bennett, J.H., Histology and the Use of the Microscope, *Lancet*, **I**, p. 517, 1845.
7. Todd, R.B., and Bowman, W., *The Physiological Anatomy and Physiology of Man*, Vols I & II. London, 1845–47.
8. Beale, L., *The Microscope in Its Application to Practical Medicine*, p. 356. John Churchill, London, 1858.
9. Lebert, H., *Physiologie pathologique*, Vol. II. p. 254. chez J.B. Baillière, London, 1845.
10. Virchow, R., *Johannes Müller, the Physiologist*, a eulogy pronounced in the hall of the University of Berlin, translated by A.M. Adam. *Edin. Med. J.*, p. 452 and 527, 1858.
11. Kölliker, R., *Manual of Human Histology*, translated by G. Busk and T. Huxley, Sydenham Society, London, 1853.
12. Bracegirdle, B., *A History of Microtechnique*. Cornell Univ. Press, Ithaca, NY, 1978.
13. Ehrlich, P., *Beiträge zur Theorie und Praxis der histologischen Färbung*, Dissertation at Univ. Leipzig, 1878.
14. Ehrlich, P., Beiträge zur Kenntnis der Anilinfarbungen und ihrer Verwendung in der mikroskopischen technik. *Arch mikr. Anat.*, **13**, p. 263, 1877.
15. Waldeyer,W. Einleitender Überlick, in Paul Ehrlich, *Eine Darstellung seines wissenschafflichen Wirkens*. G. Fischer, Jena, 1914.
16. Ehrlich, P. and Lazurus, A., *Histology of the Blood, Normal and Pathological*, translated by W. Myers. Cambridge Univ. Press, London, 1900.

17. Ehrlich, P., Über das Methylenblau und seine klinisch-bakterioskopische Verwerthung., *Z. klin. Med.*, **2**, p. 710, 1881.
18. Ehrlich, P., Die Wertbestimmung des Diphtherieheilserum., *Klin. Jb.*, **6**, p. 299, 1897.
19. Ehrlich, P., Chemotherapeutische Trypanosomen-Studien, *Berl. klin. Wschr.*, **44**, pp. 233, 280, 310, 341, 1907.
20. Hughes, A., *A History of Cytology*. Abelard-Schuman, London, 1959.
21. Rindfleisch, E., *A Manual of Pathological Histology*, translated by E. Baxter. The New Sydenham Society, London, 1873.
22. Zeigler, E., *A Textbook of Pathological Anatomy and Pathogenesis*, translated by D. MacAlister. William Wood and Co., NY, 1887.

CHAPTER VIII

> All diseases are in the last analysis reducible to disturbances, . . . of large and small groups of living units (cells), whose functional capacity is altered in accordance with the state of their molecular composition and is thus dependent on physical and chemical changes of their contents.
>
> — R. Virchow (1855)

The Contributions of Rudolf Virchow to Pathology

One of the most influential medical men of the nineteenth century was, without question, the Prussian pathologist Rudolf Virchow, who established himself as a leader in medicine as a young man and then went on to dominate medical thought until his death in 1902. Virchow was born October 13, 1821, in the little Pomeranian town of Schevelbein in Northern Germany. His character expressed itself early by the fact that his scholastic record was always brilliant but that he always ranked last in his class in behavior because of his nonconformist opinions. However, because of his anti-establishment ideas, he was popular with his classmates. He also wrote a graduation composition in which he said "A life full of work and toil is not a burden but a benediction," a theme by which he certainly abided during his lifetime. In 1843, he graduated in medicine at the University of Berlin, after which he became assistant prosector to Robert Froriep at the Charité Hospital in that city and in 1846 he replaced Froriep as chief prosector. He immediately utilized his position to open the postmortem facilities as an educational opportunity and delivered lectures on the subject of anatomical pathology to the medical students. It was during this time that he asserted his leadership qualities, because he not only knew the field of medicine, but had an incisive mind, a pugnacious temperament, a dramatic manner of speaking and writing, and a tremendous capacity for work. These assets and characteristics together with a carefully honed and often ruthless manner enabled him to become one of those political academics who, in spite of their perhaps lesser accomplishments compared with others in their fields, would be able to maintain leadership throughout their lives. In Virchow's case, although he ceased to publish original work in pathology during the last thirty-four years of his life, his opinions were always solicited by others in Germany, and for those who contradicted or threatened his ideas, there was the fear of ridicule or ostracism. Even his students and disciples were not immune, as in the case of Cohnheim, Klebs, and Haeckel. But Virchow, although not an excellent investigator, was a trailblazer not only in pathology but also in such diverse fields as anthropology, archaeology, public hygiene, and government.[1] With regard to the latter, he was one of the few individuals in the Prussian parliament to personally and dangerously challenge the veracity of the despotic Otto von Bismarck, the first chancellor of the German Empire, and was always, perhaps ironically recognizing his own dictatorial ways, a champion of democratic government.

His career to fame is a fascinating one. While prosector in Berlin at the age of 24 and essentially an unknown, at a scientific meeting he dared to verbally admonish the established physicians to stop their speculative deductions about disease, and told them to concentrate on careful gross and microscopic examinations of autopsy materials and to perform experiments on animals. His audacity is best expressed in a letter written to his father at the time:

> I like to accept (the offer of the second speech). Unfortunately the occasion to give a piece of one's mind to Geheimraeten, secretaries of state and generals arises so rarely, . . . and I hope to make myself understood. I don't deceive myself, with real knowledge and a determined language one can impress everybody, even in the highest ranks, because everything is hollow and rotten up to the top. . . . Although I have not yet published a line, people know, not only in Berlin, but in Halle, even in Prague and Vienna, that there is now a man in the Charité who takes the cause seriously. . . . It is a true work of Danaides, this medicine. Nothing has been examined properly. Everywhere one has to start from scratch again, and there is so much that sometimes one really despairs. If I had not the results in front of me that now everybody in the Charité regards me as an authority in scientific matters, and that everybody believes my statements, really I would have given up already. I, who

> have worked for such a short time, and who does not know innumerable things, I to be an authority? It is ridiculous. How little should those know who ask, me knowing myself so little.[2]

Then, as related in Chapter VII when Rokitansky published his monumental work on gross pathology and added his ideas about "crases," Virchow enhanced his reputation by severely criticizing the Viennese pathologist. In retrospect, although Rokitansky made a mistake by including his "crases" theories in his book, he probably did not deserve the severe criticism of Virchow. Jacob Henle in 1839, published his *Rational Pathology*, which in spite of Henle's important contributions to biology, was almost entirely speculations in the Natural Philosophy tradition.[3] But Henle, like Virchow, was one of Johannes Müller's favorite students, and although they would eventually become enemies, Virchow never made any reference to Henle's book, which essentially contributed almost nothing to pathology. Also from the comments made by Virchow, it is likely that there was, during those early days when Berlin was asserting itself in biology and medicine, a competition between that city and Vienna that explains Müller's "appreciation" for the Rokitansky criticism.

In 1847, Virchow found that not all editors of some of the well-known journals were willing to publish his strong points of view. The solution to this problem was simple. Along with his friend and fellow pathologist, Benno Reinhardt, he decided to publish his own journal, *Archives for Pathological Anatomy and Physiology and Clinical Medicine*, which still exists today as *Virchow's Archives.* The first volume was issued in 1847 and was to become the medium through which Virchow gave his views until his death in 1902. Regarding the new journal, he revealed his goal in a letter to his parents in which he said:

> I know now almost all German Universities and most of the German medical big shots, and, what is no less important, they know me. Our Archives have thus gained in distribution and influence, and I will be able to consciously pursue my goal of becoming the representative of a certain trend in medicine.[4]

In the first article of the first volume, Virchow clearly establishes for the first time, the guidelines for the progress of modern medicine.

The paper was entitled *Standpoints in Scientific Medicine* and the highlights were as follows:

> Scientific medicine, for its part, has as its object the investigation of those altered conditions which characterize the diseased body or various ailing organs, the identification of abnormalities in the phenomena of life as they occur under specifically altered conditions, and finally the discovery of means for abolishing these abnormal conditions . . . it will be understood that only calm, industrious, and steady work or experiment, has permanent value.[5]

At the time that Virchow was attempting to establish himself as a leader in medicine, one of the major controversies in biology was the significance of the cells and how they were produced. The idea that all living material was made up of cells traces its roots to the work of Robert Hooke[6] and Nehemiah Grew[7] in the seventeenth century, and Robert Brown,[8] who not only observed in 1828 the random motion of particles in plant tissue, but also called attention to the fact that there was an areola or nucleus in the cells of all flowering plants. But with the significant improvement in the compound microscope by Joseph Lister and the great activity of Johannes Müller and his group (as discussed in the last chapter) and others in Germany, France, and Great Britain it was simply a matter of time before revolutionary ideas would result. This was the case when Theodor Schwann (1810–1882) in 1839 conclusively established that all living organisms are made up of cells, which was thereafter known as the Cell Theory.[9] However, the mechanisms by which cells are produced was the greatest controversy after Schwann's publication. As of 1847, Schwann, Müller, Schleiden, Henle, Kölliker, and Virchow believed that cells were formed from the extravascular fluid, the cytoblastema, by a type of crystallization around a granule with the later formation of the nucleus and finally the cell membrane. Virchow stated at that time[10]:

> 1. All organization progresses through differentiation of a formless blastema.
> 2. Blastema is primarily fluid and an exudate from vessels.
> 3. Differentiation within the blastema results in the formation of cells.

Only Robert Remak, as far back as 1842 and alone in his opposition to his mentor, Müller, and his students and colleagues, was dubious about cells forming from exudative fluid. In 1852, he stated, "for myself, the extracellular creation of animal cells has been, since this cell theory was made public, as incredible as the generation equivoca (spontaneous generation)."[11] By 1854, however, Virchow decided that Remak was correct, gave him credit in his *Handbook on Special Pathology and Therapy*, and said "there is no life but through direct succession."[12]

Then, in 1855, Virchow revealed another talent, which was to take various ideas that were already stirring in a given field at a certain period of time and a particular intellectual milieu and combine them into a system, using new words and expressions in a dramatic manner. This often serves to clarify confusion that exists between new and old ways of thinking. In Virchow's case, he took the ideas of Remak and John Goodsir, a Scotsman, and, combining them with the cell theory as stated by Schwann, proposed his *Cellular Pathology*, which he confidently hoped would "become the pathology of the future."[13] It consisted of the following major statements:

1. I formulate the doctrine of pathological generation and of neoplasia in the cellular pathological sense, in simple terms; omnis cellula e cellula (all cells arise from other cells).[14]

2. Now if pathology is nothing but physiology with obstacles, and diseased life nothing but healthy life interfered with by all manner of external and internal influences, then pathology, too, must be referred back to the cell.[15]

3. All diseases are in the last analysis reducible to disturbances, either active or passive, of large and small groups of living units, whose functional capacity is altered in accordance with the state of their molecular composition and is thus dependent on physical and chemical changes of their contents.[16]

Implicit in Virchow's concept was the denial that diseases were specific entities that can be classified like plants and animals, each with its own characteristic signs and symptoms and that can be differentiated from all other diseases, as proposed by Thomas Sydenham in the seventeenth century and later Pierre Bretonneau in the early nineteenth century. Virchow rejected this idea of "ontology" and said in 1849:

> If disease is only orderly manifestations of certain phenomena of life, normal in themselves, that occur under abnormal circumstances, with deviations which are merely quantitative, then all treatment must be directed essentially against the altered conditions; moreover, when in the course of the same disease, together with continual change of conditions determined in turn by reciprocal disturbances of new organs by those already diseased, new groups of symptoms appear and still other parts come under the influence of the altered conditions, then the therapeutic procedure must of course be appropriately altered.[17]

With the development of microbiology, Virchow[18] later embraced the concept of ontology, but at the beginning of his Cellular Pathology, his dismissal of the idea of the specificity of disease was emphatic. Virchow spent much of his time defending his Cellular Pathology from the time of its inception until his death in 1902. The fact remains that the concept was stated in such a careful and clever manner that it has remained valid since it was first proposed. It was, however, the work of Pasteur that produced the most difficult period for Cellular Pathology. Some pathologists, such as Virchow's former student Edwin Klebs,[19] who followed the lead of Pasteur by working in the new field of bacteriology, used the new discoveries to attack the relevance of the Cellular Pathology of Klebs's old chief because it implied that disease was produced by an intrinsic dysfunction of certain cells, and that Virchow's concept had outlived its usefulness. In retrospect, the only error that Virchow had made was his adamant anti-ontology position. Eventually Virchow had to admit that some of the infectious diseases were specific because they were produced by specific microorganisms and that they were not due to such nonspecific factors as filth and poverty. Earlier in his career, when he was present at a typhus epidemic in 1847, he became convinced that it was sociological factors that produced typhus; but in 1871 he admitted it was most likely a contagious disease.

One of the historical paradoxes in medicine is that the idea of diseases such as plague, yellow fever, cholera, and typhus being contagious was completely discarded by almost all the most brilliant medical minds during the second quarter of the nineteenth century, with the exception of Jacob Henle. The rationale for the rejection was that there were simply too many cases in which the disease was not transmitted to a healthy person by close contact with a sick individual, and other cases in

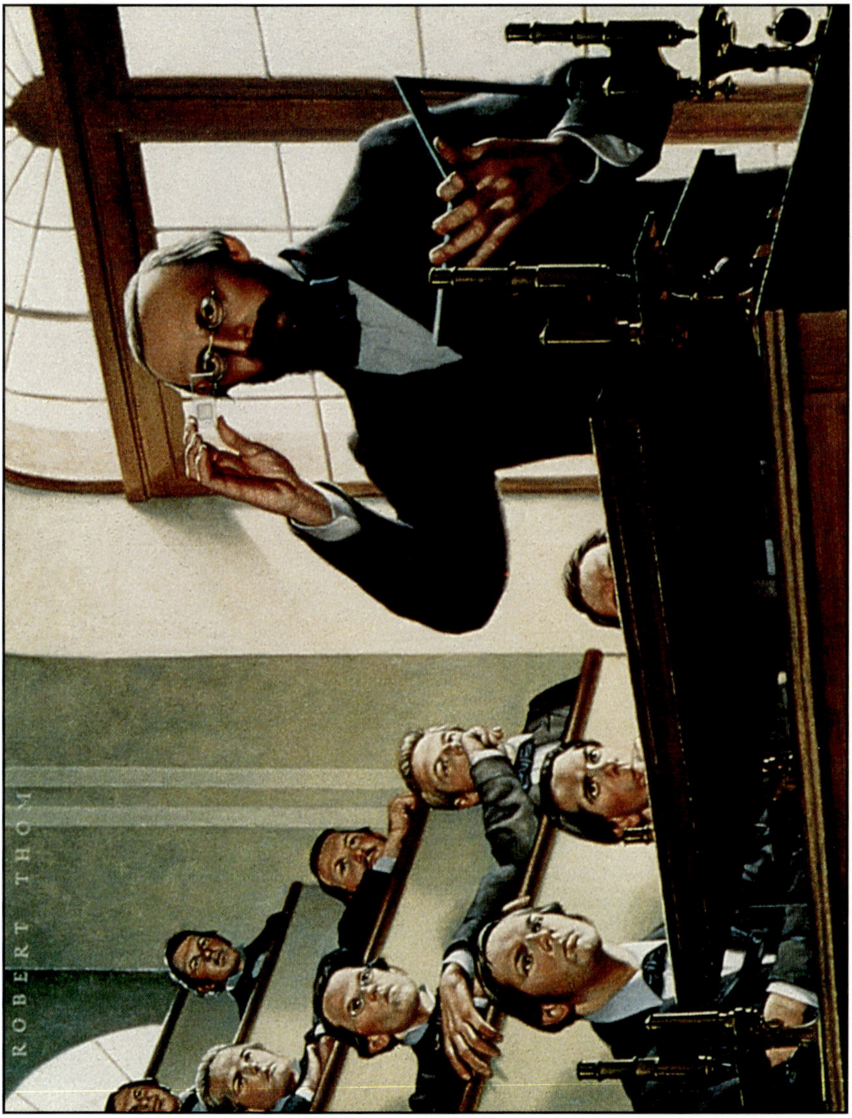

VIRCHOW AND CELLULAR PATHOLOGY

which the disease appeared in a healthy person who had no contact with a sick individual. Thus it was difficult to convince an objective physician of the validity of contagiousness. Thus the anti-ontology position of Virchow appeared valid, and it was logical to assume that disease is simply abnormal physiology in all cases. But the fact was that the anti-ontology idea, proven invalid by the microbiologists, was, fortunately for Virchow, never part of his Cellular Pathology concept. Thus Virchow, although conceding that ontology exists, could reply to Klebs by stating that his former assistant was confusing the initiating causes of disease with the disease process itself. In 1898, Virchow stated that:

> There is the necessity for distinguishing between the inciting cause, (causa) and the essential nature (essentia) of infectious diseases. Parasitic beings, specifically bacteria, are never more than inciting causes; the nature of the disease depends upon the behavior of the organs or tissues affected by the bacteria or their metabolic products. In my opinion this distinction is of cardinal importance.[20]

Today we know that Virchow's arguments were correct because even at the time of the debates, it was known that the presence of diphtheria, typhoid, or cholera organisms in a human did not necessarily produce pathological changes. It is only the body's reactions to the microorganisms that produce the signs and symptoms and lesions that the clinician and pathologist see as the disease. Since Virchow was not likely to be able to predict the above facts at the time he proposed his cellular pathology in 1855, he might be considered lucky that cellular pathology is "still alive and well" near the beginning of the twenty-first century. On the other hand, he did show remarkable vision in 1854 when he made this statement:

> The basic error of this (Rokitansky's) point of view rests in our opinion, on the confusion of the anatomical with the material. We are, as well, in no position to conceive of any kind of living process in the human being, regardless of how functional it may seem, without a material change — however must it be anatomical. . . . Every anatomical change is a material one as well, but is every material change, therefore, also anatomical? Cannot it be molecular? Can a deep-reaching molecular alteration of the inner composition of matter not

> take place with the preservation of its inner form and outer appearance? These finer molecular changes of matter are objects of physiology, not anatomy; they are functional — dynamic if one wishes to use this forbidden expression. . . . One can have the greatest respect for anatomical, morphological and histological studies . . . but must one proclaim them, therefore, the only ones to be pursued, the ones of exclusive significance? Many important phenomena in the body are of a purely functional kind, and when one attempts to explain these also with a mechanical hypothesis, in terms of fine molecular changes, it should never be forgotten that the methods for their observation and pursuit can never be anatomical.[21]

The wisdom of Virchow's statement has been borne out because today we know there are defective macromolecules in the form of genes on the DNA molecules that in turn produce genetic diseases such as Gaucher's disease, Tay-Sachs disease, phenylketonuria, Niemann Pick disease, primary gout, or tyrosinemia where a dysfunctional enzyme reflects the abnormality of the DNA.

However, Rudolf Virchow's contributions were more than his cellular pathology and his writings. He was a great teacher and his pupils and disciples were as numerous as were those of his own mentor, Johannes Müller. In pathology they were Georg Eduard Rindfleisch, Edwin Klebs, Otto Beckmann, Friedrich von Recklinghausen, Julius Cohnheim, Emil Ponfick, Paul Gravitz, Johannes Orth, Christian Baeumler, Ferdinand Hueppe, Robert Langerhans, Felix Hoppe-Seyler, William Roux, Felix Marchand, Carl Weigert, and Friedrich Martius from Germany; A.R. Simpson and Wilson Fox from England; Tommasi-Crudeli from Italy; Sergei Botkin from Russia; Axel Key from Sweden; Andre Cornil from France; and Reginald Heber Fitz and William Councilman from the United States. In anatomy he taught Wilhelm His, Sr., Ernst Haeckel, Karl Gegenbaur, and Otto Deiters and in medicine, Adolf Kussmaul, Hugo Ziemmsen, Johann Czermak, Nikolaus Friedreich, and Carl Gerhardt.

The feelings toward Virchow by his students were ambivalent. They all recognized his brilliance but they feared him because he was prone to speaking with sarcasm to those who disagreed with him. However, he did seem to enjoy bantering with some of his assistants who were on occasion willing to challenge him. In his autobiography, Carl Ludwig Schleich, who was a junior assistant of Virchow for three years, relates some of his experiences with Virchow which reveals the famous man's personality:

> Let it be said at once that Virchow was a crass mechanist and materialist who insisted that all vital phenomena could be explained by the mechanism of the cells. . . . From this we proceeded to discuss questions of faith. I expressed my doubts as to whether the universe could have come into being as a result of chance. I remember that I called chance the clown of possibilities, of whom it was inconceivable that he could have created the iron laws of Nature.
>
> Virchow: "Now in you we have just another such case of a dissolution (he actually said a colliquative condition) of the brain. You are still holding on, as all of us did when we were children, to all sorts of theistic and pantheistic fairytales."
>
> Schleich: "But does Herr Geheimrat really think a Goethe, for example, suffered from such a colliquative condition, despite his otherwise impeccable intellect?"
>
> Virchow: "Naturally the poetical way of regarding the world is quite different from the scientific. His inaccessibility to exact thinking is plainly shown in his Theory of Colors. That is clearly colliquative. You can find pages and pages in my work which will tell you what I think of all the metaphysicians and transcendentalists. But there my interest ceases!"
>
> Schleich: "Yes, but it is a remarkable fact that this is just where many people begin to be interested; that is, in the quest for God!"
>
> Virchow: "Putting all the theological simpletons aside, read in Kant what he thought of the so-called evidence of the existence of God!"
>
> Schleich: "Yet those who believe in God find themselves in very good company. I don't know of any really eminent and significant man who didn't believe in something like God or the spirit of Nature!"
>
> Virchow stood still and looked at me, and asked me, quite

ingenuously: "Don't you regard me as an eminent man?"

Schleich stammering: "Of course."

Virchow: "Well, then !"[22]

There is no question that with regard to his human relationships Virchow was conceited, arrogant, unforgiving, and had a minimum of a sense of humor. But he had a soft heart for animals. Schleich describes an incident in which:

> We wanted to make some sort of an injection under the skin of a rabbit, and owing to our lack of practice, we had fastened the rabbit very unskillfully. Seeing this, Virchow came over to us, saying angrily: "But you are hurting the beast like that! Give it to me, I'll show you!" I must confess, alas, that this was the only time one of my many teachers ever conveyed a deep and lasting impression of compassion for the living creature, of tenderness, of sympathy with suffering. How skillfully he showed us the requisite knack![23]

In a more serious vane, one of the best examples of Virchow's influence is described in a letter written by William Osler, when as a recent graduate of McGill Medical School in Canada, he was studying in Berlin during the last months of 1873:

> But it is the master mind of Virchow and the splendid Pathological Institute, which rises like a branch hospital in the grounds of the Charité, that specially attract foreign students to Berlin. This most remarkable man is yet in his prime (52 years of age) and the small, wiry, active, figure looks good for another twenty years of hard work, when one knows that in addition to the work at the Institute, given below, he is an ardent politician, evidently the leader of the Prussian Opposition, and a member on whom a large share of the work of the budget falls; an active citizen, member of the Council, and the moving spirit in the new canalization or sewerage system; an enthusiastic anthropologist as well as a working member in several smaller affairs, some idea may be formed of the comprehensive intellect of the man. On Monday, Wednesday and

> Friday from 8:30 to 11 he holds his demonstrative course of Pathological Histology, while on the fourth day at one o'clock he lectures on General Pathology. Virchow, himself, performs a postmortem on Monday morning making it with such care and minuteness that three or four hours may elapse before it is finished. The very first morning of my attendance he spent exactly half an hour in the description of the skull-cap! On Wednesday and Saturday the demonstrations take place in a large lecture room accommodating about 140 students, and with the table arranged, that microscopes can circulate continuously on a small tramway let into them. Generally the material from 10 to 12 postmortems is demonstrated, the lecturer taking up any special group and enlarging on it with the aid of sketches on the blackboard and microscopical specimens, while the organs are passed around on wooden platters for inspection. A well provided Laboratory for Physiological and Pathological Chemistry also exists as well as rooms where men carry on private investigations; and a Library and Reading room is now being fitted up.[24]

Undoubtedly inspired by Virchow, Osler, as a new professor at McGill Medical School, emphasized the importance of correlating the signs and symptoms of terminal patients with the gross and microscopic findings and with his students as observers, he personally performed more than 800 autopsies at Montreal General Hospital during the years 1877–1878.[25] He also was stimulated to stress the significance of using the clinical laboratory procedures to aid in making diagnoses.[26] It was his stated ambition to "build up a great clinic on Teutonic line . . . which have placed the scientific medicine of Germany in the forefront of the world."[27] But Osler was not alone in his admiration of Virchow. William Henry Welch, Osler's close friend and colleague when both were members of the "Big Four" at the Johns Hopkins, had studied with Virchow's most illustrious pupil Julius Cohnheim in 1877 and was thus indirectly influenced by the senior pathologist. On the occasion of Virchow's death in 1902, Welch wrote that:

> Important as was the reformatory influence upon medicine of the few leaders whose names are worthy to be placed besides his, such as Galen, Vesalius, Harvey, Hunter, and Pasteur, it may safely be said that the establishment by Virchow of the principles of cellular pathology marked the greatest advance

> which scientific medicine had made since its beginning. Upon this foundation, embedded in the solid rock of truth, medicine has built for nearly two generations, and we may confidently believe that upon this same foundation future generations will continue to build with every increasing benefit to science and humanity. Investigation will penetrate deeper and deeper into the structure and the life of cells, but there is no reason to believe that ultimate analysis will ever be able to refer the primary seats of disease to any independent, vital units outside of the cells.[28]

Therefore, for both Osler and Welch, following their training periods in Europe and especially during their leadership as professors at the Johns Hopkins Medical School and Hospital throughout the heroic period of 1893–1905, it would be fair to say that Virchow's influence on them was a contributing factor in eventually establishing the present-day high standard of medicine in the United States.

Bibliography

1. Ackerknecht, E., *Rudolf Virchow, Doctor, Statesman, Anthropologist*. Univ. Wisconsin Press, Madison, 1953.
2. Ibid, p. 10.
3. Henle, J., *A Treatise of General Pathology*, translated by H. Preston. Lindsay and Blakiston, Philadelphia, 1853.
4. Ref. 1, p. 14.
5. Virchow, R., Standpoints in Scientific Medicine, 1847, in *Disease, Life, and Man*, edited and translated by L. Rather. Stanford Univ. Press, Stanford, 1958.
6. Hooke, R., *Micrographia*. Martyn and Allestry, London, 1665.
7. Grew, N., *Anatomy Vegetables, Begun*. Hickman, London, 1672.
8. Brown, R. Observations on the organs and mode of fecundation in Orchideae and Asclepiadeae. *Trans. Linn. Soc.*, **16**, p. 685, 1829-32.
9. Schwann, T., *Microscopical Researches*, translated by H. Smith, Sydenham Society, London, 1847.
10. Virchow, R., Ueber die Reform der Pathologischen und therapeutischen Anschaungen durch die Mikroskopischen Untersuchungen. *Virchow's Arch.* **1**, p. 207, 1847.
11. Remak, R., Ueber extracellulare Entstehung thierischer Zellen und über vermehrung derselben durch Theilung. *Müller's Archiv.*, **19**, p. 47, 1852.
12. Virchow, R., *Handbuch der speziellen Pathologie und Therapie*. F. Enke, Erlangen, 1854.
13. Virchow, R., Cellular Pathology, 1855, in *Disease, Life, and Man*, p. 101, edited by L. Rather. Stanford Univ. Press. Stanford, 1958.
14. Ibid, p. 88.
15. Ibid, p. 81.
16. Ibid, p. 100.
17. Virchow. R. , Scientific Method and Therapeutic Standpoints, 1849, in *Disease, Life, and Man*, p. 59, edited by L. Rather. Stanford Univ. Press, Stanford, 1858.
18. Virchow, R., One Hundred Years of General Pathology, 1895, in *Disease, Life, and Man*, p.207, edited by L. Rather. Stanford Univ. Press, Stanford, 1858.
19. Virchow, R., Krankheitswesen und Krankheitsursachen. *Virchow's*

Archiv., **79**, p. 1, 1880.
20. Virchow, R., Recent Progress in Science, 1898, in *Disease, Life, and Man*, p. 239, edited by L. Rather. Stanford Univ. Press, Stanford, 1958.
21. Virchow, R., Specifiker und Specifisches, *Virchow's Archiv.*, **6**, p. 14, 1854.
22. Schleich, C., *Those Were Good Days*, 1922, p. 159, translated by J. Mall. W.W. Norton, N.Y.
23. Ibid p. 156.
24. Osler, W., Berlin Correspondence. *Canadian Medical and Surgical Journal*, **2**, p. 308, 1873-74.
25. Osler, W., *Montreal General Hospital Pathological Reports*, no. 1, 1877.
26. Malkin, H., The influence of William Osler on the development of clinical laboratory medicine in North America. *Ann. Clin. Lab. Sci.*, **7**, p. 281, 1977.
27. Osler, W., L'Envoi, in *Equanimitas, with other Addresses*, 3rd ed. Blakiston, Philadelphia, 1914.
28. Welch, W., Virchow, A Tribute. in *Papers and Addresses by William Henry Welch*, Vol. 3. Johns Hopkins Press, Baltimore, 1920.

CHAPTER IX

Medicine is a great humbug.

— Magendie (1856)

François Magendie and the Beginnings of Pathological Physiology

It will be remembered that, until the 1870s when the work of Pasteur and Koch showed that microorganisms could produce specific diseases in mammals, most physicians not only did not believe in contagion, but along with their spokesman, Virchow, most were convinced that disease was produced by abnormalities of physiology that in many cases finally manifested in anatomical lesions. Virchow, since the beginning of his career, did not believe in specific diseases, or *ontology* as he called it then, which was the belief of Sydenham and Bretonneau. Therefore, although he was primarily an anatomical pathologist, he was always convinced that disease essentially started with abnormal physiology and encouraged experiments to prove this idea.

But this belief had its beginnings in the thoughts and experiments of François Magendie, one of the memorable physician investigators in France during the first half of the nineteenth century. Magendie was the first modern investigator and pure mechanist in his approach to physiology. This was brought out in his 1816 *Précis Élémentaire de Physiologie,* which reads like a current textbook and is devoid of romantic and nebulous terms such as found in Johannes Müller's book. Listen to what Magendie writes in his preface:

> The natural sciences, like history, have had their fabulous period. Astronomy commenced in astrology; chemistry was

not long since alchemy; and medicine but a combination of absurd hypotheses. Strange condition of the human mind, which seems to require that it should long exercise itself in error before it dare approach the truth! Such were the natural sciences before the seventeenth century, when Galileo appeared, and discovered to mankind that to understand nature, it is not enough to IMAGINE or BELIEVE, as the ancients supposed, but to OBSERVE, and above all, to INQUIRE BY EXPERIMENTS. This was the spirit that inspired the labors of the immortal Newton, and of those men of genius, who, during the last century, annihilated the antique doctrines of the four elements. The same spirit animates the natural philosophers and chemists of the present day; guides them in their ingenious and useful researches, and forms between them a new and indissoluble bond.

Glory, then, to Galileo! In demonstrating by memorable example the immense advantages of observation and experiment; in turning the human mind from the false direction where its powers had exhausted themselves for ages in vain efforts, he really laid the foundation of the physical sciences. . . . Would that I could say that Physiology, in the language of Bacon, THE SCIENCE OF OURSELVES, has pursued the same course, and undergone the same metamorphosis as the physical sciences. But unfortunately, this is not the case; Physiology is still, in the minds of many, and in some of our books, a mere work of the imagination; it has different creeds, and opposite and contending sects; it admits the existence of fabulous beings, who, like the pagan gods, preside over the phenomena of life; the authority of authors calling themselves infallible is invoked; in a word, it may be said to be the framework of a religion strangely filled with scientific terms.
Still there are men who have successfully applied the experimental method to the study of life; great discoveries have been the fruits of their efforts; science is enriched — and by the side of the phenomena of the circulation of the blood, of respiration, muscular contraction etc. are placed, in the same line, such metaphors as the ORGANIC SENSIBILITY, or such offspring of the imagination as the NERVOUS FLUID, or such unintelligible expressions as the VITAL FORCE OF PRINCIPLE. . . . Numerous prejudices separate Physiology at present from the exact sciences; extreme repugnance to ex-

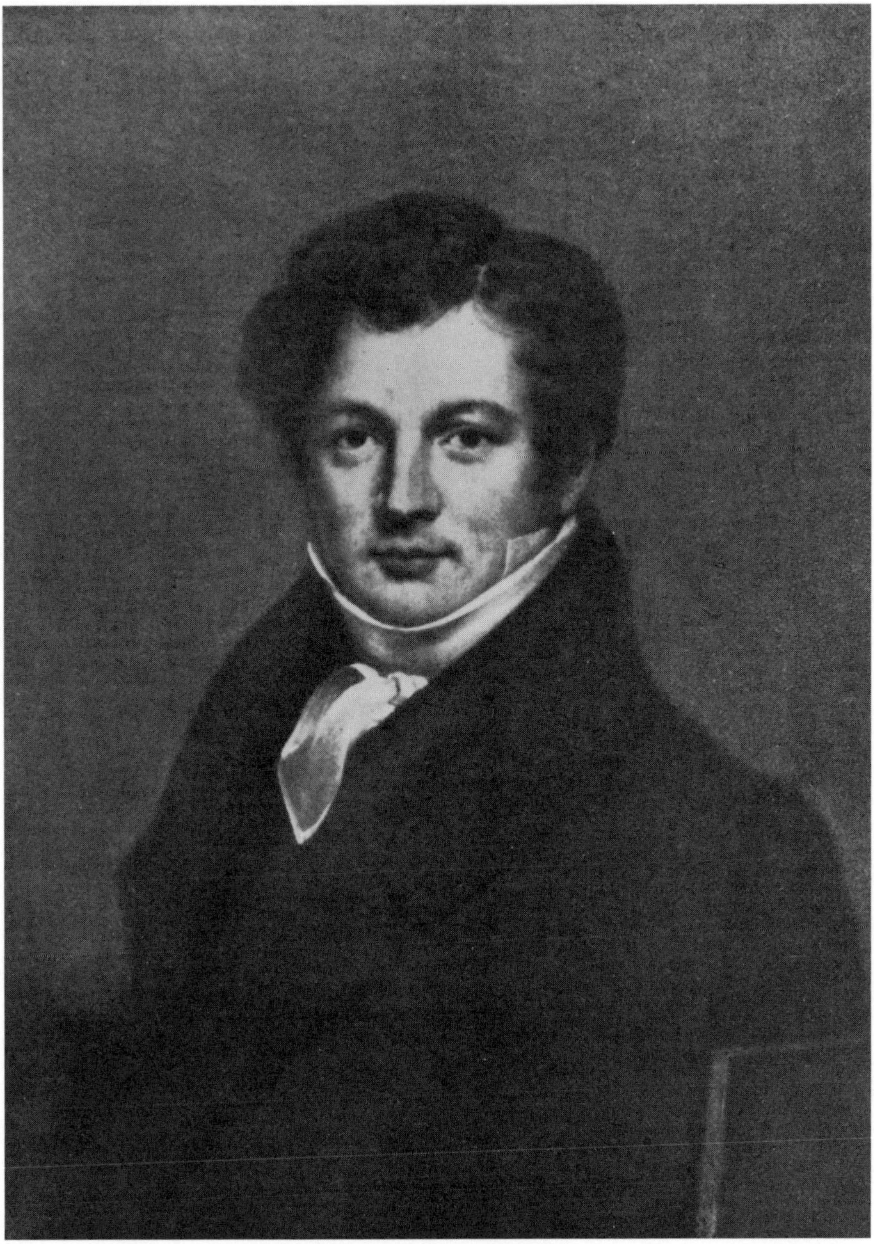

FRANÇOIS MAGENDIE

> periments on living animals; the pretended impossibility of applying these deductions to man; the almost absolute ignorance as to the method of proceeding so as to attain truth; the attachment to old ideas, always sustained by carelessness and indolence; . . . these are some of the obstacles which it will be necessary to surmount. . . . The belief, so injurious and absurd, that physical laws have no influence on living bodies has no longer the same force. It is no longer doubted that researches made on animals apply with remarkable precision to the phenomena of life in man; the vivid light that recent experiments relative to the nervous functions have thrown upon pathology, has removed all uncertainty on this point. . . . Medicine, which is but the PHYSIOLOGY OF MAN DISEASED, will not fail to follow in the same direction and attain the same height. We shall then see those erroneous explanations disappear which have misled the best minds, and disfigured it so long.[1]

And what was the personality of this man, the teacher of Claude Bernard, who liked to call himself "a scavenger, who with a rake in hand, collected whatever facts I could possibly find." He was a true mechanist, contemptuous of elaborate theories, particularly those of the vitalists, and he carried out innumerable vivisections on dogs, cats, and rabbits. Because he could not support himself as a full-time physiologist, Magendie practiced medicine, although he was a skilled surgeon. He essentially was an iconoclast and an outsider, but he was highly respected by the more enlightened medical men in Paris. He gave lectures at the College of France, but never was a faculty member of the medical school in Paris. His classes always attracted an audience, although he sometimes offended by his perceived cruelty to animals with his vivisections in class. Magendie's comments on the state of medicine were unorthodox and did not make him popular with the more establishment physicians. In a 1856 lecture to medical students he said the following:

> Gentlemen: Medicine is a great humbug. I know it is called a science — science, indeed! It is nothing like science. Doctors are mere empirics, when they are not charlatans. We are as ignorant as men can be. Who knows anything in the world about medicine? Gentlemen, you have done me the honor to come here to attend my lectures, and I must tell you frankly now, in the beginning, that I know nothing in the world about

medicine, and I don't know anybody who does know anything about it. Don't think for a moment that I haven't read the bills advertising the courses of lectures at the Medical School. I know that this man teaches anatomy, that man teaches pathology, another man physiology, such-a-one therapeutics, such another materia medica — Eh bien! et apres? What is known about all that? Why, gentlemen, at the school of Montpellier (God knows it was famous enough in its day!) they discarded the study of anatomy, and taught nothing but the dispensary; and the doctors educated there knew just about as much and were just as successful as any others. I repeat it, nobody knows anything about medicine. True enough, we are gathering facts everyday. We can produce typhus fever, for example, by injecting a certain substance into the veins of a dog — that's something; we can alleviate diabetes, and I see distinctly, as we are fast approaching the day when phthisis can be cured as easily as any other disease. We are collecting facts in the right spirit, and I dare say in a century or so the accumulation of facts may enable our successors to form a medical science; but I repeat it to you, there is no such thing now as a medical science. Who can tell me how to cure the headache? or the gout, or disease of the heart? Nobody. Oh, you tell me doctors cure people. I grant you people are cured, but how are they cured? Gentlemen, nature does a good deal. Imagination does a good deal. Doctors do devilish little when they don't do harm! Let me tell you, gentlemen, what **I** did when I was the head physician at the Hotel Dieu. Some three or four thousand patients passed through my hands every year. I divided the patients into two classes; with one, I followed the dispensary, and gave them the usual medicines without having the least idea why or wherefore; to the other I gave bread pills and colored water, without, of course, letting them know anything about it. . . and occasionally, gentlemen, I would create a third division to whom I gave nothing whatever. These last would fret a good deal — they would feel they were neglected, unless they were well drugged (Les imbeciles!) and they would irritate themselves until they got really sick, but nature invariably came to the rescue, and all the persons in the third class got well. There was a little mortality among those who received but bread pills and colored water, and the mortality was the greatest among those who were carefully drugged according to the dispensary. You ask then, what is

> the use of my lecturing. I'll tell you. We have come here to study nature, not to spin fine theories about this and that, and to anticipate brilliant conclusions — leave that to the German gentlemen. I don't say these doctrinaires fail to hit occasionally upon some brilliant truth, by the aid of their theories — for I have sometimes been astonished by their discoveries but for once they are right, they are wrong a hundred times, and by their theories they are never sure of knowing assuredly what they do know. Now what I know, I know. There can be no mistake about it. I see it with my eyes; I touch it with my fingers. I would not give that for all the theories in the world — give me stubborn facts. That's the way, gentlemen, we are going to study here![2]

There is little that Magendie said that was probably untrue, although he undoubtedly was exaggerating for a dramatic effect on the students. But he had faith in the idea that pathology was abnormal physiology, and he was an anti-ontologist and anti-contagionist as was Virchow. This evidently led him to believe that by producing some signs and symptoms similar to those of typhus by injecting some substances into dogs, showed that even the great skeptic Magendie could be misled by bias! Magendie was often criticized for his cruelty to animals, but in his defense, it should be pointed out that during most of his career, surgery was carried out on human patients without anesthesia because ether and chloroform did not become widespread in use until after 1850. Thus the early surgeons and physiologists had to be stoic and dedicated because their daily work was brutal and bloody. On the other hand, human lives were often saved because of their work, and knowledge about physiology was obtained. Magendie determined the nature and function of cerebrospinal fluid, the elasticity of the vascular system, the origin of the cardiac sounds, the nature of diastole and systole of the heart, the nature of absorption of nutrients from the intestine into the blood and lymphatic system, and that animals fed food without nitrogen or gelatin as the only protein soon died. However, Magendie is best known for his discovery with regard to the functions of the spinal cord, that the dorsal roots are for the most part sensory and the ventral roots are motor.

With regard to pathology, Magendie was the first individual to emphasize that the study of disease processes could shed light on normal physiology and that the converse was also true, that artificially produced lesions could help explain some disease processes. In 1839 he said that:

> What we do not dare to do on man, nature, a less scrupulous experimenter, takes it upon itself to do. How many diseases of the brain and spinal cord are only the faithful reproduction of our experiments! The pathology of the nervous system is thus nothing other than experimental physiology applied to men.[3]

By studying the location of various neurological lesions and their effects on various functions of the nervous system, he and his clinical colleagues were able to show that various functions of the brain were localized and that by studying conditions such as hydrocephalus he was able to understand the circulation of the cerebrospinal fluid. He was concerned that there were different types of hydrocephalus, depending upon whether the fluid was in the ventricles or on the outer surface of the brain. He then predicted that with apoplexy there would be blood in the cerebrospinal fluid, and he showed how cerebrospinal fluid abnormalities could produce brain compression. Thus with his success in showing how abnormalities or lesions in the nervous system produced certain signs and symptoms in the patient, it gave him confidence that all diseases would eventually be explained by an abnormal physiology. Claude Bernard, Magendie's most illustrious disciple, had basically the same philosophy regarding pathology, and in his famous *An Introduction to the Study Experimental Medicine*, he said the following:

> So if I were planning a treatise on experimental medicine, I should go to work by invariably making observation of disease the basis of every experimental analysis. I should then proceed with my explanations, symptom by symptom, until I had exhausted all the information obtainable from present experimental physiology, and the result would be medical observation reduced to its simplest terms. In saying above that we must explain by experimental physiology only what can be explained in disease, I do not want my idea misunderstood or taken as an admission that there are things in disease which can never be physiologically explained. My idea is just the reverse, because I believe that we shall explain everything in pathology, but little by little and in step with the development of experimental physiology.[4]

In retrospect, most everything that Magendie and Bernard said is still true. But the unexpected explosion in the knowledge of disease with

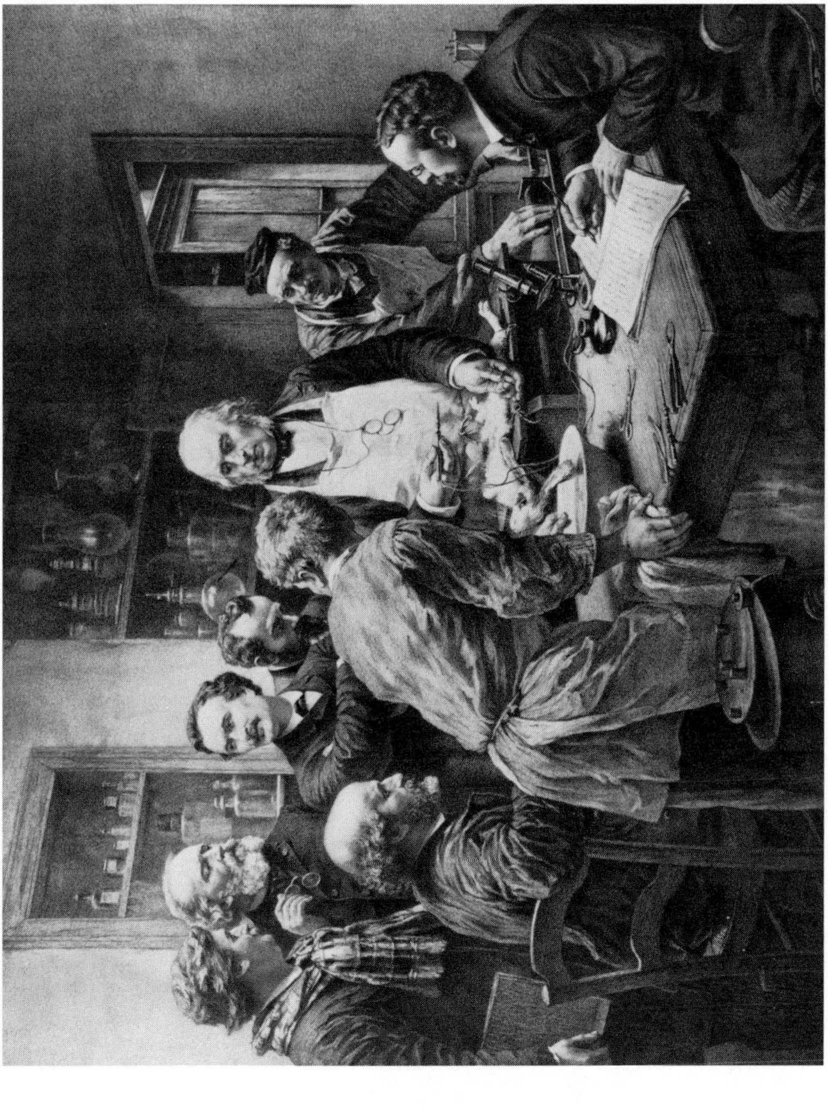

CLAUDE BERNARD

the work of Pasteur and the other microbiologists brought about a period of disorientation on the part of biological philosophers like Bernard and Virchow. Bernard was not an avid anti-ontologist like Virchow and did not seem to become involved in the problem of specificity of disease like the pathologist and his German colleagues, such as Ludwig Traube and Wunderlich. The anti-ontological polemics were directed at the old ideas of the disease taxonomists and nosologists, and became irrelevant with the discovery of microorganisms and their contagious nature. As more knowledge has accumulated, it has become obvious that the specificity of diseases is relative, that is, although the gonococcus organism produces essentially the same disease as defined by signs and symptoms and thus could be considered specific by the criteria of Sydenham, the beta hemolytic streptococcus can manifest itself as pharyngitis, erysipelas, rheumatic fever, or glomerulonephritis, all of which certainly have different disease manifestations, and, in the majority of cases when found in the throat of individuals, may produce no disease or symptoms at all. Thus Bernard was correct in that regardless of whether disease-producing factors are extrinsic or intrinsic (as in our definition of pathology), ultimately it is the dysfunction of physiology that produces the signs and symptoms of what we recognize as disease. This may be the result of the immunological or genetic system of which Bernard was unaware in 1856, but by definition how these systems function can still be considered part of the field of physiology.

However, at the time of Magendie and Bernard, it was really a question of emphasis on research into studying disease, and specifically whether pathological anatomy or experimental physiology performed on animals would be more fruitful. (At that time it was not realized that certain disease processes were species specific and that it was fruitless to attempt to produce typhus in dogs.) Although Virchow believed in the importance of physiology in studying disease, he and almost all of his followers found that, during the last half of the nineteenth century, the anatomic pathologic approach was pragmatically the most fruitful. It was not until the twentieth century that there was enough information accumulated on normal physiology to investigate such diseases as those involving the endocrine system and even later in this century abnormal functions of the genetic or immunological systems. But, nevertheless, during the nineteenth century there were a few individuals besides Magendie and Bernard who were determined to throw light on disease processes by practicing experimental physiology. Their trials and tribulations will be further discussed in the following chapters.

Bibliography

1. Magendie, F., *Précis Élémentaire de Physiologie*, 1843, English translation by J. Revere, Harper and Brothers, New York, 1855.
2. Magendie, F., Paris Correspondence, by Spiridion. *The American Medical Gazette*, **7**, p. 337, June 1856.
3. Lesch, J., *Science and Medicine in France*, p. 166. Harvard Univ. Press, Cambridge, Mass. 1984.
4. Bernard, C., *An Introduction to the Study of Experimental Medicine*, 1865, translated by H. Greene, p. 200. Dover Edition, New York, 1957.

CHAPTER X

Pathological Physiology Moves to Germany

In 1841, Carl Wunderlich (1815–1877), after many years of study in Paris, returned to Germany, enthusiastic about the approach to the study of disease that was being championed in France, particularly by Magendie and to some extent Andral. He stated in his book that

> although the idea of physiological pathology originated in France, the means and the proper understanding were lacking (and) Germany must develop them, must order and use its wealth, and a new epoch in medicine will open up.[1]

This concept was primarily a reaction to the still dominant ideas of ontology and some of the Natural Philosophy systems. For example, K.W. Stark (1787–1845) in Jena and Ferdinand Jahn[2] (1804–1859) were dedicated ontologists and proposed that diseases should be regarded as parasites, although not produced by parasites. They felt that diseases were a type of parasite with their own laws of existence and development, much as the "aliens" that took over the bodies of sleeping humans in the twentieth-century science fiction movie, "Invasion of the Body Snatchers."[3] On the other hand, Karl R. Hofmann, a follower of Natural Philosophy, believed that disease was a type of regression to a lower form of life and gave as an example that rickets were a return to molluscan life because the bones became soft. He also thought that digestive diseases showed a type of rumination that indicated a retrogression to the level of cows and that hemorrhoids were crooked animal limbs.[4]

Disgusted with such theories, Wunderlich's ideas were endorsed by Johannes Müller and the eminent clinician Ludwig Traube, and journals appeared to support "physiological pathology." The purpose was to emphasize that descriptions of diseases were no longer sufficient and that attempts should be made to understand the signs and symptoms of disease in terms of genesis, development, and abnormal physiology. The goals were certainly admirable, but unfortunately the proponents, with the exception of Müller, were clinicians and not true experimentalists, or pathologists. Before long, the movement was called "German physiological medicine" and soon received the support of the young Rudolf Virchow, who said that:

> Pathological physiology gets its questions partly from pathological anatomy, partly from practical medicine; it creates its answers partly from observations at the bedside, and thus it is a part of clinical medicine, and partly from experiments on animals. The experiment is the ultimate and highest resort in pathological physiology.[5]

But this movement was led astray. For example, Laennec had carefully described tuberculosis as a generalized disease that could affect, in addition to the lungs, many different organs such as the lymphatic glands and intestine; but Virchow rejected Laennec's ideas and stated that each organ was diseased because of local factors not part of the same generalized malady.[6] And Paul Niemeyer, following the same reasoning, stated, "Everything which Laennec has been designated as infiltrating tuberculosis is the product of chronic, especially catarrhal, pneumonia."[7] Thus clinicians were suddenly confused because what Laennec had described as beginning tuberculosis now was described as nonspecific apex pneumonia, catarrhal pneumonias, apex catarrhs, or even bronchitis. Hebra, the great Viennese dermatologist, believed that chickenpox and smallpox lesions were simply variations of the same local condition; so averse was he to admitting that each type of lesion was specific for a different disease. Thus "physiological medicine," for all of its good intentions, in many ways was a regression, and only the discoveries of specific microorganisms for specific diseases stopped this regression.

However, there were several factors that over the next fifty years helped to achieve the goals of this movement, and although the terms "physiological medicine" or "pathological physiology" are no longer used, explanations of disease in terms of physiology are still occurring today. These factors were the advancements in physiology and biochemistry and the instruments and ideas that brought about this progress. In the second half of the nineteenth century, in addition to the institutes for pathology, there were established in German-speaking countries, institutes for physiology which were centers where the Golden Age of Physiology took place until the beginning of the twentieth century. Johannes Müller and E. Dubois-Reymond (1818–1896) in Berlin, Carl Ludwig (1816–1895) in Leipzig, Ernst Brücke (1819–1892) in Vienna, Hermann

Helmholtz (1821–1894) and Willy Kühne (1837–1900) in Heidelberg, R. Heidenhain (1834–1897) at Breslau, Adolf Fick (1829–1901) at Wurzburg, Hugo Kronecker (1839–1914) at Zurich, Eduard Pflueger (1829–1910) at Bonn, Karl Vierordt (1818–1884) at Tubingen, Carl Voit (1839–1909) at Munich, Max Rubner (1854–1932) at Marburg, F. Hoppe-Seyler (1825–1895) and F. Goltz (1834–1902) at Strasbourg, Ewald Hering (1834–1918) at Prague, Wilhelm His, Sr., (1831–1904) and F. Miescher (1844–1895) at Basal, and A. Rollet (1834–1903) at Graz all contributed significant information on which others in medicine and pathology drew upon for their own advancement. New methods and instruments were developed, and the clinicians who worked for a time in these institutes soon began to utilize them in the clinic. The ophthalmoscope invented by Helmholtz initiated a flourishing period in the study of the eye and its diseases; the quantitative determination of erythrocytes, leukocytes, and hemoglobin by Vierordt, R. Thoma (1847–1923), and Hoppe-Seyler was responsible (along with the new stains of Ehrlich) for stimulating many studies on blood; and the sphygmograph and kymograph of Vierordt and Ludwig allowed the study of metabolism, respiration, muscular contraction, and the vascular system.

Additionally and just as importantly, there was major progress in physical chemistry. Such work as S. Arrhenius (1858–1927) on ionization, C.M. Guldberg (1836–1902) and P. Waage (1833–1900) on the Mass Action Law, J. van't Hoff (1852–1911) on partial pressures of gases in liquids, and E. Starling's (1866–1927) work on the osmotic pressure of proteins in blood and its effect on diffusion of crystalloids and water into the body compartments from the capillaries enabled physiologists to understand the important functions of the body at lower and lower levels of cells and molecules. A comparison of physiological textbooks written in 1861[8] with those written in 1890[9] reveals a quantum jump in knowledge greater than in all the prior centuries. Also, although the French and English physiologists did not have the great facilities as the German investigators, Magendie and his student Claude Bernard (1813–1878) and their fellow Frenchmen, C.E. Brown-Sequard (1818–1894), M.J.P. Flourens (1794–1867), J.J.C. Legallois (1770–1840), and E.J. Marey (1830–1904), all made many important contributions to physiology as did Michael Foster (1836–1907), William Sharpey (1802–1880), John Burton-Sanderson (1828–1905), Edward Sharpey-Schafer (1850–1935), Sidney Ringer (1835–1910), and others in Great Britain later in the century. These studies in addition to the new work on microbiology and immunology primarily by Pasteur and his group in France and Koch and his colleagues in Germany set the stage for the great advancements in medicine and pathology during the twentieth century.

Bibliography

1. Wunderlich, C., *Wien und Paris*. p. 22, Stuttgart, 1841.
2. Jahn, F., Die Krankheit als Afterorganisation. *Haeser's Arch. Ld. gesamte Med.*, **5**, p. 354, 1843.
3. Siegel, D., *Invasion of the Body Snatchers* (Movie), 1956.
4. Boas, J.H., *Outlines of the History of Medicine*, translated by H. Henderson, p. 948. J.H. Vail, New York, 1889.
5. Virchow, R., Standpoints in Scientific Medicine, in *Disease, Life, and Man*, and translated by L. Rather, p. 37. Stanford Univ. Press, Stanford, 1858.
6. Virchow, R., *Cellular Pathology*, 1863, Translated by F. Chance, p. 519. Dover Publications, New York, 1971.
7. Niemayer, P., quoted in Knud Faber's *Nosography in Modern Internal Medicine*, p. 78. Paul Hoeber , New York, 1923.
8. Dalton, J.C., *A Treatise on Human Physiology*. Blanchard and Lea, Philadelphia, 1861.
9. Foster, M., *A Textbook of Human Physiology*. Lea Brothers, Philadelphia, 1895.

CHAPTER XI

Etiology can be nothing more . . . than an enumeration and discussion of very different factors, having only one feature in common, namely a capacity to act as exciters of disease.

— J. Cohnheim (1877)

Julius Cohnheim — From Anatomic Pathology to Pathological Physiology

Julius Cohnheim died at the age of 44 on August 15, 1884, of kidney failure as a complication of gout. He published only 41 papers, and many were of only minor importance. But his fresh approach to pathology, with its emphasis on experimentation and the physiological alterations that occur in disease, put into practice the aims of Traube, Wunderlich, Magendie, Bernard, and Virchow with regard to pathological physiology.[1] The institutes and departments of pathology throughout the world in the last part of the nineteenth century and most of the twentieth century have been essentially morphologically oriented, and Cohnheim's approach was exceptional, and essentially not followed up after his death. Originally Cohnheim, with his training under Kölliker and Virchow, was also morphologically oriented, but his experience as an army surgeon during the war with Denmark was influential in changing his perspectives in medicine. While working as chief assistant to Virchow in 1865, he developed a close relationship with Ludwig Traube, called by William Osler "one of the greatest German clinicians."[2] Traube emphasized on the young Cohnheim the importance of asking *why* certain disease processes produce the structural changes at death, rather than simply *what* are the structural changes themselves. Traube, it will be remembered, was a member of the physiological medicine and pathological physiology movement twenty years earlier and still believed in approaching pathology from the standpoint of experimental disease produced in animals. His influence in stimulating Cohnheim to become truly the first experimental pathologist is proven by the fact that ten years after leaving Berlin he dedicated his famous *Lectures on General Pathology* to the memory of Ludwig Traube, and not to his mentor, Rudolf Virchow.[3] (His famous controversy with Virchow regarding the origin of the pus cell in inflammation, discussed in the next chapter, was most likely the key in his break with his former chief). He also became a good friend of Willy Kühne, the Berlin physiologist who had taken Hoppe-Seyler's place, and had previously worked with both Claude Bernard and Carl Ludwig. Together Cohnheim and Kuhne published a paper on carbohydrate enzymes (then called ferments).[4] The influence of Traube on Cohnheim during this period at Berlin has recently been commented on by Maulitz:

> What was critical in his influence was the emphasis on an approach to the whole organism which was vivisectional and global. Such a holistic viewpoint was instrumental in that it played a crucial permissive role in Cohnheim's manner of formulating pathological problems. Despite the pervasive localism of the pathologists around him, Cohnheim produced a hybrid model of inflammation because he was a hybrid of scientific medicine, drawing from both the localizationism of the histologist and pathologist, and the holism of the physiologist. It was this holism, rather than experimentalism per se which was critical.[5]

Also, as discussed in Chapter X, this period was during the Golden Age of Physiology in Germany, and it was natural that an imaginative investigator such as Cohnheim would have been current with all the physiological work and publications that were occurring throughout Europe at that time. In the fall of 1868, still only 29 years old, Cohnheim accepted the chair of pathology at Kiel, where he studied the effects of venous obstruction and studied more thoroughly the problems that had intrigued Virchow earlier in his career — embolism. Cohnheim showed that the varying pathological results of embolism depended upon the presence or absence of collateral circulation beyond the point of obstruction.[6] It was while he was at Kiel as a full professor that he elected to study for two months with Carl Ludwig at Leipzig, where the very latest knowledge existed regarding the vascular system. In 1872, Cohnheim went to Breslau, where he had his own institute and began to attract the most imaginative students interested in experimental pathology. Some of these individuals were William Henry Welch, Albert Neisser, Paul

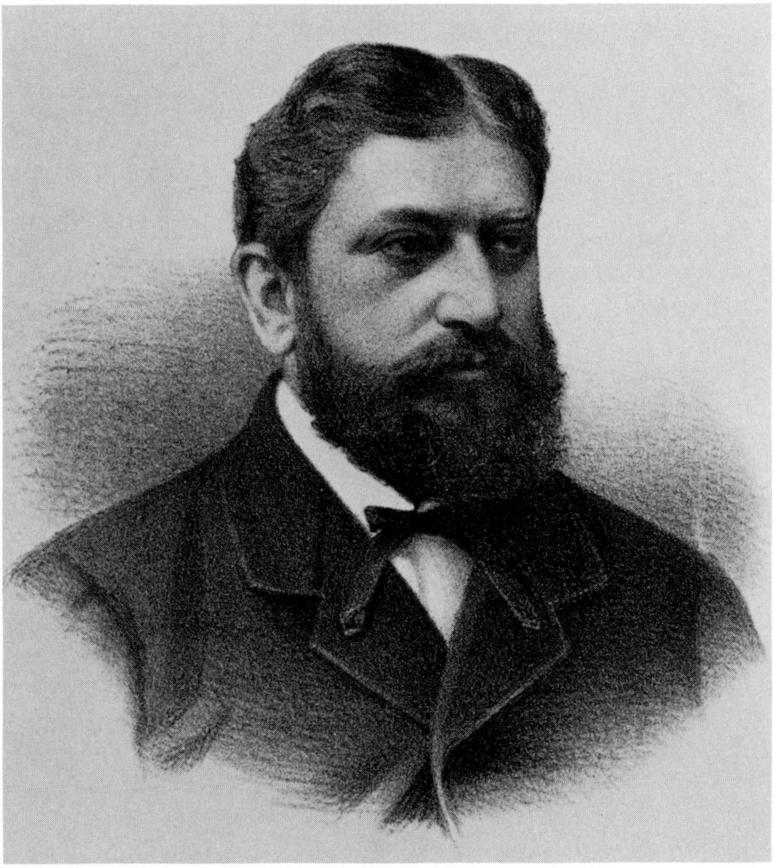

J. COHNHEIM

Ehrlich, Ludwig Lichtheim (1845–1915), Ottomar Rosenbach (1851–1907), Carl Salomonsen (1847–1924), and Charles Roy (1854–1897). Assisting Cohnheim was Carl Weigert (1845–1904), one of the most eminent anatomic pathologists in Germany, who was responsible for being the first to definitely differentiate bacteria from artifacts in tissue using HCl-glycerin-carmine stain. The relationship between Cohnheim and Weigert was described by Salomonsen in this way:

> Weigert was the real pathological anatomist of the institute, prosector as well as microscopist. Cohnheim himself was tired of the prosectorship; he had become the complete experimenter. He only entered the dissection room when all postmortems were finished; then he selected something for his courses; only once, on the first day after vacation, did we have the opportunity of admiring the elegance and skill with which he dissected and taught at the same time; otherwise he willingly left postmortem dissections and microscopic investigations to Weigert as his equal as a prosector, and as a microscopist, perhaps his superior.[7]

Cohnheim would also in a joking way chide the morphologists, particularly Paul Ehrlich. He would refer to him as being a "master dyer" and "painter," obviously not recognizing at the time the potential greatness of Ehrlich and how his experience with stains and aniline dyes would eventually lead him to discoveries in hematology, immunology, and chemotherapy. On the other hand, Cohnheim, unlike his mentor Virchow, quickly recognized the significance of the work of the country practitioner Robert Koch, who was visiting Ferdinand Cohn, Germany's most renowned microbiologist. Koch demonstrated his conclusive studies that proved that anthrax bacteria could produce disease in animals. When Cohnheim heard of the demonstration in Cohn's laboratory, he said to his staff:

> Now leave everything as it is, and go to Koch. This man has made a magnificent discovery, which, for simplicity and the precision of the methods employed, is all the more deserving of admiration, as Koch was shut off from all scientific associations. He has done everything of himself and with absolute completeness. There is nothing more to be done. I regard this as the greatest discovery in this domain and believe that Koch

> will again surprise and put us all to shame by further discoveries.[8]

Then to enable Koch to leave his medical practice and continue his work in bacteriology, Cohnheim used his influence to persuade the German government to appoint Koch to a position as a member of the Imperial Sanitary Commission in Berlin. On the other hand, although Koch's proof about anthrax was conclusive, when he visited Virchow in Berlin two years later, he was treated very coolly, and the great pathologist told Koch that the "whole business seemed quite improbable." And when Koch tried to tell him about his new studies using the new oil immersion lens, Virchow told him "anything he couldn't see with the dry lens wasn't worth looking at!" Koch supposedly left Virchow "with bitterness in his heart."[9] Undoubtedly Virchow's unreceptiveness was related to the threat that Koch's research appeared to make to Virchow's pet anti-ontology positions, and perhaps his Cellular Pathology concept. It is interesting and ironic that the young Koch eventually would become, in his later years, an even more opinionated and tyrannical person than Virchow.

Cohnheim assigned William Henry Welch the problem of attempting to determine the mechanism of the production of pulmonary edema during heart failure, and they co-authored this work in 1877.[10] Then, just as he helped Koch, Cohnheim was very influential in obtaining for Welch the deanship and head of the new pathology department for Johns Hopkins Hospital in 1884. He wrote to President Gilman of the university that

> the person best fitted for the chair of general pathology is Mr. Welch of New York. Welch, indeed, worked with me for a long time and I regard him as an astute as well as a thoughtful investigator.[11]

Because of his early death, Cohnheim's scientific discoveries were not numerous. Aside from his monumental studies on the origin of the pus cell in inflammation, his major contribution was as a catalyst for the development of experimental pathology, which was based upon contemporary physiology. This was best expressed in his *Lectures on General Pathology*, which appeared in three volumes and were translated into English by Alexander McKee for the New Sydenham Society in

1889.[12] The lectures are remarkable in their degree of modernity when compared with books by Henle, Rokitansky, and even Virchow's *Cellular Pathology* of 1858, considering the comparatively short interval of time in which they were written. Excerpts of his lectures are given here because his wisdom for the most part still applies to the understanding of disease today:

> We speak of a disease where the regulative mechanisms, acting in opposition to one or more vital conditions, are no longer adequate to secure that the various vital processes shall proceed undisturbed . . . one individual may be better able than another to adapt himself to one and the same external condition; or, in other words, that disease may be produced in one person by causes which have no effect on another. Disease is nothing more or less than a deviation from the normal vital process, brought about by the action of external conditions and the reaction of what may be called in general terms the internal regulative capabilities or the organism. . . . We regard the clinical symptoms and the anatomical changes as equally valuable factors in the estimation and termination of a form of disease. The knowledge of the symptoms gained by observation at the sick bed, and the knowledge of the anatomical changes, as revealed with but few exceptions by postmortem examination, are alike indispensable to the understanding of a disease.
>
> Neither of them alone is sufficient, just as little as in normal physiology the most minute and accurate knowledge of the conformation and structure of muscular fiber permits a surmise as to the contractile power of the muscle, or the most strict observation of its action, even when conjoined with a determination of its collective physical properties, allows of approximate guess as to its structure. To pathology this applies, if possible, in a still higher degree. It is impossible, from the postmortem appearances in case of typhoid, to sketch a picture of the course and symptoms of this disease, having even a remote resemblance to the reality, nor to take a chance example from the microscope can anyone in the least deduce the characters of the urine "intra vitam" from fatty degeneration of the renal epithelium or from amyloid degeneration of the renal vessels. . . . Etiology can be nothing more, I believe, than an enumeration and discussion of very different factors,

having only one feature in common, namely a capacity to act as exciters of disease . . .

. . . I am persuaded that it is far more to your advantage to concentrate our united energies on the other branch of general pathology, namely 'morbid physiology.' This science, as its name indicates bears the same relation to normal physiology as does morbid to normal anatomy. While in morbid anatomy we learn the modifications undergone by the morphological (or chemical) constitution of the individual organs in disease, morbid physiology teaches how the functions of the affected organs are performed under abnormal circumstances. . . . the subject matter of normal physiology is not sufficient for our purposes in general pathology. It is, of course, perfectly true that the laws of physiology fully apply to the diseased organism as well as to the healthy one; but since physiology explains the process of healthy life alone i.e. of the life under ordinary conditions, it does not without more ado help us to an insight into the processes going on within the organism when the conditions are essentially changed. Nowhere does physiology afford information as to what occurs when, in addition to the ordinary food, a perfectly foreign substance, such as phosphorus, for example, is absorbed by the body. From physiology we receive the most detailed intelligence as to the normal circulation i.e. where heart, vessels, and blood are healthy; but of the state of the circulation when the valves do not close in consequence of previous disease, or when the vessel walls are altered, or when the blood is coagulated in some part, we learn nothing from physiology. . . . Just as modern physiology has long broken with all speculative systems, and become an explanatory science after the manner of physics and chemistry, so do we banish from us in pathology all the systems which have succeeded one another in large numbers in the course of centuries. Far be it from me to deny our indebtedness to these manifold systems for many a great and important advance in pathology; but they have as such, whatever be the names they bear, a purely historical interest. . . . The method of investigation is the same in morbid as in normal physiology. You know what the most essential aid of physiology is, that one by which she has become an inductive natural science in the sense that chemistry and physics are such; it is experiment and where purely physical and chemical experiments are inad-

> equate express physiological experiment. By experiment, as is well known, the single possible factors are tested as to their performances, and the conditions in which an organ works are varied in order to obtain information as to the significance of the individual factors. The results of physiological experiment are in the first place of service to pathology; then, however, we make use of pathological experiment, which was first practiced in England by John Hunter, and in France by Magendie, yet was only raised to the rank it at present occupies as our most important fundamental aid by the researches of Traube and Virchow in the fifth decade of this century. . . . Every dead body is equally valuable so far as the anatomy of the normal lung is concerned, provided this organ has been healthy; it is otherwise with the inflamed lung. Here it is very different whether the individual has died on the second or third or as late as the eighth day; for inflammation of the lung is progressive, while anatomical examination can evidently only supply information as to the condition of the lung which prevailed at the moment of death. This gap is filled by pathological experiment. By its aid we are in a position to work out the anatomical history of many highly important processes, either following them by continuous observation, or at least subjecting them to examination at whatever intervals we please; thus our most valuable knowledge of the processes of morbid development and growth, of intoxications, of the processes of inflammation, thrombosis, and embolism, of dropsy, and of many other subjects is owing to experiment.[12]

Of particular interest is the definition of disease given in the first paragraph of the quotation. It is clear that Cohnheim was thinking of disease as a failure of what Walter Cannon was to develop and call "homeostasis," less than one-half century later.[13] It is all the more remarkable considering that the fields of bacteriology, immunology, and endocrinology, and the physiology of the autonomic nervous system were either non-existent or in their infancy.

Bibliography

1. Malkin, H., Julius Cohnheim (1839-1884), His Life and Contributions to Pathology. *Ann. Clin. and Lab. Sciences*, **14**, p. 335, 1984.
2. Osler, W., Berlin Correspondence, *Canada Medical and Surgical Journal*, **Vol. II**, p. 308, 1873-74.
3. Cohnheim, J., *Lectures on General Pathology*, translated by A. McKee. New Sydenham Society, London, 1889.
4. Cohnheim, J., Zur Kenntniss der zuckerbildenden Fermente. *Arch. Path. Anat.* **28**, p. 241, 1863.
5. Maulitz, R., Rudolf Virchow, Julius Cohnheim and program of pathology. *Bull. Hist. Med.*, **52**, p. 162, 1978.
6. Ref. 3, p. 210.
7. Salomonsen, C.L., Reminiscences of the summer semester, 1877, at Breslau, translated by C.L. Temkin. *Bull. Hist. Med.* **24**, p. 333, 1950.
8. Flexner, S. and Flexner, J., *William Henry Welch and the Heroic Age of American Medicine*, p. 100. Viking Press, N.Y., 1941.
9. Brock, T.D., *Robert Koch, A Life in Medicine and Bacteriology*. p. 82. Science Tech Publishers, Madison, 1988.
10. Cohnheim, J., and Welch, W.H., Ueber acutes Lungenodem. *Berichte der schles. Gesellsch. für vaterl. Cult.* Dec. 7, 1877, p. 593.
11. Ref. 8, p. 129.
12. Ref. 3.
13. Cannon, W.B., Organization for Homeostasis, *Physiol. Rev.*, **9**, p. 399, 1929.

CHAPTER XII

Without vessels, there is no inflammation.
— Cohnheim (1867)

The Great Pus Cell Controversy at the Berlin Institute of Pathology

In the first century A.D., A. Cornelius Celsus, not a physician but an intellectual and encyclopedist of the times, wrote *De Re Medicine.* In the form of eight books of pathology, it was based upon medical books available at the time, many of which were lost over the succeeding centuries. Celsus's books, because they were written by a lay person and not based upon personal experience, were essentially lost until they were found by Thomas of Sarzana (later Pope Nicholas V) who had them printed in 1478.[1] In Book Three, he describes the cardinal signs of inflammation: tumor (swelling), rubor (redness), dolor (pain), and calor (heat). John Hunter, in the last quarter of the eighteenth century, explained each of these signs in terms of local dilation of blood vessels and exudation and even without a microscope described the process at the tissue level. He also correctly expressed the belief that inflammation was a reaction of the body to irritants and not a disease itself and that it is the first stage in healing of a wound.

With the development of the compound microscope as an instrument for biological investigation, it was possible to examine the process of inflammation at the cellular level. The result was a major controversy, during the years 1840–1870, regarding the origin of inflammatory cells. Following Schwann's establishment of the cell as the basic unit of all living organisms, two other biological axioms came into being. The first was that of Remak and Virchow that cells can only be derived from other cells. The second was that of Müller and Henle who showed that the vascular system in higher animals was essentially closed and that, rather than being similar to rivulets in soil, the capillaries and other small blood vessels had walls that were permeable only to water and other small molecules. With regard to pus cells in inflamed tissue and white cells in the blood, they appeared, even before any stains were available, to be morphologically identical, and their relationship was unclear. There were three possible explanations:

1. The white blood cells and the pus cells were completely identical and those present in the blood migrated there, in some unknown manner, from an origin in the tissue producing a pyemia or leukocytosis.
2. The white blood cells and the pus cells were completely identical and those present in the tissue migrated there, in some unknown manner, from the blood stream.
3. The white blood cells and the pus cells were morphologically identical but they had separate origins: those present in an inflamed tissue being produced by division of local cells, and those in the blood originating elsewhere (the hematopoietic function of the bone marrow was unknown at that time).

Several investigators, including A. Waller, W. Addison and G. Zimmermann, had reported seeing blood cells pass through the capillary walls during the years before 1852, but Rudolf Virchow was dubious about these observations and wrote in 1847:

> In recent times some have even fallen from one extreme into the other, and while for a time they regarded all colorless corpuscles in the blood as resorbed pus corpuscles, now they want to interpret all cells turning up in pus as extravasated colorless blood corpuscles.[2]

and in 1858 he wrote:

> a pus corpuscle can be distinguished from a colorless blood cell by nothing else than its mode of origin. If you do not know whence it has come, you cannot say what it is. In every case of the sort of points to be considered are, where the body belongs to, and where its home is. If this prove to be external to the blood, you may safely conclude that is pus; but if this is not the case, you have to do with blood cells.[3]

Thus Virchow opted for the third theory listed above. He became convinced that the origin of pus cells in inflamed regions was due to the division of local cells in the connective tissue that were activated by irritants, and the increased blood to the inflamed area was simply to supply needed nutrients for the pus cell formation. But he needed proof. Perhaps it is true, as Maulitz[4] suggests, that Virchow thought his Cellular Pathology, with its emphasis on "localism" of pathological processes, would be better served if he could prove the local origin of the pus cells. In any case, he assigned two of his chief assistants the task of resolving the problem.

The first assistant was Friedrich Daniel von Recklinghausen (1833–1910), who received his medical degree at Berlin in 1855, and, after working with Virchow for several years, became Professor of Pathology at Konigsberg, then Wurzburg, and finally Strasbourg. He did outstanding work on neurofibromatosis (von Recklinghausen's disease), spina bifida, adenomyoma of the uterus, and diseases of the bone. But while he was with Virchow during the years 1855–1864, his work was always with the pus cell and the wandering cells of the connective tissue. His thesis *De Pyaemiae Theoriis*, written in 1855, concluded that pyemia was not always related to wounds. But he continued his work on inflammation, and in 1863 published a paper in which, using a moist chamber, he observed the amoeboid motion of pus cells and commented that in the space of a half hour they could cross an entire microscopic field. With regard to the difference between the pus cell and the colorless white cell, he stated that they were identical. Then, without definitely contradicting Virchow, he also pointed out that because pus cells could move so rapidly under the microscope that their accumulation in an area of inflammation did not necessarily mean that they had their origin there. Most importantly he found no evidence of pus cells arising from division of existing cells in the inflamed connective tissue. He them carried out further experiments in which he introduced particles of red dye and pieces of cornea into the subcutaneous lymph sacs of frogs. After fourteen days he found pus cells with dye in these pieces of corneal tissue, indicating that the pus cells and dye had migrated from outside the pieces of corneal tissue. He then could have answered the question of whether the white blood cells could have become pus cells by altering the experiment by injecting the dye into the blood stream and then examining the corneal tissue in the lymph sac. Either he did perform the experiment but did not report the result or he hesitated to perform the test, because, as Leland Rather suggests, "he may have felt that he had already come close to treading on the toes of his master."[5]

As related in the memoirs of both Ludwig Aschoff and W. Waldeyer, von Recklinghausen was always in awe of and intimidated by Virchow, even after he had become a world renowned pathologist at Strasbourg and his former master would visit him. A good description of von Recklinghausen was given by William Councilman who, prior to his career at Johns Hopkins and Harvard, had studied with von Recklinghausen in 1883:

> He was never controversial, although critical of all that seemed to lack in scientific accuracy. In all his work, he used simple methods with which he had begun his work, and it is amazing what he was able to do with scalpel, scissors and microscope. He was by nature conservative and he was essentially an anatomical pathologist, his work being based on embryology and the study of stages of processes rather than the experimental method.[6]

When Julius Cohnheim started work in Virchow's institute, he also was assigned the problem of the pus cell but based his experiments of inflammation on the serosal membranes of various organs. The results of his work were published in 1861 with the title of *De Pyogenesi in Tunicus Serosis* and concluded that the serosal membranes had comparable reactions to the loose connective tissues elsewhere and that pus in experimental inflammation produced by physical, chemical, or thermal injury in the serosal membranes was the same, regardless of the organ or animal used.[7] But starting in 1864, when he took von Recklinghausen's place as chief assistant to Virchow, he started to perform new experiments on inflammation, and in doing so, established for all time the origin of the pus cells in inflammation. These observations were published shortly before he left Berlin, and the results contradicted the long-time view of Virchow of a local origin of the pus cell, and probably more than any other factor produced his permanent break with his mentor. Because the findings were so conclusive and changed the concept of inflammation from a local phenomena to a systemic one, the experiments and observations of Cohnheim are given in detail:

> Using techniques he learned from von Recklinghausen, Cohnheim produced inflammation in the cornea of the frog in conjunction with staining with gold chloride and found that in the stromal layer, pus cells appeared. He decided that these

> pus cells either arose from preexisting wandering cells in the cornea or came in from the outside. He then injected a colloidal aniline blue dye in either the anterior chamber of the eye or the subcutaneous lymph sacs. Then he irritated the cornea as before, but only in the case of the injected lymph sacs did pus cells containing blue dye appear in the corneal stroma. The only conclusion he could make was that wandering cells from the lymph sacs had migrated to the cornea. He next injected dye into the blood stream of the frogs, induced corneal irritation and within a few his days he found the dye in the pus cells of the cornea. He expressed his conclusions as "some pus cells in the inflamed cornea were formerly colorless blood corpuscles; they forced their way into the cornea from the blood vessels."[8]

Once Cohnheim was convinced that leukocytes from the blood vessels could migrate into an inflamed area to produce pus, he was determined to visualize this phenomena, and therefore carried out observations on the mesentery inflamed by cantharides or simply dry air, of a curarized frog. His pertinent observations were as follows:

> The first thing that happens is widening of the arteries — it can be very distinct after as short a time as 10 to 15 minutes. Nothing is more frequent than to see an artery having a diameter of .14 mm increase to .22 mm. Whereas at the beginning all the arteries are extended straight or run their course with only slight inflection, in the exposed mesentery, many of them constantly develop marked tortuosity and even though this depends only on elongation of the vessel, it can be understood how much the capacity of a dilated and simultaneously contorted vessel has increased. The peripheral zone of the blood stream, the plasma layer, becomes filled with innumerable colorless blood corpuscles. Single white corpuscles push into the field of vision in the direction of the capillaries in slow and occasionally somewhat retrograde movement. The number of cells that accumulate in the marginal zone becomes increasingly greater. The final effect of this process is that after a shorter or longer time, the entire marginal zone of the vessel is filled with colorless corpuscles. . . .
>
> In the entire process of inflammation there is no phase that runs more irregularly than this extrusion of colorless cor-

> puscles at the outer periphery of veins. While in certain individuals, especially of Rana temporaris, I saw this as early as three to four hours after exposure of the mesentery, in other specimens 12 or even 15 hours and more elapsed before even faint beginnings were evident. In reality, as I must assume, the account I have given above, although it may depict the remarkable process incompletely, yet it must convince any unprejudiced person that the process consists of extrusion of colorless corpuscles from the interior of the vein through the intact wall of the vessel. For this species of inflammation the blood vessels henceforth come more and more into the foreground. Without vessels there is no inflammation. Vasodilation, injection and hyperemia are the necessary first stage. The dilatation of the arteries is followed by a similar but very much slower occurrence in the veins. At the same time in the veins, which are much more extensible than the arteries, sinuosities and curvatures are never seen to develop. At the same time that the dilatation of the vessels is developing, the speed of the blood within them is also undergoing changes, predominantly of variable character. In some vessels, both arteries and veins, a retardation of the blood current takes onset right from the beginning, together with progressive dilatation. In other vessels there is no change in the speed. One thing additional has changed; the bloodstream has lost its axial character. No longer does one see on both sides of the red blood column a colorless layer of plasma devoid of corpuscles, but the mass of blood fills the entire lumen of the vessel and the corpuscles at every place flow over the inner border of the vessel wall.[9]

Aware of the possible adverse political effects of his discoveries, Cohnheim disavowed any intent that he was replacing his master's view on inflammation. He agreed that the pus cells increased by proliferation, but said that the origin was probably neighboring lymph nodes and the spleen (the bone marrow as the origin of some of the white blood cells was not established until the following year by E. Neumann and G. Bizzozero). He attempted to placate Virchow by writing that:

> We see that it is only necessary to modify the current view so as to transfer the site of new formation from the connective tissues into the lymph glands and spleen. Virchow, himself, had for a long time insisted on the necessary relationship be-

> tween the increased number of leukocytes in the blood and the associated enlargement of lymph nodes and spleen that so frequently accompanied local inflammation.[10]

This was, of course, patronizing, which would have been recognized, not only by Virchow himself, but by other investigators throughout the world. But ten years later, Cohnheim was less timid and in his lectures said that:

> In its pure and unadulterated form, the cellular theory of inflammation is, in fact, at present maintained by no one. This being the state of affairs, the only question that can be debated at present is whether, side by side with the circulatory disturbances, Virchow's so-called nutritive and formative changes of the tissue cells at all occur in inflammation, and in particular whether by means of these changes exudation or pus-corpuscles arise. Above all, we know that pus corpuscles can wander into every part, and, in particular that they can penetrate into other cells. We accept the new formation of a pus cell as demonstrated, only where we have seen it take place directly under our eyes, or where — and this appears the utmost concession we can make — strict proof can be offered that the pus-corpuscle in question cannot have traveled from some other place. No one has so far succeeded in observing the formation of a pus-corpuscle.[11]

It should be pointed out that during this time and until Ehrlich developed his stains to differentiate the various types of white blood cells, "pus cells" and the "colorless white blood cells" were used to describe all of the leukocytes — neutrophils, eosinophils, basophils, lymphocytes, and monocytes. The drawings of Virchow and Cohnheim, done at a maximum of three-hundred magnification and without stains, indicate that most of the "pus cells" and "colorless white cells" were actually polymorphonuclear, although they also illustrated cells with round nuclei. Not only was there no evidence that these morphologically different cells had different origins but there was speculation that they were simply variations of the same cell type and that possibly they gave rise to the red blood cells.[12] But because "pus cells" are predominantly polymorphonuclear in an inflamed region and the predominant "colorless white cell" in the blood is usually the polymorphonuclear cell, the arguments of both Cohnheim and Virchow were valid for the time.

In any case, as studies progressed, it became clear that, although the polymorphonuclear cell in an inflamed area originated totally from the blood, there were local cells that were able to divide and had macrophagic functions. However, during the past forty years, it has become clear that most macrophages in an inflamed region are monocytes migrating from the blood. But the cellular pathology of Virchow survived in spite of the fact that Cohnheim showed that it could not maintain its localism with regard to inflammation, which was actually a systemic response. History has vindicated both Virchow and Cohnheim, but the master never forgave the student, although the animosity was not reciprocal. According to Ackerknecht, although he compensated his assistants fairly and allowed them to publish under their own name, he was very paternalistic and attempted to control their right to marry, teach, or to leave him.[13] Schleich describes an incident that occurred when he was at the Berlin Pathological Institute:

> Late one autumn afternoon there was a knock on the door of the general preparation room. Before it was a man of medium height, who was evidently trying to attract somebody's attention. "My name is Cohnheim" he said courteously, "and I just wanted to speak to one of the assistants". I stammered, "but not the famous Julius Cohnheim, Virchow's greatest. . . ." He smiled. "I am that Cohnheim" he said nodding. "Perhaps you can help me. I heard that Schaper had made a marble bust of Virchow. I felt that I should just like to see it. My departure from this Institute was not entirely peaceful, but before I die, which may not be too long, I should like to see, not Virchow himself, but this portrait, which I hear is admirable!" — "But of course!" — I hastened to explain that I was quite alone in the Institute, and took him to the great lecture room where Virchow's bust stood against the right hand wall. "Is old Hubner still here?" At that moment Hubner appeared. "My God! Herr Geheimrat! An honor to meet you again! Wait a moment, why it's fourteen years ago! Yes, yes! They roll by so fast, as the skittle player says! You want to see the bust? There it is. But with a curtain over it. The Geheimrat doesn't like to see it always in front of him while he is lecturing, like his own corpse. It upsets him. So I always have to cover it. But it's dusted once a week. Now just you look at it. There! Now, isn't it the very spit and image!" Julius Cohnheim stood, hat in hand, as though absorbed in his

dreams. The garrulous Hubner continued; "But you ought to see him with his glasses on! Just you look now, when I put my pince-nez on him!" He took a chair, and was actually going to fix his glasses on Virchow's nose. Cohnheim protested, but Hubner would have his way. . . . Afterwards Hubner asked me: "Shall I say anything to Rudolf about his coming? A queer thing, you know, Behind one's back, like that, in the night, so to speak, and unofficious. Pity they quarreled like that. Cohnheim was the most gifted man we had. A great light!"[14]

Cohnheim had not much longer to live.

Bibliography

1. Celsus, A., *De Re Medicine*, 3 vols. Translated by W.G. Spencer, Heinemann, London, 1935-38.
2. Virchow, R., Ueber die Reform der pathologischen und therapeutischen Anschauungen durch die mikroskopischen Untersuchungen. *Virchow's Archiv*. **1**, p. 207, 1847.
3. Virchow, R., *Cellular Pathology*, 1863, translated by F. Chance, p. 188. Dover Publications, NY, 1971.
4. Maulitz, R., Rudolf Virchow, Julius Cohnheim and the Program of Pathology. *Bull. Hist. Med.* **52**, p. 162, 1978.
5. Rather, L., *Addison and the White Corpuscle; an Aspect of Nineteenth Century Biology, Wellcome Institute of the History of Medicine*, p. 159. Univ. Calif. Press, Berkeley, 1972.
6. Councilman, W., Friedrich Daniel von Recklinghausen (1833-1910), *Proc. Amer. Acad. Arts and Sci.*, **53**, p. 872, 1917-18.
7. Cohnheim, J. *De pyogenesi in tunicus serosis*. Thesis, G. Lange, 1861.
8. Jarcho, S., Cohnheim on Inflammation. *Am. J. Cardiology*, **29**, p. 247, 1972.
9. Cohnheim, J., Ueber Entzündung und Eiterung. *Arch. Path. Anat.* **40**, p. 1, 1867.
10. Ref. 5, p. 171.
11. Cohnheim, J., *Lectures on General Pathology*, Vol.1, p.287, translation by A. McKee. New Sydenham Society, London, 1889.
12. Ibid., p. 429.
13. Schleich, C., *Those Were Good Days*, translated by J. Mall. W.W. Norton, 1936.
14. Ibid.

CHAPTER XIII

> A new scientific truth is often accepted, not as a result of opponents becoming convinced and declaring themselves won over, but rather by the opponents dying off, and the oncoming generation of scientists becoming familiar with the new truth right from the start.
>
> — Max Planck

Microbiology and Its Revolutionary Effect on Pathology

Early Ideas on Contagion

In spite of all the advances that were made during the first three quarters of the nineteenth century, the knowledge gained in the study of pathology was primarily that of secondary or tertiary structural changes in the tissues when they were present at all. With respect to etiology, except for such factors as physical trauma or poisons, no specific causes of disease were known. But this was to change dramatically, particularly for the infectious or contagious diseases. During the last quarter of the nineteenth century, the Germ Theory of Infectious Diseases was established and would dispel not only much of the mystery and terror of contagion but simplified the diagnosis of many diseases and led to the logical basis for the evolution of preventative and therapeutic procedures.

The idea in its infancy that small invisible living organisms were the cause of contagious diseases can be traced back to Columella (c. 60 B.C.) , Varro (c. 30 B.C.), Pliny the Elder (23–79 A.D.), and others during the Middle Ages, but their writings were vague and undeveloped. Then three years after Vesalius wrote his monumental book on anatomy, another alumnus of the University of Padua, Girolamo Fracastoro (1478–1553), published the book *De Contagione et Contagiosis*[1] that for the first time made a clear statement about the likely nature of contagious germ particles. He defined three fundamentally distinct classes of infections: (1) those that are transmitted by immediate contact of one individual with another, (2) those that are transmitted through intermediate material, such as clothes and bedding, that he called fomites, and (3) those that are transmitted at a distance or through the air. He astutely made an analogy illustrating the first class by describing the transfer of putrefaction of one grape to another by contact.[2] Even more remarkably, he stated that the contagion of the third class included those that cause tuberculosis and some of the fevers prevalent in Italy at the time. He also wrote that the third class of contagions differs greatly among themselves, some attacking children more often, others, elder individuals, and others, animals, and he stated that different germs attack different organs.[3] Additionally he drew a parallel between the processes of contagion and fermentation of grapes,[4] a conclusion that Pasteur proved three hundred years later. Fracastoro also hypothesized that one method of penetration of the germs into the body is

> through the breath by inspiration . . . for along with the air that is drawn in, there enter, mixed with it, germs of contagion, and once these are introduced, they do not retire as easily by expiration as they entered. . . . I have said that contagion lies in particles imperceptible to our senses . . . the difference between a simple vapor and a germ of contagion is that a vapor is a highly alterable thing made of a combination that is not strong and viscous, such as that of which the germ is made.

With regard to the propagation of germs, he said that:

> For the original germs . . . generate and propagate other germs precisely like themselves, and these in turn propagate others.[5]

On the other hand, Fracastoro believed that germs originated in individuals,[6] by a type of spontaneous generation, although he did not ever say that the germs were living organisms. He did believe that epidemics were related to the position of the planets and such natural phenomena as earthquakes and climatic conditions. However, by stating that there were specific germs for specific diseases, he was a forerunner of Thomas Sydenham and the disease taxonomists, and even Louis Pasteur three hundred years later. The problem with the concept of contagion was that, although the layman saw the truth in the idea as he watched such diseases as yellow fever spread into his community and kill his family and friends, the physicians could not explain its inconsistencies. There were too many cases in which disease occurred and none of Fracastoro's classes of contagion applied. The theory seemed to be valid in such diseases as syphilis, gonorrhea, smallpox, and measles but not with regard to yellow fever, malaria, bubonic plague, and typhus. The idea that there could be an insect vector in the transmission of the latter group of diseases did not occur to Fracastoro, and, although it might have been casually suggested with regard to house flies at times, it was not proven until Patrick Manson (1844–1922), Ronald Ross (1857–1932), Theobald Smith (1859–1934), and Walter Reed (1851–1902) did their experimental work during the years 1875–1900. However, before this time, the idea of "contagion animatus" was considered an obsolete idea. This was expressed by Ackerknecht as follows:

> It was, curiously enough, in the first half of the nineteenth century, that is shortly before their final and overwhelming victory, that the theories of contagion and the contagium vivum experienced the deepest depression and devaluation in their long and stormy career, and it was shortly before its disappearance that anticontagism reached its highest peak of elaboration, acceptance and scientific respectability.[7]

In 1840, there appeared in Germany an article by Jacob Henle, whom we have seen was never at a loss to speculate about disease. The title of his work was *On Miasmata and Contagia*, and, without mentioning Fracastoro, he essentially came to many of the same conclusions as did the Italian and in addition offered excellent reasons why the contagious "particles" were most likely living organisms. Henle concluded the following:

> 1. The ability (of the particles) to multiply by assimilating foreign material is known to us only in living, organic beings.
> 2. The action of the contagion . . . is in no relation to the quantity used. A needle dipped into diluted chickenpox material is capable of infecting. This action by a minimum depends on the ability of the agent to multiply. . . as has been demonstrated in fermentation and putrefaction and is therefore a proof of the animate nature of the contagion.
> 3. The precise, typical course of the miasmatic contagious

> diseases, and the relations in the course of the corresponding epidemics themselves seem to speak for an independent, temporal development of the disease cause, which occurs only among organic beings.[8]

But Henle still spoke of miasma or the supposition of a matter that mixes with and poisons the air, although he acknowledged that such a miasma had never been demonstrated. But, at the time of Henle's book, there was a young man in France training to become a chemist, not a physician, who was to make a series of experiments during the years 1846 until his death in 1895, that have remained unsurpassed in the annals of scientific and medical history, and who on his death, was described by William Osler as "the most perfect man who has ever entered the Kingdom of Science."[9] With his discoveries, mankind attained knowledge in three areas of the greatest importance: the true nature of fermentation, a basic information on the causes of major illnesses that had devastated man and animals throughout history, and fundamental measures that can be taken to protect the body against these diseases. The story of Louis Pasteur's work is presented here because it changed the entire nature of pathology.

Louis Pasteur

Born in 1832 in the small town of Dôle, Pasteur was stimulated and trained in the French school of chemistry that included such illustrious names as Lavoisier, Fourcroy, Vauquelin, Thenard, Guy Lussac and then his own teachers, Dumas, Balard, Biot, Laurent, and Delarosse. Pasteur first gained fame when he was able to show that there were two forms of tartaric acid, chemically identical, but with crystal structures that allowed one form to rotate light to the right and the other form to the left. His keen sense of observation while studying the crystal facets enabled him in 1849 to separate, by hand, each of the forms from a mixture of the two that did not rotate light. In 1854 as a young professor of chemistry at Strasbourg, he accidentally found that a mold that grew in a solution of the mixture of the two types of tartaric acid (a racemic mixture) fermented one form but not the other, which resulted in a solution with initially no optical rotation but developed it after fermentation took place. To any other chemist, this would have been an isolated observa-

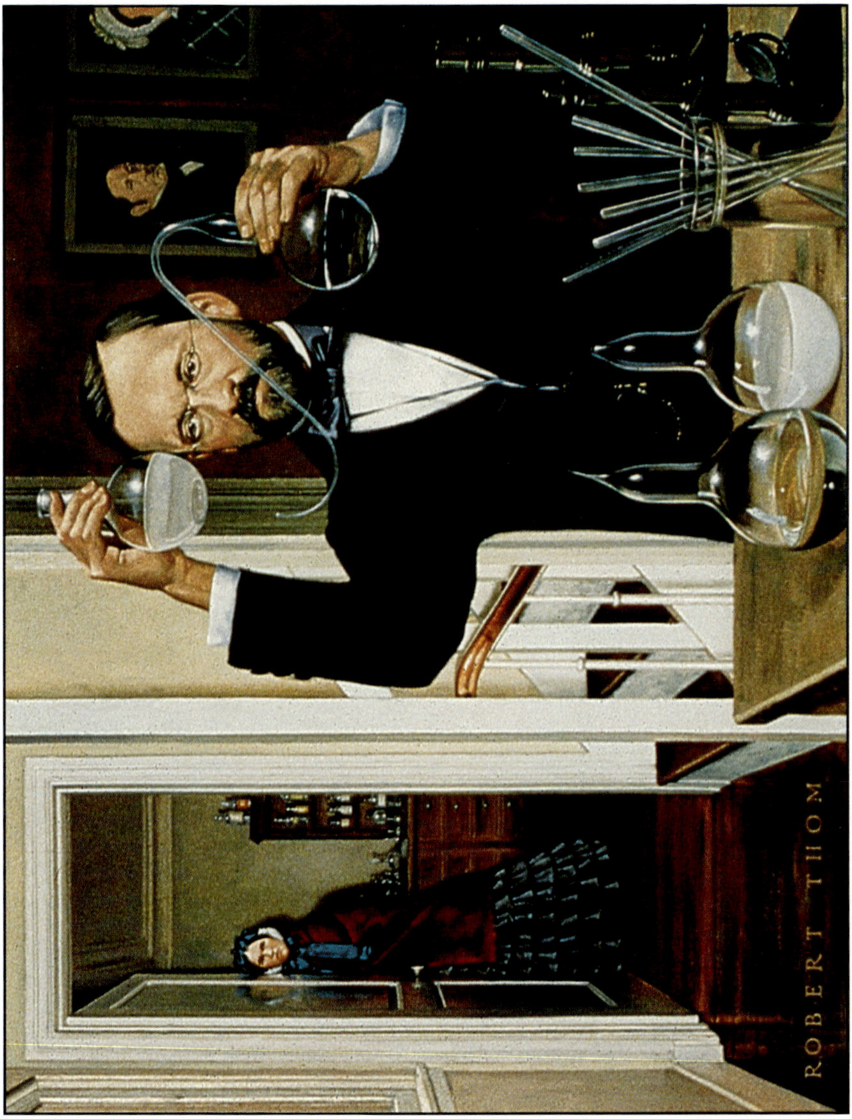

PASTEUR: THE CHEMIST WHO TRANSFORMED MEDICINE

tion and quickly forgotten, but Pasteur's intuition told him that perhaps living organisms were always important in the process of fermentation. When he later obtained a position at Lille University he had an opportunity to test his ideas. A sugar beet factory nearby was having difficulty producing alcohol from beet sugar (sucrose) when on occasion lactic acid was formed instead. Using a student's crude microscope, Pasteur studied the fluids in which the fermentations were taking place, and found that when the alcohol was produced, there were present in the vats globules of yeast, which had been described by Cagniard-Latour in 1845, but that when lactic acid was produced, the fluid swarmed with tiny elongated microorganisms. Justus Liebig, the eminent German chemist, had stated that in alcoholic fermentation, the yeast cells were incidental to the fermentation process and that the production of alcohol was an independent chemical process. He also stated that when lactic acid formed, no organisms were present, perhaps because his eye or his microscope was inferior to that of Pasteur. Then in his famous preliminary paper of 1857 entitled *Mémoire sur la Fermentation Appelée Lactique*, Pasteur not only repudiated Liebig's ideas, but with these words he expressed his manifesto regarding the nature of fermentation:

> I propose to establish in the first part of this work that, just as there is an alcoholic ferment, the yeast of beer, to be found wherever sugar breaks down into alcohol and carbonic acid, so there is a specific ferment, a lactic yeast, always present when sugar turns into lactic acid; and that if any nitrogenous plastic material is able to convert sugar into that acid, this is because it provides a favorable food for the development of that ferment.[10]

Over the next few years he not only proved his thesis, but was able to isolate the organisms, grow them in pure culture, and then put them back into specific organic solutions to produce again the same type of fermentation. There have been several biographies of Pasteur, and all of them emphasize the tremendous confidence that Pasteur had in himself and the experimental method. He also had a fearless and combative spirit that made him a devastating adversary to those who questioned or contradicted the results of his always careful and thorough experiments that he had carried out himself. He had great imagination and mental agility that enabled him to overcome difficult technical obstacles. The fact that he was a chemist and initially had no training in working with living plants and animals did not deter him. He felt it was a mistake to simply make chemical analyses on fermentation products, but rather used his eyes to attempt to see what was transpiring in the fermenting liquid. His work on crystals obviously gave him the skill of using the microscope, but the difficulties that Pasteur had to overcome to visualize and describe microorganism with a lens of no greater magnification than 300-400 × with perhaps a resolving power of a maximum of .5 microns, with the major source of light being the sun, and with no bacterial stains, can be appreciated by any microscopist today. Emile Roux, one of his assistants, related his experience in Pasteur's laboratory:

> It is necessary to have seen Pasteur at his microscope to form an idea of the patience with which he could examine a preparation. In fact he looked at everything with the same minute care. Nothing escaped his nearsighted eye; and jokingly, we used to say that he could see the microbes grow in his bouillons. (and with regard to his determination) Pasteur would say "let me tell you the secret which has led me to the goal. My only strength resides in my tenacity", and how many times, in the presence of unforeseen difficulties when we could not imagine how to get out of them, have I heard Pasteur tell us "Let us do the same experiment over again — the essential is not to leave the subject".[11]

One of the problems that Pasteur soon faced with his experiences with microorganisms was regarding the origin of these primitive organisms. With this question, he became involved in a controversy that had raged over the centuries between biologists and philosophers — that of whether organisms could arise spontaneously out of organic material, or, as it was called, Spontaneous Generation. The ancients took for granted that eels could be produced from slime in rivers, and that maggots were generated in decaying flesh although Francesca Redi (1626–1697), by placing a piece of gauze over fresh meat, had already proved that maggots were hatched from eggs left by flies.[12] But the microscopic organisms that could be found by the millions in any fermenting or putrefying material, was a different matter, and it was a common belief, even among outstanding scientists in the middle of the nineteenth century, that these tiny plants were most likely formed from the decaying material. The logic was philosophically that, with the death of an animal, during decomposition, there remained living particles that are rebuilt into such things as microscopic plants and even animals. The proof was offered by the Catholic priest John Needham in the middle of the eighteenth century, who boiled meat broth in flasks, then corked them and found in 24 hours that the broth was swarming with microrganisms, declaring that there was Vegetative Force that could produce such life.[13] However, Lazzero Spallanzani (1723–1799) thought that Needham either did not boil the liquid long enough or the corks were not secure. Spallanzani repeated the experiments, but heated the broths for a longer period of time, and found no organisms.[14] Needham said Spallanzani destroyed the Vegetative Force by heating it too long, which was a difficult argument to disprove. There were experiments done by others during the following one hundred years, and in 1858 Felix Pouchet did some experiments in which he claimed that he could produce spontaneous generation at will, by adding air to sterilized putrescible matter.[15] Against the advice of his old teachers Dumas and Biot, Pasteur had to enter the fray, because his ideas on the role of microorganisms in the economy implied that each organism was a species which was constant in its action, and to think that nonspecific organisms could be produced by some Vegetative Force violated Pasteur's entire concept about microorganisms.

He therefore set about to resolve the problem for all time, and he used all of his experimental skill to accomplish this goal. To put to rest the objection that Spallanzani had destroyed the air during his sterilization process that was essential for the Vegetative Force to work, Pasteur drew out the neck of the flask with the nutrient media in it after boiling and then turned it downward and made a loop, so that the interior of the flask could obtain by diffusion new air from the outside, but that any solid particle with bacteria would settle on the bottom of the loop but could not ascend and enter the liquid. He found in almost all cases that there would be no growth. But there were occasional failures, until Pasteur realized that certain spores (most likely *Bacillus subtilis*) could only be killed by raising the sterilization temperature to 110-112° centigrade, which was only possible by increasing the pressure to one and one-half atmospheres. When this was done, growth never occurred. In a public demonstration of this experiment in a dramatic manner he said with regard to these flasks with the nutrient fluid:

> And I wait, I watch, I question it, begging it to recommence for me the beautiful spectacle of the first creation. But it is dumb, dumb since those experiments were begun several years ago; it is dumb because I have kept it from the only thing man

> cannot produce, from the germs which float in the air, from Life, for Life is a germ and a germ is Life. Never will the doctrine of spontaneous generation recover from the mortal blow of this simple experiment.[16]

Then he would shake one of his flasks so that the nutrient liquid would touch the dust accumulated in the bottom of the loop of the flask neck. Within a day the nutrient broth would be swarming with bacteria, proving that microorganisms were present on the dust particles and that all living organisms are only derived from preexisting ones. Then armed with this knowledge he showed that in spite of similarity of appearance of microorganisms under the microscope, when isolated, each one produced a different type of fermentation. His conclusions were that each bacterial species reproduced its own kind, just as cats, dogs, or oak trees do. He then described putrefaction simply as a type of fermentation that produced malodorous gases and that were usually caused by a mixture of different microorganisms that came from the air or the soil.

In 1865, Pasteur was asked by his mentor, Dumas, to investigate a mysterious epidemic that was affecting the silk worms in southern France to the extent that the entire silk industry was on the verge of ruin. Although he had made contributions of help to the wine, beer, and vinegar industries, he was reticent to accept Dumas's request because he knew absolutely nothing about silk worms at the time and was being pushed further over into the realm of biology than ever before. He was a brilliant chemist, but he felt unprepared for the task. According to his biographer and colleague, Emile Duclaux:

> Pasteur had reached one of the turning points of his life. For a long time he had a presentiment that all the new ideas he had introduced into science might be of importance for the physiology and pathology of the higher animals. For a long time the two notions of fermentation and disease had been connected, as we have seen from our consideration of spontaneous generations. But when there was raised the question of going farther and of actually coming into contact with the higher animals, Pasteur hesitated. He was not a physiologist. To no purpose did we go to hear the course of Claude Bernard, where he took notes feverishly. It would have been nec-

> essary for him to become a new soul, and he had neither the time for it nor the patience. The insistence of Dumas had just placed him face to face with an experience which he both desired and dreaded, and if his self-distrust had made him hesitate, at the first encounter, in reality, the attraction for the unknown and a certain interior voice urged him to accept.[17]

Pasteur worked for four years on the problem, mostly in Provence where he set up a laboratory, and gained vast practical experience in studying infective diseases. His two volumes that he published in 1870 *Études sur la Maladie des Vers À Soie*[18] are without doubt the greatest accumulation of experiments of a biological nature ever produced up to that time. Although he was able to show how the silk producers could avoid the problems they were having by careful inspection and selection of disease-free worm eggs, he was never able to completely solve the problem biologically, because after working for two years in which he had almost concluded that the disease was an inherited abnormality, he finally recognized that he was dealing with two diseases that were occasionally superimposed one on the other — flacherie, which may involve a virus, and pébrine, which is produced by a protozoan with a complicated life cycle — and both diseases seem to be affected by such factors as temperature and humidity. But in spite of the difficulties, Pasteur gained the confidence and experience that was to serve him well over the next twenty-five years, and he was finally convinced that microorganisms were the causes of many specific diseases.

However, at this time the Germ Theory of Disease had few advocates especially among the clinicians, and there were good reasons for rejecting the idea. The first reason was the common knowledge that bacteria exist almost everywhere in the environment, in addition to being found in large numbers in the digestive tract, the upper respiratory tract, and on the skin. It was logical to assume that if bacteria were the cause of disease, all animals and humans would be sick or die. Second, injection of putrefying material with its massive numbers of microorganisms seldom killed experimental animals. Third, the concept of a bacteria producing death seemed unlikely because microscopists had seen "organisms" in healthy blood. (It appears now that they were seeing platelets under the influence of Brownian movement.) Fourth, smallpox or chickenpox lesions contained no visible microorganisms, although the fluid could transmit the disease. Fifth, if a disease such as yellow fever, typhus, or plague would spare individuals in intimate contact with sick ones, it seemed unlikely that these diseases could be spread by bacteria through contact or respiration (insect vectors were not known at the time). And sixth, to many physicians the proposal that microscopic organisms could make ill or kill an animal as large as a horse seemed to defy "common sense."

There was a new interest in bacteria though, and individuals with little experience started writing papers and creating more confusion. The surgeon Billroth, between operations, quickly came to the conclusion that all the round- and rod-shaped bacteria were only stages of a plant he called *Coccobacteria septica*, and in a book he stated that he did not even believe that this universal organism was the cause of septic infection but rather was a consequence of a more obscure morbid process.[19] William Osler said this book was an excellent example of the "futility of brains without technique."[20] Then there was Virchow, who was concerned about the threat the new bacteriology might be to his long-standing Cellular Pathology. Before his belittling of Koch in 1878, he had repressed the finding of one of his young assistants, Otto Obermeier, who found in 1868 that a spirochete (*Borrelia recurrentis*) was present in the blood of patients suffering from relapsing fever and wanted to publish the discovery. Only in 1873, when Obermeier found them again in a new epidemic, did Virchow allow him to submit his work for publication,[21] the same year the young assistant died of cholera at age 30. There is no explanation of why Virchow did not publish the work in his own journal.

Also, it did not further the cause of bacteriology when the famous Swiss botanist Carl von Nägeli wrote that in over ten years of work, he had been unable to distinguish even two distinct species.[22] But Pasteur had allies. Lister, the distinguished English surgeon, in spite of the ridicule of his fellow surgeons, instituted antiseptic techniques in surgery in the late 1860s. In 1867, Lister published in *Lancet* an article "On a New Method of Treating Compound Fractures" in which he wrote:

> Turning now to the question how the atmosphere produces decomposition of organic substances, we find that a flood of light has been thrown upon this most important subject by the philosophic researches of M. Pasteur, who has demonstrated by thoroughly convincing evidence that it is not to its oxygen or to any of its gaseous constituents that the air owes this

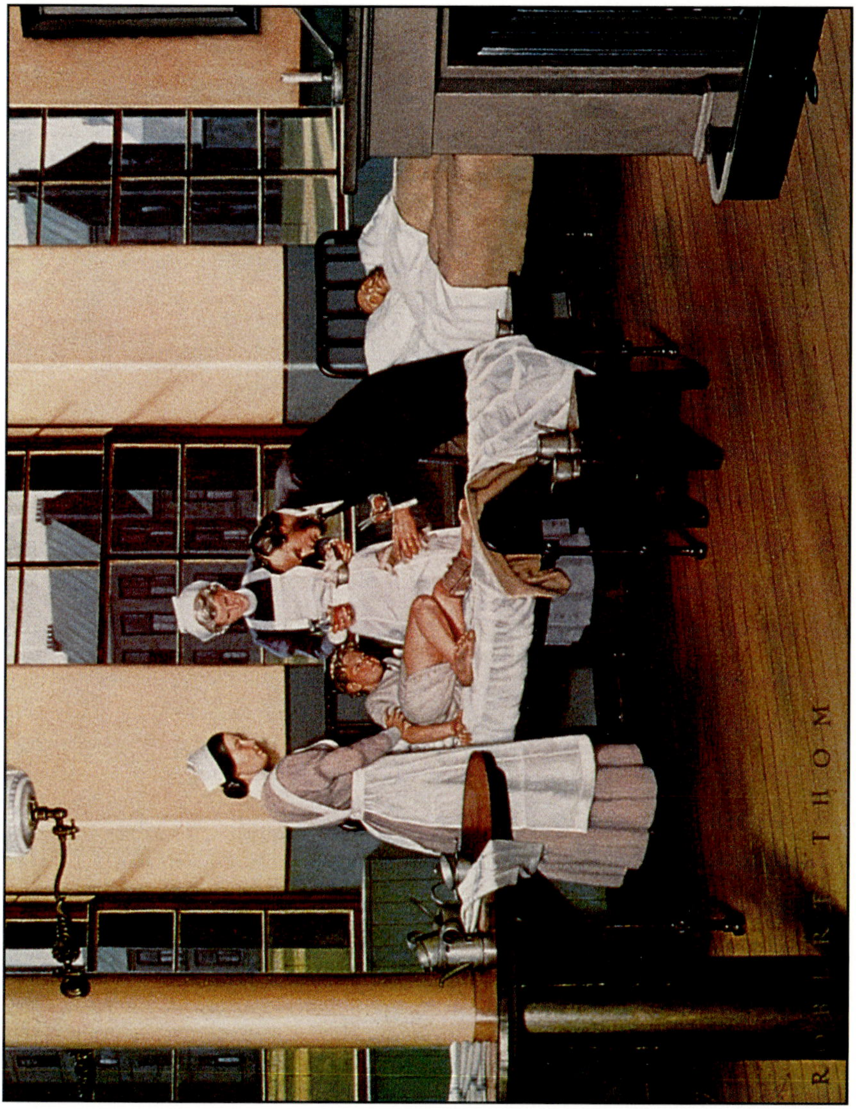

LISTER INTRODUCES ANTISEPSIS

> property but to minute particles suspended in it, which are the germs of various low forms of life, long since revealed by the microscope and regarded as merely accidental concomitants of putrescence, but now shown by Pasteur to be its essential cause resolving the complex organic compounds into substances of simpler chemical constitution, just as the yeast plant converts sugar into alcohol and carbonic acid. A beautiful illustration of this doctrine seems to me to be presented in surgery by pneumothorax . . . resulting from puncture of the lung by a fractured rib. Here though atmospheric air is perpetually introduced into the pleura in great abundance, no inflammatory disturbance intervenes; whereas an external wound penetrating the chest if it remains open, infallibly causes dangerous suppurative pleurisy . . . in case of puncture of the lung without external wound, the atmospheric gases are filtered of the causes of decompositions before they enter the pleura, by passing through the bronchial tubes, which by their small size, their tortuous course, their mucus secretion, and ciliated epithelial lining seem to be especially designed to arrest all solid particles in the air inhaled. . . . Applying these principles to the treatment of compound fractures . . . it appears that all that is requisite is to dress the wound with some material capable of killing these septic germs, provided that any substance can be found reliable for this purpose, yet not too potent as a caustic. My first attempt to use carbolic acid was made in the Glasgow Royal Infirmary in March 1865, in a case of compound fracture of the leg. It proved unsuccessful, in consequences, as I now believe, of improper management; but subsequent trials has more than realized my most sanguine anticipations.[23, 24]

By 1879 Pasteur had the only laboratory in France that had the capability of isolating and growing in liquid media a single species of bacteria, and he decided that, with the problem of anthrax devastating the animal industry, he had an obligation to attempt to understand and perhaps prevent this disease. It was the work on anthrax in which Pasteur, together with the work of Robert Koch, not only proved unequivocally the Germ Theory of Disease, but also that it was possible to prevent some infectious diseases. A survey of the various diseases to which were found a bacterial etiology before the end of the nineteenth century will be given here since they were so important in the history of pathology.

Anthrax

Franz Pollender (1800–1879) in 1849 discovered the anthrax bacteria in the blood of animals dead of the disease, but did not report this until 1855.[25] In the meantime Pierre Rayer and Casimir Davaine (1812–1882) inoculated sheep with blood of diseased animals and were able to find the bacteria in the inoculated sheep.[26, 27] Then during the years 1863–1868, Davaine was further able to show that anthrax could be transmitted to horses, mice, and guinea pigs and that the bacteria appeared in the blood 4-5 hours prior to death. He found that he could produce the disease by injecting a drop of dead-animal blood that was diluted one million times and assumed that this proved that the bacteria produced anthrax, although it was still possible that another agent caused the disease and that the bacteria was simply the carrier. It was about this time that Robert Koch entered the scene and, while a country doctor during the years 1873–1876, developed methods to establish beyond all doubt that the bacterium seen by Davaine was the etiological factor in producing the disease. Working with wild mice caught in his barn, Koch found that the anthrax bacteria could be transferred from one mouse to another at least twenty-two times with a constant replication of the same lesions. Then, using a warm microscope stage, he was able to visualize the entire life cycle of the anthrax bacterium and its different morphological characteristics that had confused prior investigators. Following this he grew them outside the animal in the aqueous humour of a cow and after inoculation of this material could again produce the disease. This was the final proof of the bacteria as the etiological factor in anthrax.[28] Fortunately, the anthrax bacteria is 4 microns in length and could be visualized under the 400 × lenses that were used in the early 1870s. In 1879 Ernst Abbe, working at the Zeiss factory, devised the oil immersion lens and the substage condenser so necessary along with the new aniline stains for study of the smaller bacteria such as the mycobacteria.

The Micrococci

The nature and causation of septicemia, pyemia, erysipelas, and puerperal fever during the 1860s was unknown. In Austin Flint's medical textbook published in 1867, he states the following:

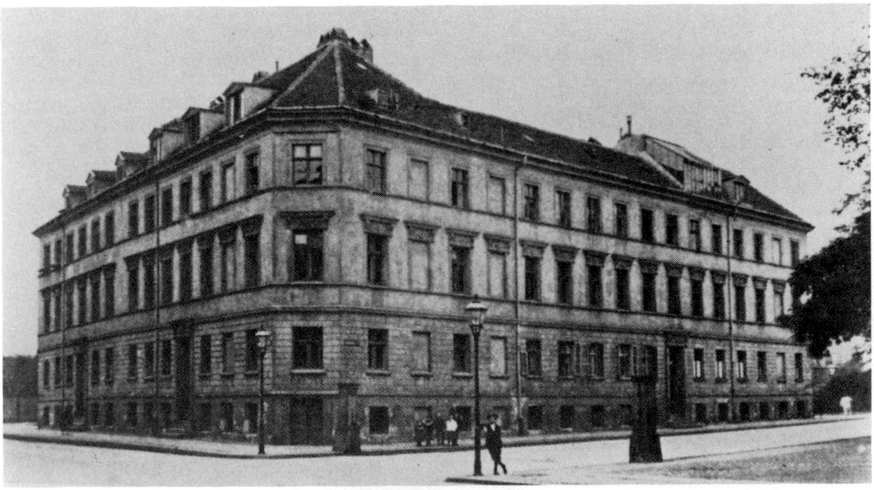
Koch Institute of Infectious Disease

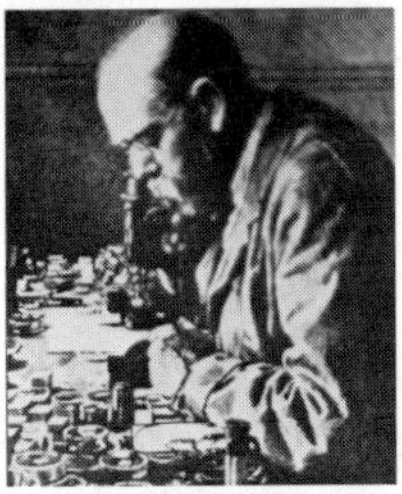
R. Koch

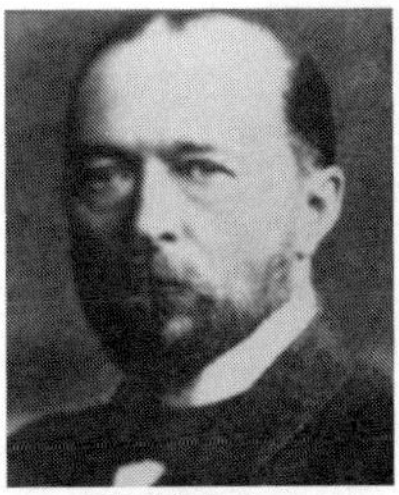
E. Behring

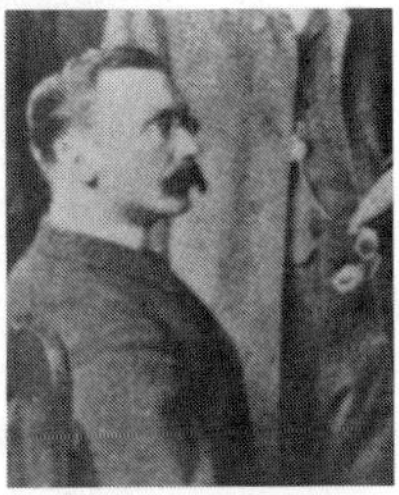
G. Gaffky

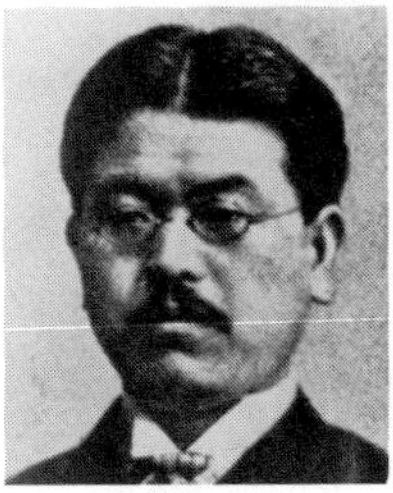
S. Kitosato

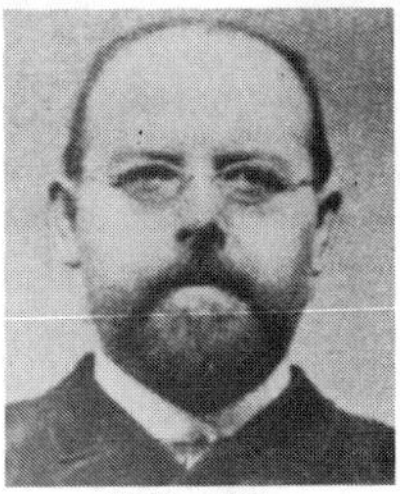
F. Loeffler

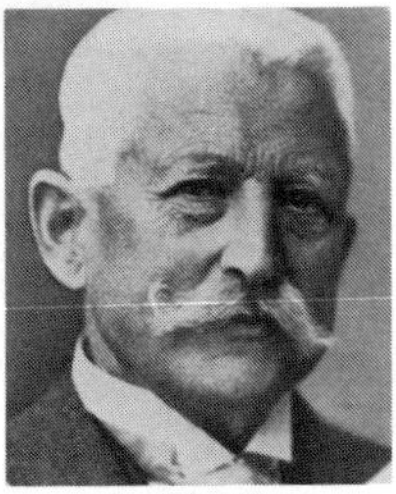
R. Pfeiffer

KOCH AND HIS DISCIPLES

> Puerperal peritonitis prevailed in conjunction with this epidemic (of erysipelas) so uniformly as to show a pathological relationship between these two affections. The opinion was generally held that the former was caused by a virus or miasm carried by the obstetrician from patients affected with the latter. Assuming this to be true in certain cases, puerperal peritonitis was by no means uniformly to be accounted for in this way. A rational explanation in many, if not all cases, is that labor acted as an exciting cause and determined the situation of the local affection in those predisposed to the disease from the action of the epidemic influence. Many, if not most, practitioners held that the disease was communicable. Its contagiousness, however, cannot be considered as established.[29]

This comment illustrates the conservatism of physicians after the work of Semmelweis in Vienna in which he concluded that puerperal fever was caused by the failure of obstetricians to wash their hands with chlorinated water following autopsies on women who had died of the disease.[30] Although the ideas of Semmelweis were supported by Rokitansky, Skoda, and Hebra during the 1850s and written about by Oliver Wendell Holmes, the Vienna obstetricians rejected them, which indicated the stubbornness with which new ideas were received at that time.

In 1866 Georg Rindfleisch (1836–1908) reported that in puerperal fever or in pyemia following surgery, small, soft metastatic deposits of the size of a pin's head were found in the muscles of the heart. These sometimes became cavities with a thick liquid pulp and under the microscope appeared to be made up of "vibrions," but, because they did not stain well, he could not tell if they were rod-shaped or spherical.[31] Then in 1871 von Recklinghausen[32] and Waldeyer independently confirmed the findings of Rindfleisch and reported these small abscesses in the renal veins, the glomeruli, and sometimes in the alveoli of the lungs. They also believed them to be bacteria because acid or alkali treatment of the sections did not affect the abscesses as the treatments usually affected cellular debris or artifacts, but without oil immersion lenses and stains it was difficult to be definitive. Birch-Hirschfeld also studied the subject in detail and came to the conclusion that the more abundant the organisms were in the tissue the worse became the appearance of the wound and the clinical condition of the patient.[33] In 1872 Edwin Klebs found bacteria he called *Microsporon septicum* in fatal wounds of soldiers, but he described them as both spherical and rod shaped and assumed that these were simply morphological variations of the same organism.[34]

Pasteur also had seen micrococci in abscesses and did not hesitate to implicate them in the causation of skin abscesses, osteomyelitis, and puerperal fever. Duclaux in his biography of Pasteur relates how Pasteur came to this belief:

> As the laboratory was not a hospital we scarcely saw diseases there; he was obliged to profit by the indispositions of the personnel. I was, just at this moment, beset by a series of boils and the first thing Pasteur did when I showed him one of them was to prick it, or rather have it pricked, for he was not fond of operating himself, and to take therefrom a drop of blood (the pustular material) in order to make a culture, in which undertaking he was successful. A second boil gave the same result, and thus the staphylococcus was discovered which since that time has been so well known. He found the same microbe made up of little aggregated granules in the pus of an infectious osteomyelitis which M. Lannelongue had submitted to him for examination and we see him, declaring immediately with a fine audacity, that the osteomyelitis and the boil are two forms of one and the same disease, and that the osteomyelitis which is a suppuration of the marrow, is the boil of the bone.[35]

A second observation was made shortly after as described by Roux:

> In the puerperal infections, the pus of the uterus, that of the peritoneum, and the blood clots in the veins, contain a microbe occurring in the form of rounded granules arranged in chains. This chaplet-like aspect is especially apparent in the cultures.[35]

Pasteur did not hesitate to declare that his microscopic organism was the most frequent cause of infections among women in confinement. One day in a discussion on puerperal fever at the Academy of Medicine, one of the most renowned of his colleagues made an eloquent dissertation on the causes of epidemics in the maternity hospitals. Pasteur from his place in the audience interrupted him: "The cause of the epidemic is nothing of the kind! It is the doctor and his staff who carry the microbe from a sick woman to a healthy woman!" And when the orator replied that he was convinced that no one would ever find this microbe, Pasteur darted to the blackboard and drew the organism with its chaplets (chain of beads), saying "There! There is its picture!" Today, one can scarcely understand the surprise and the stupefaction of the medical men and their students when at the hospital, with a simplicity and an assurance that seemed presumptuous in a man who was entering a lying-in hospital for the first time, Pasteur criticized the methods of dressing wounds and declared that all bandages should be placed in a sterilizing oven. Furthermore, he maintained that he could tell by examination of the lochia which women would have an attack of puerperal fever, and he assured them that, in a woman who was very badly infected, he could demonstrate the microbe in the blood from the finger.[36]

Then Robert Koch, fresh from his outstanding studies on anthrax undertook the problem of infections following traumatic injuries. He immediately recognized that micrococci, being so much smaller than the anthrax microbe, had been confused by others with cellular debris, which often takes spherical shapes. With regard to proving the presence, let alone the ability, of micrococci to produce septic infection Koch said that:

> All investigators who have been engaged in seeking bacteria in morbid tissue agree in regarding the undertaking as one of extraordinary, often even of insuperable, difficulty. To make up for the weakness of the anatomical proofs as to the presence of bacteria, pathological experiment has in most cases been resorted to.[37]

Armed with the new oil immersion lens, and Weigert's methyl violet, Koch started experiments on small animals. He injected purulent blood into various animals and was able to produce septicemia and death, and sometimes abscesses and gangrene. In the lesions he was often able to detect one type of micrococci that would be predominant. He found he was more likely to produce disease if the purulent material was fresh than if it was a few days old. He also agreed with Pasteur, who could not grow any organisms from blood of healthy animals, that normal blood is sterile. But until he was able to isolate and grow the micrococci in pure culture, his proof that micrococci were the cause of septicemia would not be conclusive. The results of his experiments were published in 1878 as his superb *Investigations into the Etiology of Traumatic Infective Diseases*. Some of his pertinent comments in this small book are as follows:

> According to my own experience the examination of blood, with the view of ascertaining the possible presence of bacteria, is excessively difficult. . . . I have, however, on many occasions examined normal blood and normal tissues by means which prevent the possibility of overlooking bacteria, or of confounding them with granular masses of equal size. I have come to the conclusion that bacteria do not occur in the blood, nor in the tissues of the healthy living body either of man or of the lower animals.[38]

Birch-Hirschfeld found, in cases of death from puerperal fever, micrococcus masses in vaginal ulcers, perivaginal cellular tissue, in the blood, in the spleen, and in the liver.[39] Koch states that in addition to puerperal fever other diseases produced by micrococci, indistinguishable from each other, were found. Such diseases are erysipelas, mycosis of the navel in newborns, hospital gangrene, endocarditis, scarlet fever, rinderpest, and pleura-pneumonia. Koch then says that:

> It is impossible that these diseases can be produced by one and the same parasite, and we must therefore assume either that the micrococci are in reality always the same, in which case they would be merely associated, as an accidental complication, with the diseases enumerated, or that the micrococci because of their small size, very similar and indeed apparently the same — are nevertheless different in nature, and consequently capable of giving rise to these diverse results.[40]

Such was the dilemma of Koch in 1878, and in light of our present knowledge regarding the nature of the various species and varieties of both staphylococci and streptococci and the fact that the nature of the inflammation or septicemia that they produce are sometimes the same, Koch's attempt to make an evaluation on the basis of morphology was premature. But progress in this area was to be made by both Koch and others. During the years 1880–1882, a Scottish surgeon, Alexander Ogston (1844–1929), using a small laboratory facility he built behind his house and a Zeiss microscope with an oil immersion lens, embarked on the study of the micrococci. Utilizing the techniques developed by Koch including his stains with aniline dyes, he aspirated pus from sixty-five cases of acute abscess and found two types of micrococci, those that appeared in groups like grapes that he called staphylococci, and those in chains that were already named by Billroth as streptococci. Ogston was able to grow micrococci in eggs from which he was able to produce abscesses in animals, but because he did not have available the still-to-be-discovered solid media he was not able to make any differentiation of the micrococci.[41]

In the meantime in 1880 Koch was finally given a position and facilities at the New Imperial Health Office in Berlin. He was assigned two assistants who also later achieved fame in bacteriology, Georg Gaffky (1850–1918) and Friedrich Loeffler (1852–1915). During his first years there, Koch, ever the perfectionist when it came to technique, recognized the importance of devising a simple method of isolating one species of bacteria from the other. Pasteur, working with microorganisms over many years, had always used liquid media but had developed nutrients containing metabolites that favored one species over the other. But as all microbiologists know, to grow a pure culture in liquid, it is necessary to use a solid medium for preliminary isolation, and it is likely that some of Pasteur's cultures were not always pure. Koch is usually given complete credit for devising the plate method for separating bacteria, but other investigators working with microorganisms that produced pigment had used such solid media as starch paste, bread, meat, and the surfaces of cut potatoes. Koch wanted to find a way in which to convert any type of media into solid, which would give him greater versatility and selectivity than any of the solids already available. He published his method in 1881, and it is given below almost in its entirety because it revolutionized microbiology because of its simplicity:

> I devoted my attention to discover how well known nutrient solutions could be converted into the solid condition, and I found the best way of accomplishing this was to mix gelatine with the nutrient liquid. The mixture of nutrient fluid and gelatine, which I shall call "nutrient jelly" is prepared by dissolving gelatine in water by heat; to it is added nutrient fluid. . . . Meanwhile a flask plugged with wool is disinfected by heating . . . and into it is poured the nutrient jelly. . . . It is plugged again and heated to the boiling point . . . to kill the microorganisms in the jelly . . . It is poured into flat watch glasses . . . in streaks . . . about 2 mm thick, and then when the jelly solidifies, the slides are laid on glass . . . so that two or three slides (are) lying side by side and placed in a moist chamber. .

> . . A small quantity of the fluid . . . containing the organism is taken by means of a previously heated platinum wire and then drawn in several crosslines across the surface of the jelly. . . . The cultures grow best at 20-25 degrees centigrade (because) . . . at temperatures above 30 degrees the gelatine melts.[42]

It should be mentioned here that Walter Hesse, working with Koch in 1881 and taking a suggestion from his wife to use agar instead of gelatin for the solid media, solved both the problem of gelatin melting at 30 degrees and also the fact that gelatin is liquefied by some bacteria whereas agar is more inert. Then in 1887, Richard Petri[43] designed a dish for the agar which made it more convenient than the flat slides kept under a bell jar. The importance of the development of solid media cannot be overemphasized because it allowed the rapid separation of easily destroyed pathogens from nonpathogenic saprophytes that usually overgrow them in liquid media. The reader can thus realize that by 1887 bacteriological methodology was essentially complete, except for the discovery of selective and enriched media and immunological procedures. The result was that in 1884 Friedrich Rosenbach, using solid media containing serum and meat peptone nutrient, was able to confirm Ogston's work and proceeded to differentiate micrococci into several groups on the basis of the nature of the color of the colonies. He differentiated *Staphylococcus aureus* and *albus*, and *streptococcus pyogenes*.[44]

In the same year Fehleisen, at Wurzburg, who had also identified microscopically the presence of streptococci in erysipelas lesions, by placing pieces of erysipelas skin into liquefied "nutrient jelly" and then allowing it to harden, was able to find colonies of streptococci growing in contact with the skin. He gave the cultures to Koch and his group who were able to continue the growth on coagulated serum. In any case Fehleisen, using organisms from the isolated colonies, was able to produce erysipelas-type lesions in rabbits, which essentially proved the etiology of this skin condition which as late as 1851 was considered to be caused by such things as "irritation of the bile, disturbance of the function of the liver, accumulation of gastric impurities, obstruction of the portal system, and a peculiar prevailing wind and condition of the weather."[45]

The micrococci, including pneumococci, staphylococci, and streptococci, however, continued to present problems with regard to their activity in producing lesions. Even in the first half of the twentieth century, it was realized that classification on the basis of cultural characteristics would not be sufficient. As a result, there have been numerous revisions of their classifications, and at the present time immunological and genetic factors are utilized. But in spite of all these advances, the pathogenicity of the micrococci appears to have changed over the years, particularly the group A beta hemolytic streptococci. The incidence of scarlet fever, rheumatic fever, acute glomerulonephritis, and erysipelas has diminished dramatically over the past century and particularly during the second half of this century. There has been no satisfactory explanation. With the discovery of at least seventy different group A streptococci based upon the immunological difference in a surface M protein on the bacteria,[46] it was hoped that it could be shown that certain organisms with specific M proteins were responsible for either rheumatic fever or acute glomerulonephritis. This was not the case, and there has been no good correlation of the M protein with the clinical diagnosis, so the mystery still remains. Although some medical people believe that the widespread use of antibiotics since 1945 is a factor, and others believe that the host factors have changed, in light of the many mutations that can occur in microorganisms (and the fact that new pathogens such as HIV suddenly appear), it is more likely that the particularly virulent streptococci have not competed well with less-virulent strains, and therefore they are less prevalent in the community. It should not be forgotten that a parasitic relationship between a bacteria and a human is best served if the human does not become ill. When the host becomes sick, it is an aberration of nature because the bacteria is eliminated by antibiotic therapy or, if the patient succumbs, so does the particularly virulent bacteria. From an evolutionary standpoint, in the case of a group A streptococcus, its virulence would be a disadvantage for its survival, and its less-virulent brethren would then become more prevalent in the human population, with the result that rheumatic fever, scarlet fever, and acute glomerulonephritis have diminished in incidence. This subject is further discussed in the next chapter in relation to Pasteur's ability to increase or decrease virulence of some microorganisms in the laboratory.

The work on micrococci had its somewhat humorous moments in that two young men who were working together in 1882 and were to achieve immortality in bacteriology did so through errors or misinterpretations of their own work. These two individuals were Carl Friedländer (1847–1887), a student of von Recklinghausen, and Hans Gram (1853–1938). Both of these investigators were attempting to find a microorganism that could be the causative factor in the production of lobar pneumonia, a disease that was very common in the nineteenth century and caused many fatalities after following a classic clinical course. Although a diplococcus had been described by both Pasteur and George Sternberg in 1881 as being present in the saliva of humans, these two individuals did not know its significance in producing lobar pneumonia.[47] But Friedländer and Gram, studying lung tissue of patients dead of this disease, found enormous numbers of "diplococci" in the alveoli and the bronchioles. Then they grew the organisms on solid medium, and, by inoculating the resulting pure cultures into mice, Friedländer stated that the mice developed lobar pneumonia.[48] Other investigators, interested in Friedländer's work asked for cultures of his "diplococci." This was his downfall, because among his cultures was a slightly different organism, a short rod with a capsule that Friedländer and Gram did not recognize as different from the other cases. Koch received a culture of the short rod, and George Sternberg, visiting Koch at the time, immediately saw that it was different from the diplococci that he had seen in saliva.[49] Albert Fraenkel (1848–1916) was able to culture the true diplococci first seen by Pasteur and Sternberg, and reproduced the lesions in the lungs of rabbits.[50] He ridiculed Friedländer for his misobservation and called his organism Friedländer's bacilli. For a while some of the bacteriologists thought that the bacillus was a saprophyte. The irony of the situation was that Anton Weichselbaum (1845–1920) in 1886 concluded that in a small percentage of cases Friedländer's bacilli was the etiological agent in lobar pneumonia.[51]

While Friedländer was working on lobar pneumonia, Hans Gram was attempting to find new stains for detecting bacteria in tissue. Gram was using methyl violet, and, according to an old bacteriology anecdote, he accidently spilled an iodide-iodine solution on the section, and in attempting to wash it off with alcohol, he noted that the tissues and some of the bacteria were decolorized while other bacteria did not. Supposedly he was upset because some of the bacteria were decolorized, but a few years later, other bacteriologists started differentiating bacteria on whether or not they were decolorized with the alcohol, and the expressions "Gram positive" and "Gram negative" bacteria has remained in the field for more than one hundred years.[52] It was unfortunate that Gram did not attempt to differentiate the organisms of his colleague, Friedländer, since they could have become aware that the true pneumococci was gram positive and the similar appearing "Friedländer's bacillus" would have been gram negative. Eventually the bacillus would be called *Klebsiella pneumoniae*, but Friedländer's name is still associated with it, and the clinical term "Friedländer's pneumonia" is still used in the latest medical textbook.

Typhoid Fever

There are now only about 500 cases of typhoid fever each year in the United States, but, until the isolation of the bacteria and the mechanism of its transmission was solved, this disease devastated armies and brought sudden and unexpected tragedy to families because it was a disease of young people, was painful, long lasting, and often fatal. (At different times during his life, Pasteur lost two young daughters to this disease, and possibly a third at two years of age). At least one in every twenty-five individuals contracted the disease during the last decade of the nineteenth century. Its importance was emphasized in that Osler made it the first subject of the first chapter in his famous 1892 textbook, and its conquest and control is a shining episode in the history of medicine. Although William Budd (1811–1880),[53] on the basis of studying the epidemiology of the disease during an epidemic in England in 1856, became convinced that it was transmitted through the water supply contaminated by human feces, his ideas were not accepted. However, in 1880 Carl Eberth (1835–1926), who was professor of pathology at Zurich, examined mesenteric nodes, the spleen, and intestinal ulcers in patients dead of typhoid fever and found bacteria in his sections. He could not stain them in the sections but was able to do so easily if he expressed fluid from these tissues, dried it on a slide, and then stained it with methyl violet.[54] Then Gaffky, in 1884, taking pieces of spleen at autopsy of typhoid patients, was able to grow the microorganism on nutrient gelatin and was able to characterize the colonies. He tried to grow the typhoid bacteria from the feces of patients with typhoid, but saprophytic organisms liquefied the gelatin and he could not obtain positive blood cultures. He attempted to produce the disease in monkeys and other animals but failed. However, weighing his evidence with that of Eberth, he concluded that

> the bacteria were observed in 26 out of 28 cases of enteric fever which I examined (and) one must admit that now we have every justification in assuming the presence of these organisms in enteric fever as constant. As soon as we admit

> that a typical form of microorganism is invariably present in enteric fever, which is never present in other diseased processes . . . we may regard these organisms as the cause of the disease with quite as much justice as is now the case with the spirochete of relapsing fever and leprosy bacilli in leprosy.[55]

However, it was not enough to identify the typhoid bacillus in the lesions of fatal cases. To be of clinical value, it was necessary to detect the organism in living cases and in asymptomatic carriers. The problem was that the pathogen was morphologically identical and, initially, identical in culture to the normal colon bacteria. Then in 1889, a series of experiments by Theobald Smith, studying the biochemical characteristics of intestinal bacteria, revealed that whereas the normal colon bacteria utilized both lactose and glucose with the production of gas, the typhoid bacillus fermented glucose but not lactose and without the production of gas. These findings led to the development of differential media by such individuals as Loeffler,[56] Drigalski and Conradi,[57] and A.J. MacConkey,[58] during the first few years of this century. But the confirmatory procedure to positively identify the typhoid bacillus was based upon the phenomenon of agglutination of the organism when mixed with serum of an immune human or animal. This procedure was pioneered by Widal[59] and Gruber and Durham[60] and conversely was used to determine the immunity of humans to the disease following infection or immunization. Unfortunately during the first week of typhoid, both the Widal test and stool cultures will be negative, and it was not possible to make an early diagnosis until it was found that blood cultures were often positive.

Discovery of the Organisms Responsible for Leprosy, Gonorrhea, and Meningitis

The first bacteria that was believed to be the etiology of a human disease was that which causes leprosy, a disease common in Norway in the last century and believed to be hereditary. Armauer Hansen (1841–1912) in 1874 found the bacilli in the giant cells associated with that disease, but without the benefit of stains, the demonstration was not conclusive.[61] Albert Neisser (1855–1916), however, used the new bacterial stains methyl violet and fuchsin to conclusively demonstrate the bacilli.[62]

This was the same year that Neisser, as a young assistant in the dermatology clinic at Breslau, first stained with methyl violet the urethral pus from several patients with gonorrhea. He also saw the organism in exudate from cases of ophthalmia neonatorum and was able to describe the characteristic kidney-bean shape of the diplococcus and to note its predominantly intracellular position in the polymorphonuclear cells. Neisser attempted to grow the organism in several different media, but he was not able to find any colonies in which he could infect humans.[63] It was not until 1885 that Ernst von Bumm, professor of gynecology in Basel, was able to culture the organism and transmit it to a woman.[64]

In 1887 Anton Weichselbaum (1845–1920), professor of pathology in Vienna, in six fatal cases of meningitis found diplococci in the cerebrospinal fluid that resembled those of gonorrhea and that did not stain with Gram's method (Gram negative).[65] However, because the Gram stain was not completely accepted as a valid way of differentiating bacteria, many investigators were still convinced that it was the pneumonia diplococci that was the usual cause of meningitis. However, during the years 1896–1897, there was an epidemic of meningitis in Boston, and W.J. Councilman, F.B. Mallory, and James Wright did a careful survey of the cases and found that in over a hundred of them the Gram negative diplococci of Weichselbaum was the etiological agent.[66]

Plague

Historically, plague has affected humankind more than any other disease. Since the beginning of the Christian era, there have been three major pandemics. The first, known as the plague of Justian, occurred in the sixth century A.D., lasted approximately fifty years, and extended over the entire Roman Empire, but primarily around the Mediterranean. Estimates have been made that one hundred million people died. The second pandemic, which was known as the Black Death (and included both the pneumonic and bubonic forms of the disease) began in the Crimea during the middle of the fourteenth century and spread throughout Europe and Great Britain, with estimates of twenty-five million deaths over a three-hundred-year period. The third pandemic, which was essentially confined to Asia started in 1894 on the border of China and Burma, spread through Hong Kong to India where the mortality was twelve million people during the period 1894–1948. The organism that causes plague was identified by Alexander Yersin (1863–1943) from material taken from excised buboes in 1894.[67] Yersin had studied medicine in Lausanne, Marburg, and Paris where he was the assistant to Cornil at the Hotel Dieu. In 1887 he went to Robert Koch's laboratory where he learned the German's latest techniques, after which he returned to Paris where he worked on diphtheria with Roux in Pasteur's laboratory. He was a very shy man but adventurous, and he went to Indochina as part of a mission in 1894 to investigate the plague in Hong Kong.[68] Eventually he became Director of the Pasteur Institute established in Saigon and remained there until his death during World War II. But on his arrival in Hong Kong in 1894, Yersin found Koch's former student sent by Japan, S. Kitosato (1856–1931), already at work on the plague. Independently they both found the causative agent — a small, rod-shaped organism — but Yersin was more successful in growing the bacterium in culture media. He quickly satisfied Koch's postulates, which were finding the microorganism in all cases of the disease, culturing it outside the body, and then inoculating the colonies into rats and mice and reproducing the disease at will. Yersin also noted that there were always dead rats to be found around human cases, and these rodents also contained the same organism. In 1895, he showed that it was possible to produce a vaccine against the bacteria. It was in 1897 that M. Ogata, working in Formosa, proved that it was the flea on the rat that was the principal vector in carrying the bacteria of plague.[69]

Tuberculosis

With his techniques and equipment worked out and in place, Robert Koch, during the period 1881–1882, undertook to prove that tuberculosis was produced by a bacterium. This disease during the nineteenth century was the cause of death in more than 10% of the population in Europe. However, its course, chronicity, and that it appeared to be selective in choosing its victims and did not become epidemic like the pestilences gave rise to many theories about its pathogenesis. Many physicians were convinced it was a hereditary condition that manifested itself later in the life of the victim. However there were clues that it could be transmitted from one person to another. Philipp Klencke (1813–1881)[70] in 1843 succeeded in producing extensive tubercular lesions in rabbits by injected material from pulmonary and miliary tubercles in humans. Then in the 1860s, Jean Villemin (1827–1892) carried out careful experiments[71] inoculating into guinea pigs and rabbits not only sputum and caseous material from tubercular lesions from humans but also those from cows. He showed that he could produce the same severe tuberculosis in the experimental animals, which not only proved it was transmissible but that the diseases in human and cows, if not identical, were closely related. Cohnheim and Salomonsen, in the late 1870s, injected caseous material in the anterior chamber of the eye of rabbits and were able to watch the development of the tubercles over a period of time. In this way they separated an immediate general inflammation that could occur with nonspecific bacteria from that of the slower tubercular process.[72] Koch, however, was interested in finding the organisms that he believed were producing the tubercular process but that no one had yet visualized. He was fortunate that the microorganism was not a submicroscopic virus, which he would not have been able to identify, and that he had the microscopic skill he had developed studying the large anthrax bacteria to be able to find the much smaller and more difficult to visualize bacteria of tuberculosis. Although he was soon able to see small, delicately thin bacteria in caseous tubercular material using an alkaline methylene blue stain, he soon used Ehrlich's new stain of aniline oil and methyl violet dissolved in alcohol, followed by washing and decolorization with dilute nitric acid. He counterstained with Bismark brown, and only the tubercular organism, called the *Mycobacterium tuberculosis*, kept its blue color. This characteristic of acid fastness of the waxy bacterium made the identification of the tubercular organism simpler because no other organism other than those of leprosy in its own respective lesions was also acid fast. The stain that became standard over a period of years was the Ziehl-Neelsen preparation, which in 1883 replaced fuchsin for methyl violet and carbolic acid for aniline oil with methylene blue as a counterstain, which colors the mycobacterium red against a blue background.[73] In any case, Koch was able to find the organism in every case of tuberculosis if he took the care of looking long enough. However, because there always existed the possibility that the mycobacterium was produced by some other material with which it is associated, he wanted to isolate the organism and grow it on artificial medium. In his monumental paper on tuberculosis,[74] Koch expressed his concern in this manner, and reiterated his famous postulates:

> From these three facts, that tubercle bacilli are always present in tuberculosis and occur nowhere else, that they precede, both

> as to place and time, all the peculiar pathological changes, and their number, appearance and disappearance are in direct relation with the course of the disease, the conclusion may be drawn with great probability that the tubercle bacillus is not a chance accompaniment of tuberculosis, but stands in the position of the direct cause of the disease. Such far reaching consequences depend on this question, however, that it was impossible to be content with a probable solution of it without endeavoring to obtain perfect certainty. . . . The only possible way of attaining this end lay in following the same method adopted in the investigation of other diseases. It was necessary to isolate the tubercle bacillus from the diseased organs, to cultivate them outside the body and study their behavior under these conditions, and finally to produce tuberculosis artificially by inoculations with the bacilli thus freed from all admixture with the products of disease.[74]

Koch was able with some difficulty to devise a coagulated serum medium that would grow small colonies after several days of incubation from caseous tubercular material where there was a minimum of other extraneous microorganisms. Then he took these tiny colonies and either inoculated them intraperitoneally into guinea pigs or had the guinea pigs breathe a spray prepared from one of the colonies. In all cases, typical tubercular lesions appeared giving testimony that all of his postulates had been satisfied. This accomplishment immediately allowed the medical community to make the correct diagnosis of the disease and such concepts as "phthisis, progressing into consumption" was eliminated from the medical writings. Koch then became very famous, and the German government over the years gave him increasingly more elaborate facilities for research. The Institute for Infectious Diseases became a mecca for aspiring investigators throughout the world.

Cholera

In spite of the fact that many physicians believed that cholera was produced by a "miasm" from soil that spread from community to community through a poison by winds and variations in the temperature and barometric pressure,[75] Koch, after his success with anthrax and tuberculosis was confident that he could find an etiological bacteria. Cholera had made its first appearance as a pandemic in India in the early 1800s, and by 1832 it had killed as many as 60,000-100,000 people in

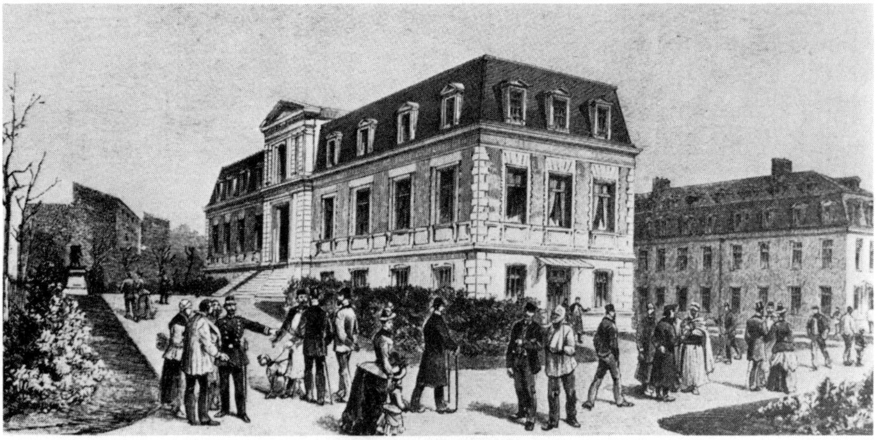

Pasteur Institute

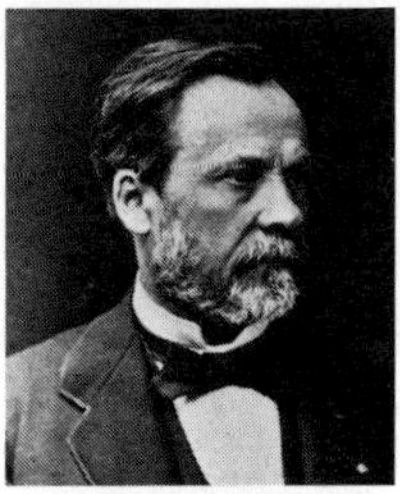

L. Pasteur

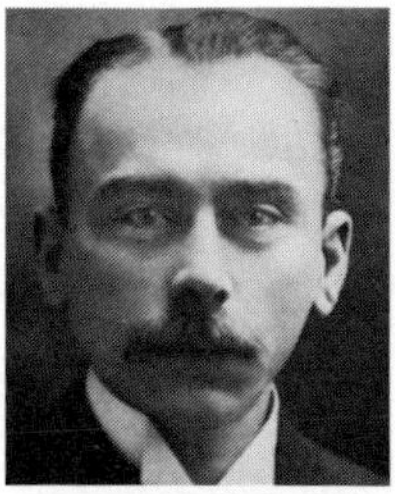

J. Bordet

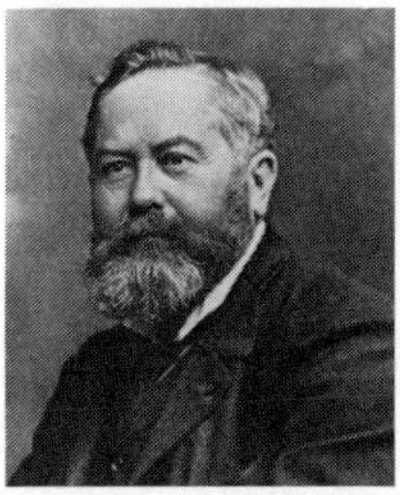

C. Chamberland

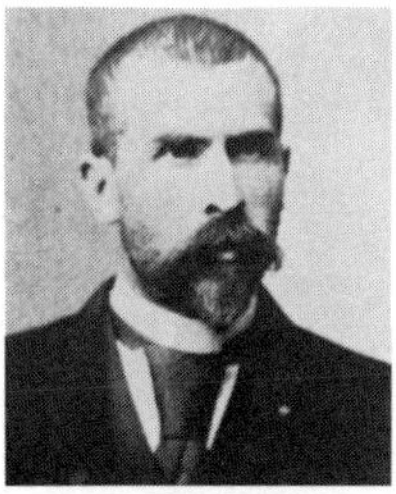

E. Duclaux

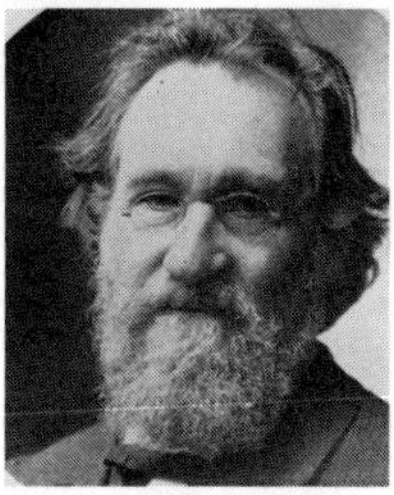

E. Metchnikoff

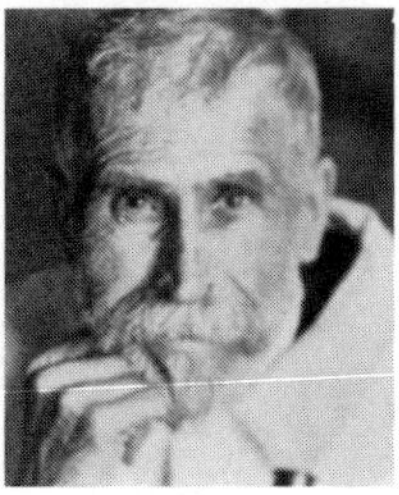

E. Roux

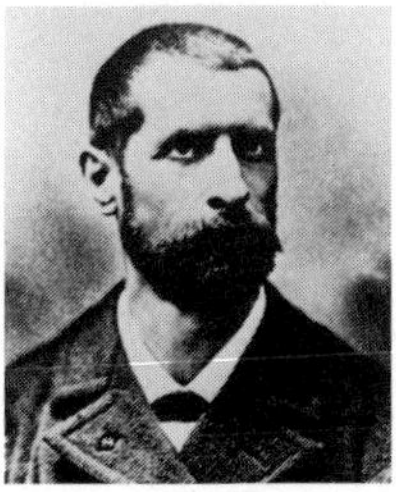

A. Yersin

PASTEUR AND HIS DISCIPLES

Egypt. It made its appearance in Poland in 1831, brought in by the invading Russians, and from there spread throughout Europe and Great Britain. Irish immigrants carried it to Canada from where it established itself in the United States. After 1837, it disappeared from Europe and North America for ten years. In 1846 it appeared again and ravaged much of the world, until 1863, when it subsided. In 1865 another pandemic occurred that lasted until 1875. However, when it appeared again in Egypt and the Middle East in 1883, concern that the scourge would cross the Mediterranean and devastate the northern countries again, caused both Germany and France, after the success of both the Koch and Pasteur groups in microbiology, to persuade Koch and Pasteur to go to Egypt to study cholera. Koch, therefore, set out with a team that included his able assistant, Georg Gaffky. Pasteur, who because of his age was discouraged from going himself, sent some of his best assistants, Roux, L. Thuillier, M. Straus, and M. Nocard. Both groups set up laboratories in Alexandria in competition with each other. Although the epidemic had almost disappeared from that city, Thuillier, only 27 years old, contracted the disease and died within two days, and Pasteur back in Paris, overcome with grief, called his group home. Koch, however, after attending Thuillier's funeral, went to Calcutta, which was believed to be the home of the disease where cholera was still raging. He was given excellent facilities by the British Government and within a short time identified a comma-shaped bacteria in the intestinal mucosa of victims, which was the same bacteria he saw in Egypt.[76] He also saw large numbers of the bacteria in the flecks of mucus that give the stools of cholera patients the appearance of "rice water." He was able to grow the organism on gelatin, and in spite of the heat in Calcutta, which on occasion melted the gelatin, he was able to demonstrate the characteristic liquedation of gelatin by the cholera bacteria, which leaves a funnel-like pattern when the gelatin is in test tubes. He found the organism in all the victims of cholera but not in the stools of healthy individuals. Unfortunately he was not able to transmit the disease to experimental animals to satisfy his postulates. He did find the organism in a water tank that was used for bathing and drinking and that was contaminated with human excrement, which led him to believe that cholera was spread through drinking water. In as much as he was unable to find the organism in the mesenteric glands or the blood, he hypothesized that the cholera bacillus produces illness by forming a poison during its growth, which produces the signs and symptoms. History has shown that he was correct, but there was great skepticism in the medical community at the time. When Koch demonstrated his work to Max von Pettenkorfer, the famous hygienist refuted the pathogenicity of the comma bacillus by swallowing one milliliter of a broth sent to him by Gaffky that supposedly contained one million organisms. The only reaction he had was a mild case of diarrhea in which the bacillus was isolated.[77] Our understanding of the disease today is that for every case of cholera there are 25-100 cases of mild or asymptomatic infections, which probably explains Pettenkorfer's survival. In any case the comma bacillus, or *Vibrio cholera,* of Koch is still considered the etiological organism and is still prevalent and dangerous in areas where excreta contaminates drinking water.

Diphtheria

The occurrence of diphtheria in epidemic form probably dates far into antiquity. Although Pierre Bretonneau placed the clinical diagnosis on a reasonably firm ground, it was not until the etiological organism was found and identified that the specific nature of the disease could be established. The problem was similar to that found in working with cholera and typhoid — the anatomical parts affected are normally populated by many non-pathogenic microorganisms that are very similar morphologically and in culture to the pathogens. Klebs in 1883 was the first to describe bacilli in typical pseudomembranes characteristic of diphtheria.[78] This brilliant assistant of Virchow was a pioneer in bacteriology and a polemic critic of his former mentor, and in a sense an itinerant pathologist. Klebs was professor of pathology at many medical schools — Bern, Wurzburg, Prague, and Zurich in Europe — after which he came to the United States and settled in North Carolina and then Chicago where he was professor for a short time at Rush Medical College. In 1900 he returned to Europe where he worked in a private laboratory in Hanover. Then, at 71 years of age, Klebs went back to work with Virchow's successor, Johannes Orth, and finally ended his career back at Bern. His work was always imaginative, but seldom definitive, and he seemed to rush to publish his work before it was technically flawless. Garrison states that he was a "man of irascible, precipitate disposition,"[79] which probably explains not only why he made so many geographical changes in his career but also why his research was marred with an impatient quality.

Friedrich Loeffler, on the other hand, starting as one of Koch's first assistants and was a consummate experimentalist, like his mentor. After working with Koch from 1879 to 1884, Loeffler became Professor of Hygiene at Greifswald, and eventually succeeded Gaffky as Director of the Institute for Infectious Diseases in Berlin. His work with diphtheria was definitive, showing that the diphtheric membrane was often made up of colonies of bacilli, which he was able to stain with his alkaline methylene blue stain. He inoculated a small part of the membrane onto the surface of coagulated lamb serum enriched with veal and glucose. He wrote that:

> On the following day numerous small, separate colonies were evident on the blood serum; most of these proved to consist of micrococci, but some were composed of the bacilli in question. . . . The diphtheritic bacilli are non-motile, and are very quickly and deeply stained with methylene blue; some of them are straight, and some slightly curved. They vary considerably in length . . . and the longer ones are composed of several members, and where these are connected there is a slightly knotty enlargement. . . . Frequently the pole of the bacillus is more deeply stained than its substance.[80]

Loeffler inoculated the bacilli into many different animals — rats, mice, rabbits, monkeys, pigeons, and hens — by means of subcutaneous injections, inoculation on almost every type of mucous membrane, and inhalation. He was never able to produce the same type of lesion as in humans, and no animal ever developed the diphtheric paralysis which is often the complication in humans. He therefore never felt he had fulfilled Koch's postulates. However, in 1888, Roux and Yersin, working at the new Pasteur Institute in Paris, were able to produce paralysis in pigeons and rabbits using a filtrate of liquid cultures of the Klebs-Loeffler bacillus and made these conclusions:

> . . . The paralysis following inoculation with the Klebs-Loeffler organism completes the resemblance of the experimental disease to the natural disease and establishes firmly the specific etiologic role of this bacillus. We have already seen that the diphtheric bacillus is not disseminated through the organs of humans or animals suffering from diphtheria, but is localized in the diphtheritic membranes or at the site of inoculation. . . . It has been postulated that a very active poison was

> elaborated at the site of localization of the bacilli, and from that point spread throughout the body.[81]

Emile Roux, the primary investigator of the diphtheria-toxin work was one of France's most notable bacteriologists and was one of the first of Pasteur's assistants. Although he attended medical school, he was primarily interested in chemistry and started with Pasteur as a media maker in 1878. (Pasteur did not like physicians working in his laboratory, since he thought that "physicians are inclined to engage in hasty generalizations . . . endowed with a quick intelligence, and elegant and facile conversation . . . the more eminent they are . . . the less leisure they have for investigative work. . . . Eager for knowledge . . . they are apt to accept too readily attractive but inadequately proven theories."[82]) Roux also did excellent work on anthrax and its use in vaccinations, but his work on diphtheria toxin was distinguished and was the starting point for Ehrlich developing, along with E. von Behring, an antitoxin that can still be used today for individuals who contract the disease but have not been vaccinated.

David Bruce and Malta Fever

In 1884, David Bruce (1855–1931), a young British Army doctor with essentially no knowledge of the new microbiology, was sent to take care of soldiers stationed on the island of Malta in the Mediterranean Sea. (According to Paul de Kruif, he joined the army after medical school simply to obtain enough money to marry the woman who would become his life-long helper in microbiology.) When he arrived there, he found there was a long-standing mysterious disease, clinically similar to typhoid, that attacked the inhabitants with aches and pain, fever, and weakness over a long period of time, although few died. Then in 1886, the disease was fatal for nine soldiers, and Bruce, just having read about the bacteriological methods of Koch, began to look for a bacteria that might account for the illness. He knew nothing of microbiology, but he managed to find a small building where he could work, and was able to obtain the material for carrying out bacteriological work and an oil immersion lens for his microscope. From the spleen of one of the dead soldiers, he made sections and stained the material with both methylene blue and Gram's stain. He luckily found large numbers of a single type of micrococci. He went back to Great Britain in the spring of 1886, where he showed his slides to Sims Woodhead, who had experience as a bacteriologist and thought that Bruce had actually found the definitive organism for Malta Fever. When Bruce returned to Malta, he prepared some nutrient agar in test tubes, made a stab culture with splenic material from a patient dead of Malta fever, and in sixty-eight hours found tiny pearly white colonies along the path of the platinum needle.[83] A short time later, he was able to transmit the disease to a monkey which developed a fever, splenomegaly, and died; the proof was complete.[84] Bruce called the organism *Micrococcus melitensis*. Then the next year, Almroth Wright prepared an antiserum which could be used to differentiate Malta fever from typhoid fever by agglutination of the organisms.[85]

In 1905, goats on Malta were found to have antibodies to Bruce's bacteria, which led to the conclusion that goat milk was the source of Malta fever and that slaughtering infected goats and boiling all goat milk would prevent the disease.[86] The problem became more complicated, when in 1918 Alice Evans, a microbiologist working for the agriculture department in Washington, D.C., found in the milk of cows that were aborting their calves a microorganism that had been found by Bernhard Bang in 1897 to do the same thing in cows in Denmark. He called this microorganism *Bacillus abortus*.[87] Evans was asked by the chief of the pathology division of the bureau whether she had ever compared the coccus of Bruce with the bacilli of Bang, because he had heard that Bruce's organism in addition to producing Malta fever also produced abortions in goats. From the American Museum of Natural History and the Bureau of Animal Industry she obtained cultures of Bruce's organism that had been subcultured for more than 20 years. She found that in culture and morphologically they were identical and that they could be interpreted both as cocci and bacilli and both forms were intermingled. She then was able to demonstrate agglutination of both organisms with antiserum to Bang's bacilli, and thus prove their identical nature or close relationship. The result was that over a period of years, Malta or undulant fever (now called brucellosis) can be produced in humans by any one of four organisms, *Brucella melintensis*, *Brucella abortus*, *Brucella canis,* or *Brucella suis*, although the first is most pathogenic for humans.[88] With control of livestock and pasteurism of milk, the disease has almost been entirely eliminated in the United States (154 cases reported in 1982), although according to the WHO there are approximately 500,000 cases each year worldwide.[89]

Tetanus, Bacillary Dysentery, and the Japanese Influence

Oriental medicine before the nineteenth century had essentially not progressed for more than a thousand years. Religion and custom prohibited the types of advancements that occurred in Western civilization as a result of the dissection of the human body and the experimental method. But the ideas of Western medicine gradually exerted their influence in China and Japan by the settling of European physicians there. In 1857, a Dutch medical school was established in Yedo, and shortly thereafter the more modern-thinking Japanese quickly recognized that German medicine was the most advanced in Europe. Many German medical texts were translated into Japanese, and soon young men from Japan went to Germany to study. This was at the time that Robert Koch was establishing microbiology, and the diligent, patient work required in that field was appealing to the Japanese character.

The first one of the many students who went to Germany was Shibasaburo Kitosato (1856–1931) who went to Berlin in 1885 where Koch assigned him to work on typhoid fever, cholera, and glanders. With his increasing knowledge, he was finally asked by Koch to study tetanus on which Gaffky and Loeffler had done some equivocal work. Kitosato found that the tetanus organism required anaerobic conditions. He published a paper in 1889 that revealed these facts about the tetanus organism:

> Properties of the tetanic bacilli are as follows; They are obligate anaerobes. They grow well under hydrogen, but not carbon dioxide. The bacilli propagate in weakly alkaline peptone agar and gelatine. . . . The tetanus bacilli is stained with aniline dyes. They held the Gram stain. . . . Mice inoculated by puncture with a platinum needle placed in pure culture developed tetanus after 24 hours and died in 2-3 days. . . . No bacilli or spores were seen in smears from the site of inoculation or the different tissues or organs in the body. Tissues taken from the various organs did not produce tetanus in different animals and did not propagate the bacilli in culture. . . . The following deductions can be made; (1) Tetanus is an infectious disease produced by a specific bacillus. (2) The etiological agent of human tetanus and experimental tetanus is the bacillus reported by Nicolaier. (3) This bacillus is present in the pus of

man and experimental animals with the symptoms of tetanus. The bacilli produce spores in the pus. (4) The bacilli can be cultured from tetanus cases and these pure cultures can create tetanus in experimental animals.[90]

The discovery that the paralytic effect of both the tetanus bacilli and the diphtheric bacilli were caused, not by a bacteria, but by the local production of a toxin that was carried through the circulation to the neuromuscular system to produce paralysis, encouraged Kitosato to work with Emil von Behring (1854–1917) to produce antitoxins to both diphtheric toxin and tetanus toxin.[91] In 1892, Kitosato returned to Japan to aid in the development of the field of microbiology, and as a result of his work on plague in Hong Kong, the government in 1889 built a facility in Japan fashioned after the Pasteur Institutes in Paris and Saigon with Kitosato as the director. One of Kitosato's assistants was Kyoshi Shiga (1870–1957) who was the first to identify a bacterium as a cause of dysentery, which produced thousands of deaths in Japan every year. He isolated a bacilli in 1898, now known as *Shigella dysenteriae*.

He described it as follows:

The bacillus of dysentery bacillus is a short rod with rounded ends similar to the typhoid bacillus, and *E. coli*. The bacteria usually occur singly but occasionally in pairs. With methylene blue, the rods are stained greater at the ends. They are decolorized with the stain of Gram. They are somewhat motile, but flagellae have not been shown with certainty and no spores are formed. The bacillus was hard to isolate at the beginning of the disease, but almost pure colonies can be easily produced during the peak of the diarrhea. When the stool becomes normal, the amount of the other bacteria increased and the number of dysenteric bacilli decreased. I could cultivate ten kinds of bacteria from dysenteric stools, but the specific bacillus was dominant. The dysenteric bacillus was cultivated from all cases of the series and was the only one that was agglutinated by the serum of dysenteric patients. The dysenteric bacillus was not found in the stools of healthy individuals or in patients having typhoid fever, acute diarrhea, chronic diarrhea, tuberculous diarrhea or beri-beri."[92]

The significance of this advance in identifying a specific bacteria with a disease by the procedure of Widal could be considered another possible postulate of Koch. This is a major confirmation that the organism isolated is the same one that produces the disease and antibodies to that disease.

Salmonella Pathogens

August Gaertner (1848–1934), Professor of Hygiene at Jena, in 1888 was called upon to investigate an epidemic of gastroenteritis among a group of people who had eaten beef from a cow that had been ill. He found in the tissues of the cow and one of the victims who had died, an organism that he called "*bacillus enteritidis*."[93] A year later, De Nobele reported the first isolation of *S. typhimurium* in another food-poisoning outbreak. Nothing more was accomplished until 1898 when the English bacteriologist Herbert Durham (1866–1945) found in several cases of "meat poisoning" the same bacillus as Gaertner determined by the new agglutination test, which had also been used for confirming cases of typhoid disease.[94] Then there began to appear cases with the signs of typhoid, but the organisms isolated did not agglutinate with typhoid antibodies. These organisms were called by Hugo Schottmuller (1867–1936) "*bacillus paratyphosus*." Durham then made a study of the enterics, including *E. coli*, the typhoid, paratyphoid, and food-poisoning organisms, using the agglutination tests and found cross agglutinations although at varying dilutions of the antisera.[95] It should be mentioned that it was this investigator that invented the "Durham tube," which was a small inverted test tube in the culture tube to detect the production of gas during the fermentation of the various bacteria.[96] During the twentieth century there have been extensive studies on the enterics, and the classifications have been based on such factors as motility, metabolism in various media, and serological testing.

At the present time[97] there are more than 1600 different serotypes of the Salmonella group, of which about 150 have been isolated from humans in the United States. This would have probably surprised D.E. Salmon from the U.S. Department of Agriculture, who, with his famous assistant Theobald Smith, isolated the organism in 1886 that produced cholera in pigs and is now known as *Salmonella cholera-suis*. Most of the cases at the present time are those due to *S. enteritidis*, *S. typhimurium*, and *S. cholera-suis*.

This chapter thus describes the major discoveries of bacteria that produced some of the major diseases in humans during the years 1878–1900, which was the Golden Age of Bacteriology, and changed Man's understanding of infectious diseases forever.

Bibliography

1. Fracastoro, G., *De Contagione et Contagiosis Morbid et Gorum Curatione*, Libri. III, 1546. Translated by W.Wright, Putnam, N.Y., 1930.
2. Ibid, p. 9.
3. Ibid, p. 39.
4. Ibid, p. 41.
5. Ibid, p. 35.
6. Ibid, p. 53.
7. Ackerknecht, E.H., *Anticontagionism between 1821 and 1867*. Bull. Hist. Med., 22, p. 562, 1948.
8. Henle, J., Von den Miasmen und Contagien, In his *Pathologische Untersuchungen*, 1840, Translated by G. Rosen, Bull. Hist. Med. 6, p. 911, 1938.
9. Osler, W., In the Introduction to R. Vallery Radot's *The Life of Pasteur*, Translation by R.L. Devonshire, Doubleday, Page and Co., Garden City, N.Y., 1926.
10. Pasteur, L., *Mémoire sur la fermentation appelée lactique*. Comptes Rendue Hebdomadaires Des Sciences de I'Academie des Sciences, 45, p. 913, 1857.
11. Dubos, R., *Louis Pasteur, Free Lance of Science*, p. 63, Little Brown, and Co. Boston, 1950.
12. Redi, F., *Esperienze intorno alla generazione degl'insetti*, Firenze, 1668.
13. Needham, J. T., A summary of some late observations upon the generation, composition, and decomposition of animal and vegetable substances. *Phil. Trans.* no. 490, p. 615, London, 1749.
14. Spallanzani, L., *Opusculi di fisica animale e vegetabile*, 2 vols. Modena, 1776.
15. Pouchet, F., *Hétérogénie ou traité de la génération spontanée, basé sur de nouvelles experiences*, Baillière, Paris, 1859.
16. Vallery-Radot, R., Translation by R.L. Devonshire, Doubleday, Page and Co., p. 108, Garden City, N.Y., 1926.
17. Duclaux, E., *Pasteur, The History of a Mind*, Translation by E. F. Smith, p. 45, W.B. Saunders Co., Philadelphia, 1920.
18. Pasteur, L., *Études sur la maladie des vers à soie*, 2 vols., Gauthier-Villars, Paris, 1870.
19. Billroth, T., *Untersuchungen über die Vegetationsformen von*

Coccobacteria septica und den Antheil, Berlin, 1874.

20. Cushing, H., *The Life of Sir William Osler,* Vol. 1, p. 114, Clarendon Press, Oxford, 1926.
21. Obermeier, O., Vorkommen feinster, eine Eigenbewegung zeigender Faden im Blute von Recurrenskrankheiten. *Zbl. med. Wiss.* 11, p. 145, 1873.
22. von Nägeli, C., *Die niederen Pilze in ihren Beziehungen zu den Infectionskrankheiten und der Gesundheitsspflege*, Munich, 1877.
23. Lister, J., On a new method of treating compound fractures, abscesses, etc., with observations on the condition of suppuration, *Lancet* 1, p. 326, p. 357, p. 387, p. 507, 1867.
24. Lister, J., On the antiseptic principle in the practice of surgery. *Lancet*, 2, p. 353, p. 668, 1867.
25. Pollender, F., Mikroskopische und mikrochemische Untersuchung des Miltzbrandblutes sowie über Wesen und Kur des Milzbrandes. *Vjschr. gerischtl. öff. Med.*, 8, p. 103, 1855.
26. Rayer, P., (with C. Davaine), Inoculation du sang de rate, *C.R. Soc. Biol.*, Paris, 2, p. 141, 1850.
27. Davaine, C., Recherches sur les infusoires du sang dans la maladie connue sous le nom de sang de rate., C.R. Acad. Sci., Paris, 57, p. 220, 1863.
28. Koch, R., Die Aetiologie der Milzbrand-Krankheit begründet auf die Entwicklungsgeschichte des Bacillus anthracis, Beitr. Biol. Pflanzen, 2, p. 277, 1876.
29. Flint, A., *A Treatise on the Principles and Practice of Medicine*, p. 819, Henry C. Lea, Philadelphia, 1867.
30. Semmelweis, I., *Die Aetiologie der Begriff und die Prophylaxis des Kinderbettfiebers*, C.A. Hartleben, Pest, Wien, and Leipzig, 1861.
31. Rindfleisch, G.E., *A Manual of Pathological Histology*, Vol. I, p. 278, English Translation by E.B. Baxter, The New Sydenham Society, London, 1872.
32. von Recklinghausen, F.D., Vortrag in der Würzb. *physik-med. Gesell*, June 10, 1871.
33. Birch-Hirschfeld, F., *Unter. üb. Pyemia,* Leipzig, 1873.
34. Klebs, E., *Beiträge zur pathologischen Anatomie de Schusswunden*, Vogel, Leipzig, 1872.
35. Ref. 17, p. 269.
36. Ibid, p. 270.

37. Koch, R., *Investigations into the Etiology of Traumatic Infective Diseases*, p. 7, Translation by W. Cheyne, The New Sydenham Society, 1880.
38. Ibid, p. 15.
39. Ref. 33, p. 799.
40. Ref. 37, p. 19.
41. Ogston, A., Report on Microorganisms in Surgical Diseases. *Brit. Med.* J. 1, p. 369.
42. Koch, R., *On the Investigation of Pathogenic Organisms*, 1881. Translation by V. Horsley, in *Microparasites in Disease*, Edited by W. Cheyne, p. 40, New Sydenham Society, London, 1886.
43. Petri, R.J., Eine kleine Modification des Koch'schen Plattenverfahrens, *Centralbl. f. Bakteriol. etc.*, 1, p. 279, 1887.
44. Rosenbach, F.J., Microorganisms in Human Traumatic Infective Diseases, in *Microparasites in Disease*, edited by W. Cheyne, p. 261, New Sydenham Society, London, 1886.
45. Fehleisen, F., On Erysipelas, 1882. Translation by L. Ogilvie, in *Microparasites in Disease*, edited by W. Cheyne, p. 261, New Sydenham Society, London,1886.
46. Krause, R.M., Streptococcal Disease, p. 1519, in *Textbook of Medicine*, edited by J.B. Wyngaarden and L. H. Smith, Jr., W.B. Saunders Co., Philadelphia, 1985.
47. Sternberg, G., A fatal form of septicemia in the rabbit produced by the subcutaneous injection of human saliva, National Board of Health Bulletin, Vol. 2, Washington, 1882.
48. Friedländer, C., Ueber Die Schizomyceten bei der acuten fibrinösen Pneumonie, *Virchow's Archiv.*, 87, p. 319, 1882.
49. Sternberg, G., The Etiology of Croupous Pneumonia. *The Medical Record*, New York, 35, p. 281, 1889.
50. Fraenkel, A., Die Mikrococcen der Pneumonie. *Z. klin. Med.*, 10, p. 426, 1886, and 11, p. 437, 1886.
51. Weichselbaum, A., Ueber die Aetiologie der acuten Lungen und Rippenfellentzündungen. *Weiner Med. Jahrbucher*, n. F. 1, p. 483, 1886.
52. Gram, H.C., Ueber die isolirte Färbung der Schizomyceten in Schnitt- und Trockenpräparaten. *Fortschr. Med.*, 2, p. 185, 1884.
53. Budd, W., *Typhoid Fever; Its Nature, Mode of Spreading, and Prevention*. Longmans, London, 1873.
54. Eberth, C.J., Die Organismen in den Organen bei Typhus

abdominalis., *Virchow's Arch.*, 81, p. 58, 1880.
55. Gaffky, Georg, On Etiology of Enteric Fever, in *Microparasites in Disease*, p. 247, Edited by W. Cheyne, New Sydenham Society, London, 1886.
56. Loeffler, F. *Deutsche medicinische Wochenschrift*, No. 39, p. 158, 1908.
57. Drigalski, and Conradi, Zeit. f. Hygiene und Infectionkrankh., 39, 1902.
58. MacConkey, A.T., Bile salt media and their advantagesin some bacteriological examinations. *J. Hyg.*, 8, p. 322, 1908.
59. Widal, F., Sérodiagnostic de la fière typhoide, *Bull. et mém. Soc. méd. d'Hôp. de Paris*, 3rd ser. 13, p. 561, 1896.
60. Gruber, M., and Durham, H.E., Eine neue Methode zur raschen Erkennung des Choleravibrio und des Typhusbacillus, *Münch. med. Wschr.*, 43, p. 285, 1896.
61. Hansen, G.H.A., *Norsk. Mag. f. Laegevidensk*, 4, 9Heft, p. 1, 1874.
62. Neisser, A., Über die Ätiologie des Aussatzes, *Jber. akad. nat. Vereins Breslau* , 57, p. 65, 1879.
63. Neisser, A., Ueber eine der Gonorrhoe eigentümliche Micrococcusform. *Zbl. med. Wiss.*, 17, p. 497, 1879.
64. Bumm, E. von, Der Mikro-organismus der gonorrhoischen Schleimhaut- Erkrankungen, Gonococcus- Neisser. *Dtsch. med. Wschr.*, 11, p. 508, 1885.
65. Weichselbaum, A., Ueber die Aetilogie der akuten Meningitis cerebrospinalis. *Fortschr. Med.*, 5, p. 573, p. 620, 1887.
66. Councilman, W.T., Mallory, F.B., and Wright, J.H., *Epidemic Cerebrospinal Meningitis and Its Relation to Other Forms of Meningitis*, Boston, 1898.
67. Yersin, A.E.J., La peste bubonique. *Ann. Int. Pasteur,* 9, p. 589, 1895.
68. Howard-Jones, N., Kitosato, Yersin and the Plague Bacillus, *Clio Medica*, 10, p. 23, 1975.
69. Ogata, M., Ueber die Pestepidemie in Formosa. *Zbl. bakt.*, 21, p. 769, 1897.
70. Klencke, P.F., *Ueber die Ansteckung und Verbreitung der Scrophelkrankheit bei Menschen durch den Genuss der Kuhmilch.*, Kollmann, Leipzig, 1846.
71. Villemin, J., *Etudes sur la tuberculose; preuves rationalles et expérimentalis de sa spécificité et de son inoculabilité*, Baillière,

Paris, 1868.
72. Cohnheim, J., *Die Tuberkulose vom Standpunkte der Infectionslehre.*, A. Edelmann, 1880.
73. Ziehl, F., Zur Färbung des Tuberkel bacillus., *Dtsch. Med. Wschr.*, 8, p. 451, 1882.
74. Koch, R., The Etiology of Tuberculosis, 1882, in *Microparasites in Disease*, Translated by S. Boyd, p. 74, New Sydenham Society, London, 1886.
75. Hirsch, A., *Handbook of Geographical and Historical Pathology*, Vol. 1, p. 394. Translation by C. Creighton, The New Sydenham Society, London, 1883.
76. Koch, R., Ueber die Cholerabakterien., *Dtsch. med. Wschr.*, 10, p. 725, 1884.
77. Brock, T.D., *Robert Koch, A Life in Medicine and Bacteriology*, p. 332, Science Tech Publishers, Madiso, 1988.
78. Klebs, E., Ueber Diphtherie, *Verh. Congr. inn. Med.*, 2, p. 139, 1883.
79. Garrison, E., *An Introduction to the History of Medicine*, 4th Edition, p. 1581, W.B. Saunders Co., Philadelphia, 1929.
80. Loeffler, F., Investigations as to the Significance of Microorganisms in the Production of Diphtheria in Man., 1884, In *Microparasites in Disease*, Translation by T.W. Hime, p. 447, New Sydenham Society, London, 1886.
81. Roux, P., and Yersin, A., Contribution à l'étude de la diphtherie, *Ann. Inst. Pasteur*, 2, p. 629, 3, p. 273, 4, p.385, 1888-1890.
82. Ref. 11, p. 61.
83. Bruce, D., Notes on the Discovery of a Microorganism in Malta Fever. Practitioner, 39, p. 161, 1887.
84. Bruce, D., The Micrococcus of Malta Fever, *Practitioner*, 40, p. 241, 1888.
85. Wright, A.E., and Smith, F., On the application of the serum test to the differential diagnosis of typhoid and Malta fever. *Lancet*, 1, p. 656, 1897.
86. Horrocks, W. H., Preliminary note on goats as a means of propagation of Mediterranean Fever. in *Reports of the Royal Society of London*, Mediterranean Fever Commission, Part III, Harrison and Sons, London, 1905.
87. Bang, B., Die Aetiologie des seuchenhaften ("infectiösen")

Verwerfens., *Z. Thiermed.*, 1, p. 241, 1897.
88. Evans, A., Further studies on Bacterium abortus and related bacteria. II A comparison of Bacterium abortus with Bacterium bronchosepticus and with organisms which cause Malta fever. *J. Infect. Dis.*, 22, p. 580, 1918.
89. Bennett, J., Brucellosis. In Wyngaarden, J. B., and Smith, L., *Textbook of Medicine*, p. 1614, W.B. Saunders, Philadelphia, 1985.
90. Kitosato, S. Ueber infectiosen Tetanus. *Dtsch. med. Wschr.*, 10, p. 842. 1884.
91. Behring, E.A., von, and Kitosato, S., Ueber das Zustandekommen der Diptherieimmunität und der Tetanus- Immunität bei Thieren., *Dtsch. med. Wschr.*, 16, p. 1113, 1890.
92. Shiga, K., Ueber den Dysenteriebacillus., *Zbl. Bakt.*, 24, p. 817, and p. 870., 1898.
93. Gaertner, A., Ueber die Fleischvergiftung in Frankenhausen, A.K. und dem Erreger derselben. *Korrespbl. ärztl. Ver. Thüringen*, 17, p. 573, 1888.
94. Durham, H.E., On an epidemic of gastroenteritis associated with the presence of a variety of the Bacillus enteritidis and with a positive serodiagnostic evidence. *Brit. Med. J.*, 2, p. 600, 1898.
95. Durham, H.E., Some theoretical considerations upon the nature of agglutinins together with further observations upon Bacillus typhi abdominalis, Bacillus enteritidis, Bacillus coli communis, bacillus lactic aerogenes and some other bacilli of allied character. *J. Exp. Med.*, 5, p. 353, 1900-01.
96. Durham, H.E., *Brit. Med.*, 1, p. 1397.
97. Hornick, R.B., Salmonella Infections other than Typhoid Fever. In Wyngaarden, J.B., and Smith, L., *Textbook of Medicine*, p. 1589, W.B. Saunders, Philadelphia, 1985.

CHAPTER XIV

In the field of experimentation, chance favors only the prepared mind.

— Pasteur

Pasteur and the Prevention of Disease

Whereas Robert Koch and his group were initially concerned with isolating, identifying, and proving that specific bacteria with unvarying virulence were the cause of certain diseases and developed elegant methods for doing this, Louis Pasteur, who had been studying microorganisms long before Koch, always had a broader perspective. He had little interest in the intrinsic properties of bacteria, such as their morphology, staining, or even their intricate properties in culture. Rather he was interested in the relationship of bacteria and their environment, whether in a wine vat or in a host animal, and whether it was possible to control their activity. He had always been intrigued by the fact that certain individuals who recovered from certain infectious diseases never contracted the disease a second time. He carefully studied the work of Jenner, who had used an inoculum of cowpox to prevent smallpox. And although he had helped the wine and beer makers solve the problem of "sick" beverages, and showed the silk growers how to minimize infections in their silkworms, he had in the back of his mind hopes of preventing certain maladies in man and animals. The first clue to accomplishing this task started almost as an accident.

Pasteur and his group had been studying chicken cholera, a disease that was killing flocks of chickens in France. He isolated a bacillus in which one drop of the bouillon, in which it had been growing, inoculated into a chicken would kill it in a few hours. These experiments were done in the spring of 1879, and with the interruptions of work due to the university's summer closure, the cultures were not renewed until fall. At that time when the cultures were transferred to new broth and examined under the microscope, there did not appear to be any change in their appearance. However, when a drop was inoculated into a chicken, the animal, which formerly would have quickly died, became only slightly ill and then recovered, which indicated a diminution of virulence. Then when he inoculated this chicken again with bacteria from a newly dead chicken, it did not die or even become ill. Pasteur also found that the bacterium that had lost its virulence did not regain it regardless of the number of times it was subcultured.[1] With regard to the chicken cholera, the following were his conclusions:

> 1. Fowl-cholera is, in the highest degree, an infectious disease.
> 2. The virus is a microscopic parasite which can easily be multiplied by cultivation outside of the bird's body. Hence the possibility of obtaining the virus in a condition of perfect purity, and an irrefutable demonstration that it is the sole cause of the disease and death.
> 3. The virus occurs in conditions of variable virulence. Sometimes the disease is followed by death; sometimes, after producing morbid symptoms of varying intensity it is followed by recovery.
> 4. The differences which can be shown to exist in the power of the virus are not merely the result of observation grounded in natural facts; the experimenter can produce them at will.
> 5. As is commonly the case with infective diseases, fowl cholera does not recur, or rather the severity of the recurrence is in inverse proportion to the greater or less severity of the first attack of the disease, and it is always possible to push the protection so far that no effect of any kind is produced by the inoculation of the most virulent virus.
>
> The time has come for me to offer an explanation with regard to the main assertion upon which the greater part of the preceding propositions is founded, namely, that there are variable degrees of virulence in fowl cholera; assuredly a strange result, when we reflect that the virus of this disease is a microscopic organism which can be worked with in the perfectly pure state in the same way as the yeast of beer, or the mycoderma of vinegar. And yet if we calmly consider this mysterious property of variable virulence, it will be quickly seen that it is probably common to the various species of the group of infective diseases. . . . Do we not also see virulent epidemics die out little by little, again reappear at a later date, and again die out?[2]

These facts caused Pasteur to return to the organism with which he had much experience — anthrax. He had the goal of preparing a vaccine capable of producing immunity in sheep and cattle, which were being devastated by this disease throughout Europe. He was able to attenuate the anthrax bacillus by either growing it at 43 degrees or by putting phenol in the culture medium. These cultures were then used to inoculate herds of sheep, and Pasteur quickly showed that he was able to reduce the incidence of anthrax. Each animal was injected twice, the first time with a lower virulence bacilli, and then twelve days later with a more virulent culture. In 1882, 79,392 sheep were inoculated, and of these only 0.65% contracted anthrax and died compared with an average death rate of 9% in unvaccinated sheep. The vaccine was also very effective in horses and cows.[3]

Pasteur next undertook to study the erysipelas-like disease of hogs called "rouget," which was killing the swine in France. He was able to isolate a bacteria, attenuate it by passing it through rabbits, and then using the less-virulent organism to produce immunity.[4] (This organism, now known as *Erysipelothrix rhusiopathiae*, can be transmitted to meat handlers, but, for economic reasons, no vaccinations are given to animals or humans.)

However, it was the development of the rabies vaccine[5] that was the culmination of Pasteur's brilliant career. It has been speculated that his interest in this disease had its origins in his childhood memories of a rabid wolf charging through his village biting both man and beast, with resulting human fatalities. Although from a purely scientific standpoint, the rabies program was probably no more important than his studies on fermentation, silkworm disease, spontaneous generation, chicken cholera, and anthrax, it was the nature of the rabies work that made the name Pasteur almost a household word in 1886. Rabies did not have the quantitative devastating character of the black plague, cholera, typhus, or yellow fever, but there were very few diseases that had as much drama associated with almost every case, considering the initial violence and trauma by the rabid animal, the anxiety of waiting during the long incubation period, and finally, perhaps, the terrible signs and symptoms leading to death in all cases.

For a period of five years, starting in 1880, Pasteur and his two assistants, Emile Roux and Charles Chamberland carried out a series of experiments that could be considered one of the most brilliant and imaginative in the history of biology. The program had as its goal the attenuation of the rabies virus for use in therapy. The difficulties were enormous compared with the anthrax work. Pasteur, by then almost 60 years old and paralyzed from a stroke, undertook a crusade against a viral disease when most medical people still did not accept the idea that microorganisms were etiological factors in any infectious disease. In addition, the natural course of rabies was unpredictable; incubation periods varied from weeks to months, and not all individuals bitten by rabid animals developed rabies. There was no way of knowing whether a vaccine could be produced to give protection against rabies, particularly after the patient had been bitten by a rabid animal. During the first years of work, all attempts to isolate a causal organism that could be seen microscopically or grown in bacteriological media failed. In retrospect this failure was not surprising, because, as more modern research was to show, the rabies virus was too small to be seen with the light microscope, and it was not possible to grow viruses in non-living media. However, characteristic of Pasteur, his intellectual agility and his mastery of the experimental method always enabled him to devise new techniques when his intuition made him aware that current methods would no longer be fruitful. He eventually developed a method of growing the agent and consistently producing rabies in 6 days by inoculation of nervous tissue from a rabid dog into the brains of rabbits. This being accomplished, he was then able to solve the problem of attenuation of the virus by serially desiccating the brains of rabid rabbits. By inoculating this material into dogs and then allowing these animals to be bitten by other rabid animals, he was able to produce immunological protection against a pathogen he had failed to prove even existed, except indirectly. He presented his data at the International Medical Congress in August 1884, after which great public pressure developed to use the vaccine on humans. In July 1885, against the advice of his chief assistant, Roux, Pasteur released his vaccine to be used on Joseph Meister, a 9-year-old boy who had been severely bitten by a rabid dog. The little boy's life was saved, and by 1886, Pasteur's laboratory was inundated by patients from all over the world. A description has recently been given of those times.[6] During the years 1886–1934, 34,111 individuals bitten by confirmed rabid animals were treated at the Pasteur Institute with a mortality rate of only 0.5%, compared with an average mortality rate of 16% of cases without vaccine treatment.

It is of interest that Robert Koch, who was always an adversary of Pasteur, attempted to minimize the Frenchman's immunization pro-

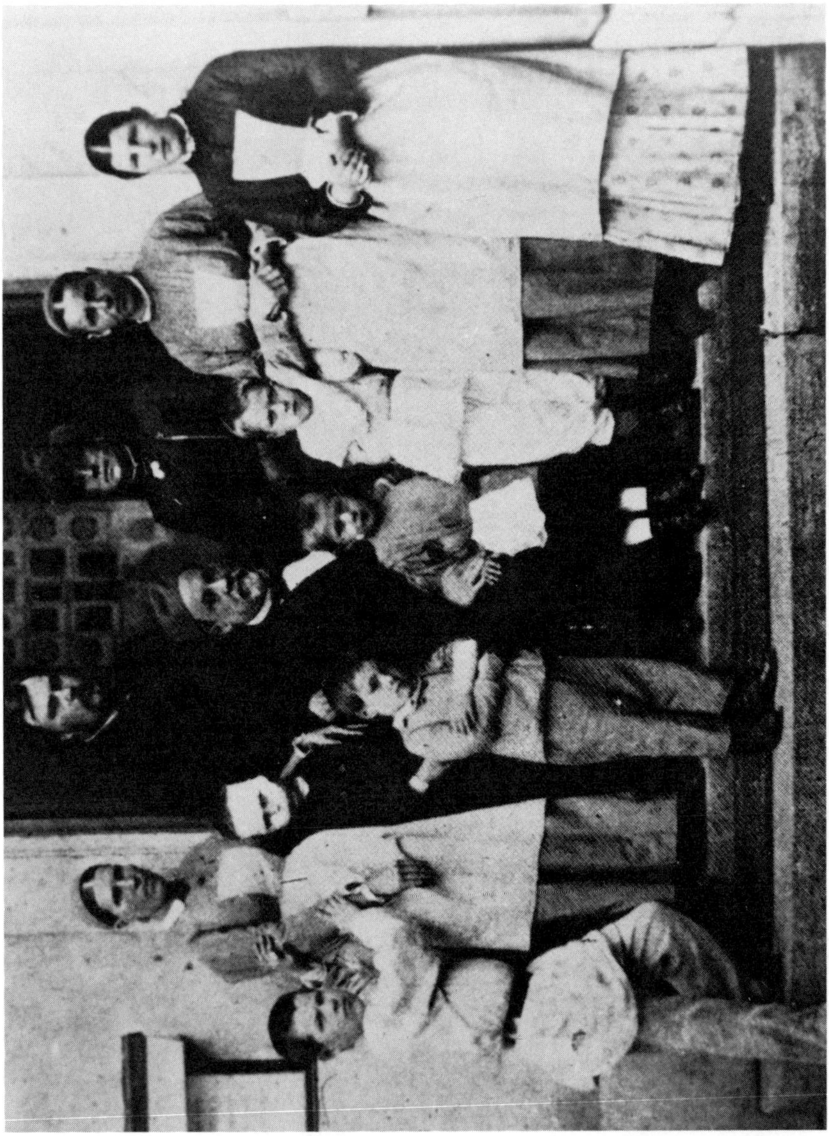

PASTEUR WITH RABIES VICTIMS

grams. As the scientist who worked out the life cycle of anthrax, it upset him that he was not the one to develop the vaccine for anthrax, and for several years minimized the value of Pasteur's anthrax vaccine, stating that it was unreliable and that his cultures of anthrax were impure. Koch also stated in 1881 that "Up to now, Pasteur's work on anthrax has led to nothing."[7] He criticized Pasteur for being optimistic about preparing vaccines for other diseases, and Koch emphasized and pointed out that an episode of gonorrhea, erysipelas, and intermittent fever (malaria) did not preclude the occurrence of another infection. But at the same time Koch embarked on a secret preparation of an extract of the tubercle bacillus, which he called "tuberculin," and was claimed by the German government as a "cure" for tuberculosis. Congratulations were sent from all over the world, including those from Pasteur, who was apparently willing to overlook Koch's denigration of him. But after some clinical trials in 1890, tuberculin was shown to be useless therapeutically, and only of use in diagnosis.[8] This was certainly a humiliating experience for Koch, especially following the successful work of Pasteur on rabies a few years before.

One great significance of Pasteur's work is that he illustrated for the first time that Man, by careful scientific investigations, could intervene effectively and change the course of some of the illnesses against which he had formerly been so helpless. He showed the path of immunotherapy to others, because after his work, preventative vaccination against typhoid, cholera, pertussis, tetanus, diphtheria, plague, and yellow fever followed. Thus of the great enemies of the human species — War, Famine, and Pestilences — the latter has certainly been minimized in most of the highly developed nations of the world. For example, the longevity for a child born in the United States in 1900 was approximately 50 years and at the present time it is more than 70 years.

Historically it is important to restudy the thinking of Pasteur during those early days of microbiology because they reveal a true understanding of the nature of Man and animals in relation to microorganisms. Although in current medical circles, there has been expressed surprise at the activities of new viruses such as HIV, Marburg fever, acute hemorrhagic conjunctivitis, Lassa fever, São Paulo encephalitis, Sudan-Zaire hemorrhagic fever, Creutzfeldt-Jakob disease, and respiratory syncytial disease, and that older diseases such as acute glomerulonephritis, rheumatic fever, scarlet fever, and even tuberculosis has diminished, this would not have surprised Pasteur at all. In fact he would have been puzzled if these transformations of microorganisms had not occurred. He essentially spent most of his life studying the relationship between microorganisms and their hosts and early on recognized and found he could produce a microecological shift in the parasite–host relationship, particularly with regard to virulence. He made these astute observations that:

> (regarding) the possible return of the virulence of a virus which has been attenuated or extinguished, we have obtained, for instance, a bacterium of anthrax, which has lost all virulence for the guinea pig, the rabbit and the sheep. Can it be again rendered active with regard to those species? In the same way we have prepared the microbe (regarding) the possible return of the virus of fowl cholera deprived of all virulence for fowls. At the present time the secret of their return to a virulent condition is merely their growth in the body of certain animals in series. Our bacterium innocuous to guinea pigs is not innocuous to these animals at all ages; but how short is the period during which it is virulent? A guinea pig several years old, one year, six months, one month, a few weeks, . . . and finally just a few days old will not be affected, but one just one day old is killed by inoculation. If now we pass from the first guinea pig one day old, to another, by inoculation of the second with the blood of the first, and then from the second to a third, the virulence increases until any guinea pig regardless of its age can be killed as can a sheep. This return to a virulent condition is of greatest interest in its bearing on the etiology of infective diseases. . . . Thus infectivity appears to us in a new light, which in truth is disquieting humanity, unless, indeed Nature in her evolution through ages past has already met all the opportunities for the production of infectious or contagious maladies, which is exceedingly improbable. A microorganism innocuous for man or for a particular animal, what is it? It is a being which cannot develop in our body, or in the body of that animal; but there is nothing to prove that if this microscopic being penetrates into some other of the thousands and thousands of species in creation, it may not be able to invade it and to render it diseased. Its virulence, strengthened by successive passages through individuals of that species, might pass into a state in which it could attack such or such an animal of larger bulk — man, or some of the domestic animals. In this way new virulences and con-

> tagions might be created. I am very much inclined to believe that it has been in this way that during past ages smallpox, syphilis, plague, yellow fever, etc. have appeared, and that it is owing to phenomena of this kind that from time to time certain great epidemics, such as those of typhus . . . appear.[9]

With these prophetic comments, Pasteur to a great degree was taking a similar point of view of more sophisticated microbiologists one hundred years later. From an anthropocentric position, the production of a deadly infection by a microorganism to an individual or his loved ones is a tragedy, but to Nature it can be a capricious and indifferent aberration of a host–parasite relationship.* Even a missionary devoured by a lion could as easily be regarded as part of the food chain of nature instead of an unfortunate and sad event. Except for green plants, which obtain their energy from the sun and can synthesize amino acids from inorganic minerals, all other living organisms subsist by their ability to gain from other living organisms the requirements for their energy, growth, and reproduction. In this struggle for existence, different stages of behavior are encountered, varying from that of a predatory animal such as Man, who devours plants and animals to survive, to a relationship called symbiosis, where two different organisms live together for mutual advantages. These behavior patterns can be regarded as stages in the general concept of parasitism, which is part of Nature's scheme of things. Ideally the parasite must be of a nature that it can be tolerated by the host to allow the survival of both organisms. If the parasite is poorly adjusted, it may ravage its host or its environment to an extent that neither survives. It is also possible that the microbe produces an immune response in the host that destroys the invader. Teleologically this violates the reproductive intent of Nature. The most efficient parasite is one that lives in harmony with its host so that both can propagate themselves. Although, for the survival of each species, both the parasite and the host must reproduce themselves, and the parasite must also have the additional means of transferring its progeny to another host. This can be done through: fluids emitted from the host such as droplets from the respiratory tract, as in measles, influenza, and the common cold; contact

*The existentialist Camus, in the last paragraph of his novel *The Stranger*, would call this "the gentle indifference of the world," but perhaps in this case the indifference could better be described as "lethal."

with an exudate that touches the skin of another host, as in scabies and impetigo; the mucous membranes, as in gonorrhea, syphilis, herpes, chlamydia, and AIDS; the ingestion of food or water contaminated by excreta and containing the parasite or its larval form, as in typhoid, cholera, amoebic dysentery, and hookworm disease; an intermediate vector or host such as an insect, as in malaria, yellow fever, dengue, or typhus; the placenta, as in AIDS ; needles, as in AIDS, malaria, or hepatitis B.

On the other hand, the production or nonproduction of pathological changes or disease by a given organism can be looked upon as the result of the product of the virulence of a microorganism and the susceptibility of the host ($V \times S$ = constant). These two factors, in turn, depend upon other variables. For example, the virulence can depend on the particular strain or mutation of a microorganism, which can be modified artificially by investigators using such devices as tissue culture, inoculating various animal or different organ systems, or even, in the case of viruses, chemically manipulating their various constituent nucleic acids or proteins (this, of course, is the manner in which immunity without producing severe disease is accomplished). Likewise, the amount of inoculum and the duration of time of exposure of the host, is also able to influence the result. Susceptibility, the other major variable, also varies according to a number of subfactors such as host species, strains of species, genetic factors within a species or individual, age, sex, and the anatomical and physiological condition of a given individual at the time of the infection. With regard to the pathological changes and the signs and symptoms of disease and their duration in a particular situation and individual, these are the result of a race between the ability of the microorganism to propagate and produce damage to specific tissues and cells, and the ability of the defense mechanisms of the host to adapt, neutralize, or otherwise eliminate the microorganism from the body.

The human body has evolved anatomically and physiologically so that infection and destruction is minimized. Man is, for the most part, protected over most of his body by a dry, relatively impermeable skin, which acts as insulation from the external world. However, because of necessity, the following orifices and systems are exposed to the outside world: (1) the mouth for the bringing in of food for energy for the human machine, and the anus for eliminating the unusable food residues; (2) the respiratory passage, mouth and nose, for bringing in oxygen for burning the food and for removing the resulting carbon dioxide and water; (3) the excretory system for the removal of nitrogen waste products from the body cells by way of the blood, for water balance, and, in the case of the male urethra, for the release of sperm cells necessary for propagation of the species; (4) the vagina, or opening to the reproductive tract of the female; (5) the eye, covered by the cornea and sclera but necessary for vision; (6) the nose, which is needed for the sense of smell; (7) the auditory canal for hearing. These openings are avenues of entry for harmful microorganisms, but each has its own mechanisms for minimizing significant invasions. The upper digestive tract has acid, mucus, and bile that can inhibit the growth of microorganisms, and the lower intestinal tract has non-pathogenic organisms such as *E. coli* that will usually overgrow any pathogens. The respiratory tract is lined with cells that have cilia that push the bacteria into the digestive tract, and there are also mucous cells that coat the bacteria and allow the white blood cells to phagocytize them. The excretory system is flushed with normally sterile urine, which keeps bacteria from ascending from the urethra to the bladder and kidneys. The eyelid motion together with the tear glands wash any bacteria that attach to the conjunctiva, cornea, or sclera into the corner of the eye or down the tear ducts into the nasal cavity. The auditory canal has cerumen to keep bacteria to a minimum, and the tympanic membrane blocks entry into the middle ear. These are the primary barriers to invasion by microorganisms. It is true that some pathogens, such as group A streptococci, *staphylococcus aureus*, pneumococci, diphtheria organisms, meningococci, and *H. influenza*, can sometimes inhabit the upper respiratory tract and remain in a microecological balance with the human until resistance diminishes and the pathogens can multiply. Clinical signs appear as the pathogens multiply and extend into areas that are normally sterile, or they produce toxins, which are absorbed into the lymphatics or blood and produce systemic effects. It is then that the secondary defenses or the cellular and humoral immune system in the form of polymorphonuclear cells, T type lymphocytes, along with monocytes (macrophages), can attack the microorganism directly. B type lymphocytes, producing soluble antibodies to inactivate the pathogens, join with the complement system to sometimes aid in the process. The result of this secondary defense in the case of bacteria is inflammation, and, in other cases such as virus invasion where inflammation is minimal, the result is systemic symptoms. The brilliance of Pasteur's experimental work allowed him to utilize the mechanism of immunity for the benefit of Mankind, but as discussed before, the French worker did not seem to have much patience with esoteric theories that did not lead to practical experiments. It seems that his idea of the mechanism of immunity was quite simple, either the microorganism permanently depleted an essential nutrient in the host and could no longer grow, as in the case of exhaustion of a substrate in a test tube, or a new poison was produced by the body to prevent a second invasion of the virulent microorganism. The latter idea had some validity if the later-discovered antibodies could be considered a poison to the microorganism, but the possibility of a permanent loss of an essential substance necessary for the growth of a pathogen, considering the length of time of immunity was not realistic, even though Pasteur thought it could be a trace element such as cesium or rubidium that might take a long time for the body to replenish. With the work of rabies and the resulting administrative responsibilities that went with this discovery, and the fact that he was in poor health and in the last stages of his career, Pasteur was not able to investigate the mechanism of immunity. Had he had the time, there is little doubt that with his chemical training he would have been exchanging important experimental results with his counterpart in Germany, Paul Ehrlich. But he died a hero, not only to France, but to the entire world.

Bibliography

1. Duclaux, E., *Pasteur, The History of a Mind*, p.280, English Translation by R. Smith and F. Hedges, W.B. Saunders Co. Philadelphia, 1920.
2. Pasteur, L., De l'atténtuation du virus due choléra des poules. Comptes Rendus, 91, 1880. Translated in *Microparasites in Disease* by D. Williams, p. 551, New Sydenham Society, London, 1886.
3. Chamberland, C., and Pasteur, L., Le charbon et la vaccination charbonneuse, Tignol, Paris, 1883, Translated in part by D. Williams in *Microparasites in Disease*, p. 560 New Sydenham Society, London, 1886.
4. Pasteur, L., and Thuillier, L. La vaccination du rouget des porcs à l'aide du virus mortel atténué de cette maladie, Comptes Rendues, 97, 1883. Translated by D. Williams in *Microparasites in Disease*, p. 619, New Sydenham Society, London, 1886.
5. Pasteur, L., Méthode pour prevenir la rage après morsure. *C.R. Acad. Sci. (Paris)*, 101, p. 765, 1885.
6. Malkin, H.M., Louis Pasteur and "La Rage"- 100 Years Ago, *Persp. Biol. and Med.*, 30,1986.
7. Ref. 3, p. 590
8. Koch, R., Weitere Mittheilungen über ein Heilmittel gegen Tuberkulose. *Dsch. Med. Wschr.*, 16, p. 1029, 1890.
9. Ref. 3, pp. 566-568.

CHAPTER XV

> Medical discovery . . . requires two rather rare qualities — an acute instinct for the right direction, and a burning perserverance in following it up.
>
> — Ronald Ross

Animal Parasites in Pathology

Besides bacteria, it is necessary to consider another group of extrinsic factors in the production of human disease — the animal parasites. In the last decade of the twentieth century, it has been estimated that of these animal parasites malaria and schistosomes each infect 600 million people and ascaris and trichuris each inhabit one billion individuals.[1] As population and poverty increase, particularly in Africa and Asia, it is likely that these numbers will increase.

The ancient physicians were aware of the existence of macroscopic parasites, such as *Ascaris lumbricoides*, the beef tape worm, the pork tapeworm, and the pinworm. They also knew of the guinea worm, *Dracuncula medinensis,* which could be removed, according to Moses, by winding it around a stick, and of schistosomiasis, which was recognized as an entity although its parasitic nature was more obscure. The liver fluke, *Fasciola hepatica,* was found in 1379 by Jehan de Brie in the liver of a sheep, and Spallanzani later studied it in more detail. Francesca Redi (1626–1697) wrote the first textbook on parasitology in 1684[2] in which he described the genital organs of ascaris and its ova and also described more than 100 different species of parasites in different animals. On the basis of this work, he is fairly called the "father of parasitology." In the eighteenth century Johan Goeze, a German pastor, wrote a book[3] that consisted of almost 500 pages with many drawings of parasites. He divided the parasites in Man into eleven groups, was able to differentiate the beef and pork tapeworm, and also found a scolex of the *Echinococcus* organism. However, it was in the nineteenth century that parasitology made its most significant advances.

Karl Rudolphi, the teacher of Johannes Müller, made a major improvement in the classification of and described over 900 different species in his two-volume book[4] published in 1808–1810. He described three species of vesicular hydatid, was the first to use the name "echinococcus," and also used the term "trematode" for a group of parasites that he characterized as being "pierced with holes." In 1842, Johannes Steenstrup (1813–1897) noted for the first time and described "an alternation of generations" in the life cycle of liver flukes in water birds,[5] in which the progeny of a parasite does not resemble the parent but does undergo a transformation before reverting morphologically to the form of the adult parent. F. Dujardin in his *Histoire naturelle des helminthes* (Paris, 1848) gave detailed descriptions of flatworms and used the term "proglottides." In 1851, Bilharz found the dwarf tapeworm, *Hymenolepsis nana* in the small intestine of a boy in Egypt and also the *Schistosoma haematobium* as the cause of hematuria. Then, C. Davaine, who also worked on anthrax, showed the importance of the microscopic examination of the feces for ova in diagnosing helminthiasis in 1860.[6] A little later, T.S. Cobbold (1828–1886), England's distinguished helminthologist, published a large book[7] that summarized all of the animal parasite work up to 1864. As pointed out by Foster,[8] it is interesting that the early work on parasites was done by zoologists and that the field of parasitology was well established by the 1860s, almost twenty years before that of bacteriology. Such problems as the complex life cycle of *Echinococcus granulosus* required the type of study of such zoologists as R. Leuckart (1823–1898)[9] and F. Kuchenmeister (1821–1890).[10] The facts were also that animal parasites usually produced chronic, sporadic, or isolated disease in humans in Europe and did not produce the acute, dramatic pestilences as those whose etiologies were bacterial, viral, or rickettsial. Therefore, the animal parasites did not gain as much attention. Also, it was in the tropics that many of the animal parasites did their major harm, and, until the European countries colonized this area, there was little concern. There were a few exceptions, and these will be discussed along with some of the important parasites likely to affect the future history of the struggling countries of Africa and Asia.

Trichinosis

Trichinosis was without doubt present for thousands of years, not only as a disease entity but also with regard to etiology since there are biblical prohibitions against the eating of pork by the Hebrews. The first description of the microscopic worm is usually attributed to James Paget (1814–1899) when he was a medical student performing dissections in London, and Richard Owen (1804–1892) in 1835, although Peacock in

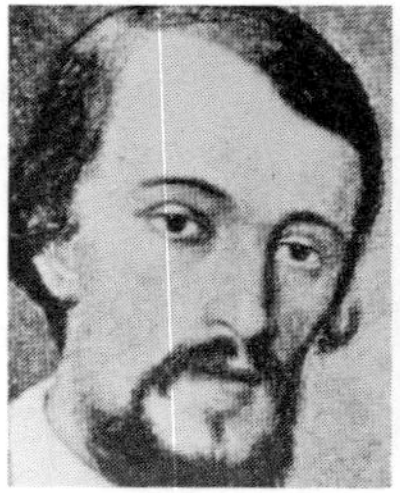
T. Bilharz

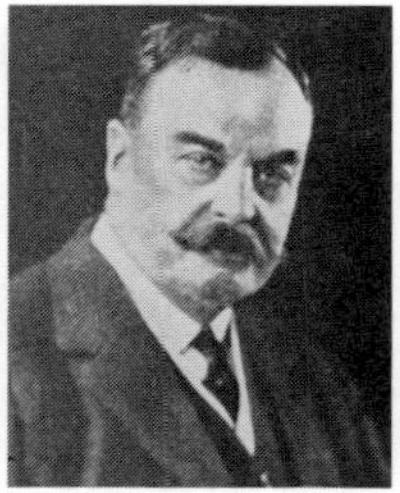
D. Bruce

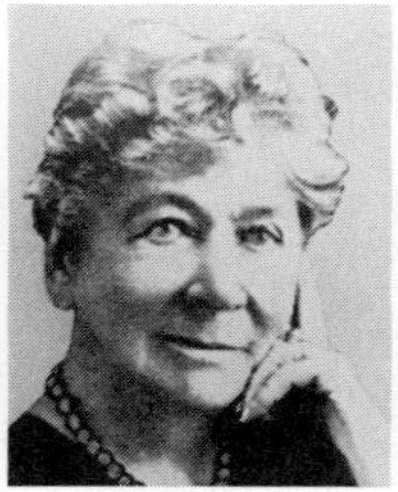
M. Bruce

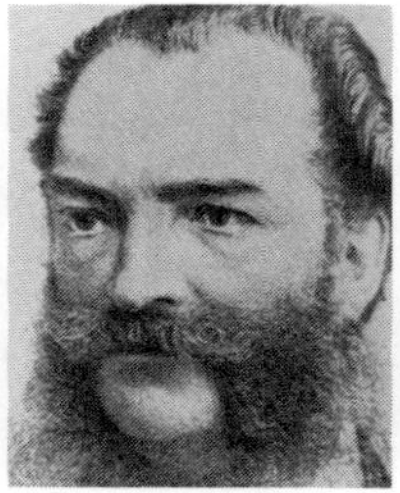
T. Cobbold

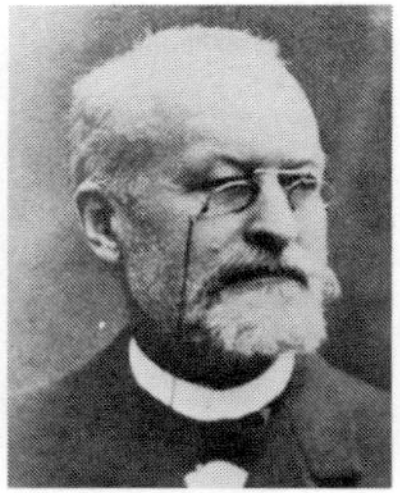
A. Laveran

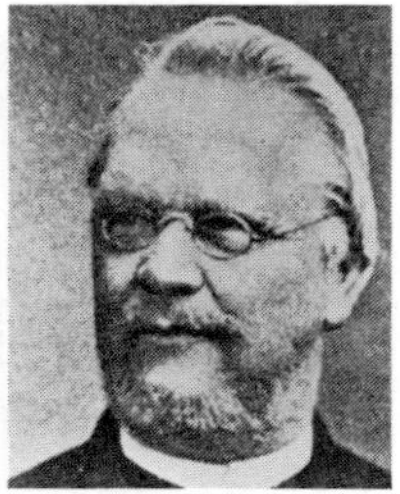
R. Leuckart

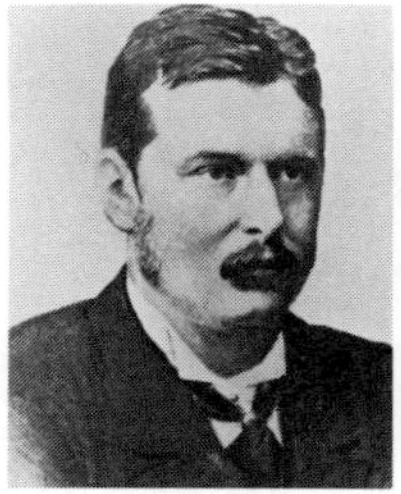
P. Manson

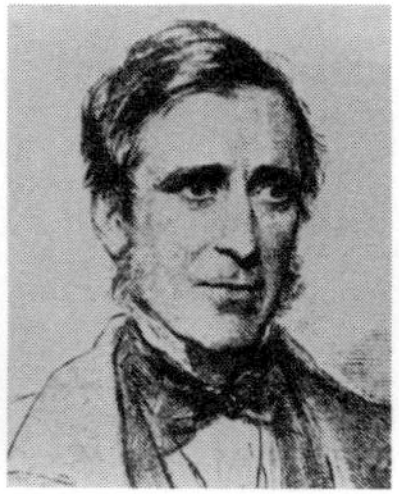
J. Paget

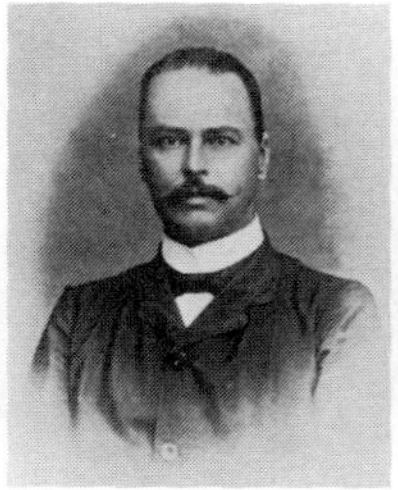
R. Ross

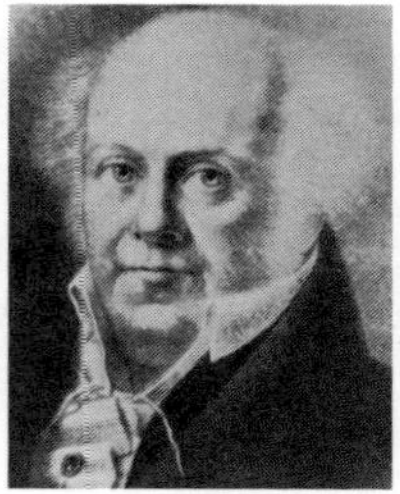
K. Rudolphi

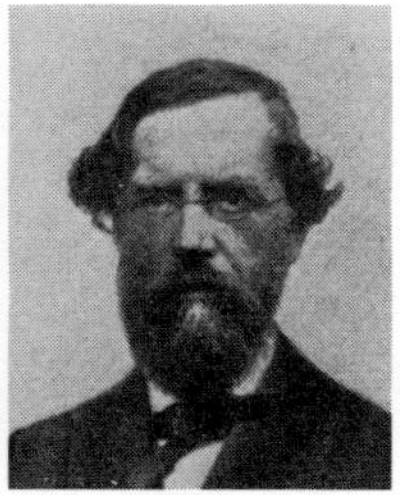
O. Wucherer

FAMOUS PARASITOLOGISTS

1828 and Hilton in 1832 had made macroscopic observations of the parasites in the muscles of cadavers. Paget, however, was interested in natural history, and, whereas his teachers and fellow students saw these hard white particles in the muscles of their anatomical specimens and simply complained about them dulling their scalpels, Paget took some of the specimens to the British Museum. There, he was first referred to Robert Brown, the botanist and discoverer of the nucleus of the cell and Brownian movement, who, in spite of telling Paget he had no interest, "Thank God," in animal parasites, allowed Paget to use his microscope and quickly draw sketches of the encysted worm. Paget presented his discovery to the Abernethian Society. Shortly after this Richard Owen, the famous comparative anatomist, studied the worm in more detail and, while giving credit to Paget for the discovery, gave a more detailed description of the parasite to the Zoological Society and gave it the name of *Trichina spiralis,*[11] which was changed in 1896 to *Trichinella spiralis*. However, the organism was not associated with any disease until Henry Wood, an English practitioner, a few months later attended a man who became acutely ill with muscle pain and died three weeks later. He had the characteristic encysted worms as described by Owen, leading Wood to the conclusion that "the presence of the animal is as consistent with an acute disease as with a chronic."[12] This work was generally ignored, and the next several years were spent by zoologists studying the internal structure of the parasite. Then in 1846, Joseph Leidy (1823–1891) found the parasite in the muscles of pigs,[13] and G. Herbst[14] in 1852 found that by feeding the muscle of an infected animal to uninfected ones (young puppies) he could find worms in large numbers in the muscles after a few months. R. Leuckart[15] was the first to elucidate the life cycle of the trichinosis parasite, finding that adult worms, which are less than 4 mm in length, mate in the intestine of the host. Over the many decades that followed, the consensus of investigators was that the female parasite produces larvae that then invade the small lymphatic and blood vessels in the walls of the duodenum and jejunum, move to the heart, and then from the arterial system are able ultimately to infect all of the muscles of the body. In 1860, F. Zenker (1825–1898) found many unencysted trichinosis larvae in the muscles of a girl who died after an acute illness with severe muscular and abdominal pain and edema; shortly before her illness, she had eaten raw pork while preparing sausages.[16] Zenker examined the sausages and found encapsulated trichinosis larva present. This pathologist thus proved conclusively that trichinosis in humans is transmitted by eating infested pork and that the result can be a severe acute illness leading to death. Rudolf Virchow[17] in a careful systematic study of trichinosis clarified some of the details of the infection, not only from a study of the life cycle of the parasite but also the histological changes in the tissues.[17] Most importantly, however, he was able to implement a preventative program for meat inspection in Germany in 1872 that over a period of time essentially eliminated trichinosis as a problem in that country. In the United States, it has been estimated that approximately 150,000–300,000 individuals are infected each year and that there are 1.5 million presently infected. On the other hand, the incidence of clinical trichinosis has diminished to less than 100 per year, with only 2–4 resulting deaths.[18] This has come about, not only because of meat inspection techniques, but also because hogs are primarily corn-fed and not allowed to eat scraps of meat from any of one hundred different possible animal hosts.

Schistosomiasis

Calcified eggs of *Schistosoma haematobium* have been found in the kidneys of Egyptian mummies, proving that the disease was prevalent in 1200 B.C. However, the first known Europeans to become infested with the parasites were the soldiers of Napoleon's army in Egypt during the years 1799–1801 during their ill-fated campaign there. There were many cases of hematuria, which, although the etiology was not known at the time, undoubtedly was related in many cases to the schistosome parasite. New light was shed on the problem by a young German parasitologist, Theodor Bilharz (1825–1862), who went to Egypt in 1850 as the assistant of Wilhelm Greisinger (1817–1868) to study hookworm disease but also to take advantage of the opportunity to discover other parasites. In 1851 Bilharz found the parasite in the mesenteric nodes of an individual from Cairo, and shortly after found ova in the urine of patients.[19] It is interesting that following Bilharz's observation, other prosectors found the parasite in as many as 30% of bodies, and others began finding the eggs in urine, indicating that, just as in the case of James Paget, it is only a few individuals who discover the significance of what many others have probably seen but chose to ignore. Cobbold, in 1870, studied the hatching of the urinary ova, noted the similarity of the larvae to those of the liver fluke, and proposed an intermediary such as a mollusc, but was not able to identify one.[20] In any case, the parasite was named *Bil-*

harzia haematobium in honor of Bilharz who died at 37 years, but the name was later changed to *Schistosoma haematobium.* It was first thought that schistosomiasis was transmitted by drinking or swallowing the larva, but, in 1894, the physician G.S. Brock in South Africa noted that boys who played in water pools where the disease was common exhibited itching and redness of the skin after a short period of time, and he suggested that perhaps the parasite entered through the skin.[21]

In the meantime there had been noticed in Japan throughout the century a disease characterized by bloody diarrhea, cirrhosis, ascites, enlarged spleen, and generalized wasting. Then, with autopsies becoming more common in Japan in the 1890s, characteristic ova were found in the liver of victims of the disease, which led to a belief that a parasite was the etiological factor in the disease. Then in 1904, Katsurada found identical ova in the feces of individuals with the disease; by dissecting cats found in the same locality, he was able to demonstrate, in some of them, the same ova in the portal veins.[22] In addition, he was able to produce the disease in cats by immersing their legs in pools of water where individuals were thought to have acquired the condition. He called the parasite *Schistosoma japonicum*, and, shortly after in 1905, Catto found the parasite in humans.[23] However, there developed much confusion among parasitologists because initially the adult form of *S. japonicum* and *S. haematobium* appeared to be almost identical, but the ova of *S. japonicum* had no spine and those of *S. haematobium* had a terminal spine. Some of the more renown parasitologists were reluctant to state that the two ova came from different organisms because they thought the spines could be artifactual. However, Patrick Manson, working in 1903 with material from the West Indies, identified, from another schistosome, ova that had a lateral spine and noted that the patient did not have the typical hematuria associated with *S. haematobium*, but rather had intestinal symptoms, and he suggested that the parasites were different.[24] Over the years it became clear that there were three common types of schistosome; *S. haematobium*, found by Bilharz in Egypt, characterized by hematuria, primarily affecting the urinary tract, and primarily located in Africa; *S. mansoni*, which produces intestinal and liver disease and is primarily a disease of the Western hemisphere; and *S. japonicum*, which also produces intestinal and liver damage but is primarily confined to the Far East. Then on the basis of the early work of Katsurada, two Japanese investigators during the years 1913 through 1915 were able to elucidate the life cycle of *S. japonicum* through the small snail, *Katayama nosophora*, along with cutaneous transmission into the animal host.[25] With this information, the British War Office sent R.T. Leiper (1881–1961) in 1915 to Egypt to clarify the problem because of the danger of schistosomiasis to the troops in Africa during World War I. Leiper accumulated as many fresh water molluscs as possible in an area where *S. haematobium* was known to have a high incidence in the population. He placed these molluscs in water and either examined it periodically for free swimming cercariae or dissected the liver of the snails looking for the parasite as sporocysts. This investigator was able to show that there were two different snail host species, one of which gave rise to adults parasites whose ova had lateral spines (*S. mansoni*) and another that produced ova with terminal spines (*S. haematobium*).[26] This confirmed Manson's concept of two distinct species producing different diseases. Thus, sixty years after Bilharz's discovery, the mechanism of the production of schistosomiasis in Egypt and in Japan was almost completely elucidated. The final proof that the *S. haematobium* entered through the skin was made by the heroic parasitologist Claude H. Barlow in Egypt during the 1940s. Barlow allowed cercariae to enter his skin and then noted the characteristic development of the disease when the ova appeared in his stools after 77 days and in his urine after 106 days.[26a]

Hookworm

It is estimated that 600 million people are infested with hookworm in the world and approximately 700,000 in the United States. The clinical disease was recognized in antiquity in Egypt and in China. However, it was less common in Europe and consequently not studied from a scientific standpoint until the eighteenth century when it was common among the slaves in the New World. Although it produced anemia just as malaria did, the characteristic fever and enlarged spleen of malaria quickly distinguished it from hookworm infestation. Also, although it was not known at the time, the anemia in hookworm disease is hypochromic and caused by blood loss from the tiny lesions produced by the worms in the intestine. Angelo Dubini (1813–1902), a physician in Milan, discovered the hookworm in 1838 in the intestine of a peasant and gave it the name *Ancylostoma duodenale*, but he did not relate it to any clinical signs or symptoms.[27] In 1850, when Greisinger and Bilharz were in Egypt studying the hookworm there, they suggested that it might be the cause of anemia but could not establish any proof. Then in 1866,

Otto Wucherer (1820–1873), a physician in Bahia, examined a negro slave who was suffering from severe anemia.[28] Being one of those unusual practicing physicians who was not satisfied with a superficial diagnosis, he read some current literature and found the work of Greisinger in which he suggested that "Egyptian chlorosis" might be caused by hookworm infestation. The patient died the next day, and Wucherer persuaded the authorities to allow him to perform a postmortem examination on the abdomen. On opening the duodenum he found the ancylostoma. He followed up this observation by performing autopsies on twenty other severely emaciated patients; in five, who were severely anemic, he found the hookworm. He sent specimens to both Greisinger in Germany and Cobbold in England who confirmed the parasite. In 1878, Grassi showed that a hookworm infestation in a living patient could be determined by finding the ova in the feces.[29] This was an important finding because shortly after, it was found that Italians working on the St. Gotthard tunnel in the Alps developed severe anemia and it was found that there were always hookworm ova in their feces. The same situation occurred in both German and English mines where there were no measures taken to prevent fecal contamination of the soil and mud. The incidence of hookworm infestation in some instances was as high as 50%, and only preventing these individuals from working in the mines lowered the incidence. At that time it was believed and proven that the parasite could be transmitted from individual to individual by ingestion of the ova. However, it was found by Arthur Loos, a student of Leuckart, that newly hatched larvae could enter the body through the skin where it produced redness and itching.[30] This was confirmed by some elegant studies of medical officer C.A. Bentley in Assam in 1902. Bentley, like Wucherer and Robert Koch, showed that natural curiosity, initiative, and keen observation combined with well-planned but simple experiments can result in monumental discoveries. He proved that the well-known "ground itch" was produced by hookworm larvae penetrating the skin.[31]

In 1902, Allen J. Smith, a comparative pathologist from the University of Pennsylvania, saw a case of hookworm disease in a patient in Galveston, Texas, in which he thought that the adult worm appeared to be different from the *Ancylostoma duodenale* and sent the specimen to Charles W. Stiles of the U.S. Public Health Service. Stiles agreed with Smith and named the hookworm *Necator americanus*, and it was realized that this parasite was the one that was predominant in North and South America.[32]

It was recognized at that time that there were thousands of cases of anemia in Puerto Rico, and Walter W. King of the U.S. Public Health Service and Assistant Surgeon B.K. Ashford of the Medical Corps of the U.S. Army, working together in 1903, attempted to determine if this anemia was due to hookworm disease. They not only found the hookworm ova of the new *Necator americanus* in most of those with severe anemia, but they were able to elicit from more than 90% of these patients that they also had suffered from small lesions of the skin with redness and itching.[33] These men then implemented a program not only to treat these patients by eliminating the hookworms but also to teach prevention of soil contamination with human feces. Before this program, it was estimated that hookworm was one of the major causes of death in Puerto Rico. The success of the Puerto Rico program was called to the attention of the Rockefeller Foundation, and one million dollars was given to attempt to eradicate hookworm in the southern United States over a five-year period starting in 1909. Traveling clinics visited almost every rural community in the area, performing fecal examinations for ova, educating the populace on prevention, and treating worm-infested persons with thymol.[34]

Filariasis

The human is the major, definitive host for seven species of filarial nematodes. *Wuchereria bancrofti* and *Brugia malayi* are the principal causative agents for "filariasis," which is a disease of the lymphatics and is present throughout the tropics. These organisms were the cause of the "elephantiasis" known to the ancients. The other important member of this group is *Onchocerca volvulus*, which produces the skin and eye lesions of onchocerciasis in Africa, Central America, and parts of South America. It is important to note that the filarial nematodes in some areas may infect most of the inhabitants, but only some individuals show severe disease whereas others may only have minimum symptoms or be asymptomatic. This, of course, is Nature's manner of keeping both the parasite and the host alive and reproducing, although the parasite appears not to care about keeping the hosts in optimal health. Jean Demarquay (1811–1875) first saw microfilaria in the hydrocele fluid of a patient in 1863, while practicing surgery in Havana.[35] Then, Otto Wucherer, the same Brazilian practitioner who found that hookworm was responsible for severe anemia, was looking for the ova of the schistosome parasite in the urine of a patient with chyluria and found filarial worms instead. Over the next two years he found more patients with filaria in their urine and finally published his findings in the *Bahia Medical Gazette* in 1868.[36] Shortly after, T.R. Lewis (1841–1886) in Calcutta found the same microfilaria in blood and urine.[37] Then in 1876, Joseph Bancroft (1836–1894) in Brisbane sent specimens from chylous urine to England, where Cobbold recognized them as embryos and encouraged Bancroft to look for the adults. Eventually, he found them in a lymphatic abscess and sent them to Cobbold who named them *Filaria bancrofti*.[38] But the life cycle was still a mystery, as were the reasons for the "elephantiasis," and, most importantly, the nature of the transmission of the parasite from one person to another was still completely unknown. This was the problem that Patrick Manson endeavored to solve.

Patrick Manson (1844–1922) received his medical degree in 1866 at Scotland's Aberdeen University. Interested in adventure, he obtained an appointment as a British medical officer in Formosa and later in Amoy, China, where for the next 17 years he gave medical care to the ship crews that arrived. He also had a private practice of surgery and medicine for the Chinese and Europeans there. The exception was the year 1874–1875 when he returned to London and spent a good deal of time studying what was known regarding chyluria and elephantiasis at the British Museum. It was there he learned of T.R. Lewis's observations of microfilaria in the blood and decided that he would try to solve the problem of the life cycle of the parasite and the mystery of its transmission. Armed with a new microscope, he went back to Amoy in 1876 where he discovered that microfilaria occurred in the blood of 9% of the Chinese and that the incidence among older Chinese was as high as 33%, but because so many of these individuals were not ill, he concluded that in most cases no clinical disease was present, and stated that:

> And so with chyluria, lymph–scrotum, varicose glands and elephantiasis of the scrotum — they are the result of the presence of the parasite, but by no means the necessary consequence.[39]

Manson guessed that the clinical disease was the result of the adult blocking the lymphatic circulation, but, because of the prohibition of performing autopsies in Amoy, it was Joseph Bancroft who found the adult worm in 1877, and Lewis also recovered it a few months later in a case of scrotal elephantiasis. Although Cobbold had suggested naming the new nematode *Filaria bancrofti*, fellow physicians from Brazil championed the work of Wucherer, who first found the filaria in chylous urine, and the name ultimately adopted was *Wuchereria bancrofti*. But it was Manson who was intrigued by the question of how the parasite went from one individual to another. Because it did not inhabit the intestine, it was unlikely that it was expulsed through the digestive system, and because it did not always produce chyluria, it was not likely that the urinary tract was the system through which the parasite left the body. However, because the blood and lymphatic system was the major site of the microfilaria, Manson concluded that it was likely that they escaped from the blood through some common bloodsucking insect, and his first guess was a mosquito. He then fed mosquitoes on a patient whose blood had many microfilaria and studied the mosquito, killing them in sequence until he thought he had seen all the stages in the larval production. In 1878, he reported his findings in *The Daily Telegraph*:

> . . . after many months of work, often following up false scents, I ultimately succeeded in tracing the filaria through the stomach wall into the abdominal cavity, and then into the thoracic muscles of the mosquito. I ascertained that during the passage the little parasite increased enormously in size. It developed a mouth, and alimentary canal and other organs. . . . Manifestly it was on the road to a new human host.[40]

This monumental discovery at first was treated with great scepticism on the part of other investigators, and Leuckart, the most eminent German parasitologist, did not believe Manson's observations. Manson, himself, thought that the larva left the mosquito when it drowned in water after laying its eggs, which was understandable because at that time it was not known that the female mosquito needed to feed on animal blood for the maturation of her eggs before laying her eggs in water. Also it was not known that the life span of the female mosquito was as long as fifteen weeks, which would have been a long enough period for her to transmit the larva to a new host during her bloodsucking period. But it was not until sixteen years later that this was shown to be the case by Thomas Bancroft,[41] and Ronald Ross proved that this was the manner in which malaria was transmitted. In 1884, Manson went to Hong Kong where he was appointed the dean of a new western-style medical school. He also developed a large practice there, and, by 1889 and a comparatively wealthy man, he returned to London with hopes of retiring, but financial setbacks made it necessary for him to practice again. He soon became a popular lecturer on tropical diseases and became the principal physician to the Seaman's Hospital Society, dealing with diseases that were brought back to England from all the tropical colonies of its empire. Soon after, under his leadership, the London School of Tropical Medicine began to evolve in 1897.

Malaria and Ronald Ross

Malaria for centuries was thought to be produced by poisonous emanations from marshes and damp ground. Hippocrates, in his book on epidemics, described periodic fevers and divided them into types: quotidian, tertian, quartan, and subtertian. Speculations that malaria could be produced by small parasites can be found in the literature going back 2000 years ago to Varro and Columella. Then during the eighteenth century, it was discussed more frequently. Lancisi (1624–1720) believed that the "animalcula" arose from putrefaction of vegetable matter in swamps, which were inhaled and spread to the blood, where they multiplied.[42] During the first part of the nineteenth century this concept had its supporters, although others believed that the effluvia was simply a poison rather than a living material. The first clue to the etiology of malaria came in 1847 when Meckel recognized that the dark color of the spleen in malarial cases was due to a pigment.[43] Virchow then noted that the pigment was intracellular in some of the white blood corpuscles.[44] It was Klebs and Tomassi-Crudeli in 1879 who excited the medical community when they reported a bacilli in the soil of malarial districts that they were able to culture and produce malarial symptoms in inoculated animals.[45] Their findings were accepted as valid although many other microbiologists were unable to repeat their results. Then, in 1880, Charles Louis Laveran (1845–1922), a French army surgeon stationed in Algeria, was looking at fresh blood from a malarial patient and made an unusual observation:

> In 1880, as I was trying to account for the mode of formation of the pigment in the palustral blood, I was led to see that besides melaniferous leukocytes, spherical hyaline corpuscles without nucleus could be seen, and also very characteristic crescent shaped bodies. I had proceeded thus far with my

> researches, and was still hesitating whether these elements were parasites, when on November 6, 1880, on examining the pigmented spherical bodies mentioned above, I observed, on the edge of several of these elements, movable filaments or flagella, whose extremely rapid and varied movements left no doubt as to their nature.[46]

When the unknown Laveran published his findings together with his drawings of these organisms, he initially received scant attention, although it was subsequently confirmed by E. Richard.[47] The astute, self-trained American microbiologist George Sternberg, who had not been able to confirm the work of Klebs and Tomassi-Crudeli, was also dubious about Laveran's work and wrote that:

> We cannot doubt that a true account has been given in both cases [Laveran and Richard] of what the observers believe they have seen. But there is a wide field of doubt as to the deductions made from the various observations recorded; for in microscopical studies of the blood made with high powers there is a great liability of error and to misinterpretation of what is seen.[48]

But at a meeting of the Association of American Physicians in 1886, the eminent physicians William Osler, George Sternberg, and William Councilman had this historical discussion following a paper given by Councilman, in which he described observations similar to those of Laveran and Richard and later Italian protozoologists Marchiafava and Celli in patients with malaria. The conversation is given in its entirety since it reveals the difficulty of the acceptance of new ideas in medicine:

> **Osler:** I have had the opportunity of examining six cases of acute malaria. . . . There were present within the red corpuscles such bodies as are represented (here). The number of the corpuscles containing them was variable, sometimes four or five in a single field of a one-twelfth immersion, sometimes many more. . . . I am not prepared to give a positive opinion as the nature of these bodies. They look to me more like vacuoles or areas of hyaline transformation than definite organisms. Secondly, there appear in certain of these vascular spaces solid bodies. . . . That these bodies actually represent organisms, I am sceptical."

> **George Sternberg:** I have seen the body in question, and have observed its amoeboid movements in the blood of a patient . . . at Rome. . . . I can hardly conceive that I was looking at a vacuole as suggested by Dr. Osler, and moreover, the fact that there is something in the red corpuscles which is differentiated by staining seems to exclude the idea of vacuoles.
>
> **Councilman:** I think that Dr. Osler would have received a more definite idea of the bodies if he had examined the stained specimens under the microscope. Frequently one finds in the stained preparations apparently several bodies . . .[49]

The skeptical Osler went back to Philadelphia General Hospital, where malaria was common in those days, and spent the sweltering summer of 1886 over his microscope examining the blood of approximately 70 patients suspected of having malaria. He confirmed the work of Laveran and Councilman and went on to write several papers on malaria[50] but always referred back to his discussion following Councilman's paper as "speaking in the fullness of my ignorance." As a clinician, he emphasized the importance of making the diagnosis of malaria by the examination of the blood, since at that time every fever was generally called "typho-malaria" and treated with quinine. To the physicians of the 1880s and those for hundreds of years before, fever with severe shivering was considered caused by a mysterious nocturnal miasm, and it took years to convince physicians that in malarial regions, the examination of the blood would prove the most valuable method of diagnosis of malaria. A few years later at Johns Hopkins, the regulation was put into effect that no diagnosis of malaria could be made without a microscopic demonstration of the parasite. It is of interest to describe Osler's technique for examining the blood:

> The layer of blood . . . should be very thin and uniform, the corpuscles as far as possible isolated and not aggregated in clumps of rouleaux. It is well to surround the cover with paraffin if the examination is prolonged. Cover slip preparations may be made and stained in methyl blue or fuchsin and mounted in balsam. Osmic acid preparations may also be employed. Although these bodies may be seen with a power of 500 to 600 diameters, it is essential for the satisfactory study of the changes to use higher power.[51]

This description is given only to emphasize the difficulties that the early workers must have had, since today the improved Wright and Giemsa stains make the microscopic search for malarial parasites so simple. It would scarcely occur to any clinical pathologist to look for living malaria organisms in unstained preparations.

In Osler's 1892 *The Principles and Practice of Medicine* he emphasized the importance of looking for malarial parasites in blood by writing that:

> To be able, everywhere and under all circumstances, to differentiate between malarial and other forms of fever is one of the most important advances which has been made of late years in practical medicine, one which will revolutionize the study of fevers in tropical and subtropical countries, and should, within a short time, bring some order out of the chaos which at present exists regarding the different forms which there prevail. . . . There are still many gaps in our knowledge. We do not know how the parasite enters or how or in what form it leaves the body; how and where it is propagated; under what outside condition it develops, whether free or in some aquatic plant or animal.[52]

However, progress was soon to be made. Patrick Manson was back home in London practicing tropical medicine and studying in his home the organisms of Laveran with the new stains of Ehrlich. Then on April 9, 1894, a young English doctor, Ronald Ross, who had unsuccessfully attempted to find Laveran's parasite in India, called on Manson asking for proof of their existence. Ross states in his memoirs:

> Within a few minutes he showed me the Laveran bodies which are technically called crescents in a stained specimen of malaria blood, and I recognized at once that no such bodies exist in healthy blood. My doubts were removed, and in a few days Manson demonstrated the other forms of the organisms to me in a patient lying in a Charing Cross Hospital . . . and made me acquainted with translations of the illuminating monographs on malaria by Mannaberg and by Marchiafava and Bignami . . . He treated me with great kindness, and I visited often and learnt all he had to tell me. In November, I called upon him again and found him just starting for the Seamen's Hospital. I went with him, and remember distinctly that as we were walk-

> ing along Oxford Street at about 2:30 PM, he said to me, "Do you know, I have formed the theory that mosquitoes carry malaria just as they carry filaria."[53]

At that time Ronald Ross was 37 years old, ambitious, and frustrated because he had written plays, novels, poetry and was an outstanding mathematician but none of these activities gave him the fame he sought. He decided that he would try his luck at scientific research. He selected Manson as his mentor, and after returning to India as a British Army doctor in March of 1895, he started his four years of arduous work, which ultimately resulted in the proof that the Anopheles mosquito was the intermediate host for the malarial parasite. His specific task was to trace the malarial parasites from the blood of a victim into the body of the mosquito, looking for transformations in its metamorphosis that could ready it for the reinfection of another human being. Ross worked under appalling conditions — alone, with a portable microscope that he carried like a pair of binoculars when he traveled to malarial areas, no knowledge about the anatomy of the mosquito so necessary in his dissections, abominable heat, becoming infected with malaria and dysentery himself, and with no assurance that any mosquito was actually involved in the transmission of malaria, except for both his and Manson's hunch. During his four years of work, he wrote 110 letters to Manson, of which each was about 1000 words in length, explaining his findings, and Manson wrote back 85 letters which were always full of encouragement and suggestions when Ross became discouraged. Initially he had trouble catching mosquitoes, keeping them alive, and then trying to persuade them to bite malarial victims. Later he found other parasites in his mosquitoes that he eventually found were unrelated to malaria but caused him significant confusion. In his own words from his diary notebook:

> I dissect each mosquito with the utmost care and then search every micron of it with an oil immersion lens which takes up to two hours. . . . But the things are there and must be found! It is simply a matter of hard work. . . . At first I toiled comfortably, but as failure followed failure, I became exasperated and worked till I could hardly see my way home late in the afternoon. . . . Swarms of flies and little insects which try to get into ones ears and eyes tormented me at their pleasure, while an occasional mosquito revenged herself on me for the death of her friends. The screw of my microscope was rusted with

> sweat from my forehead and hands, and its last remaining eyepiece was cracked.[54]

However on August 16, 1897, a series of events occurred that rewarded Ross for all of his difficult times. An assistant brought him about a dozen big, brown, mosquitoes with tapered bodies and dappled wings, a type he had not noticed before. These are Ross's words:

> Immediately my patient, Husein Khan, a man with fairly numerous crescents (and also filaria) was stripped and put on the bed under the mosquito net. This was at 12:25 PM by my notebook; and in five minutes ten of the new mosquitoes had gorged themselves on him and were caught by the Hospital Assistant, each in its separate test tube with a drop of water to drink and a loose lump of cotton to prevent escape — Husein Khan received one anna for each. At 12:40 and 12:50 PM I dissected two of the insects at once in order to watch the crescent sphere flagella metamorphosis in them. The next day, 17 August, two of my new beauties (*A. stephensi*) were dead, but I dissected two of the survivors, mosquitoes 32 and 33. They are described in my notebook as "large legs, proboscis and anterior border of wings, spotted dark brown, and white-brown spots on tail joint of body. Back of abdomen and thorax light brown, belly dark brown. Wings nearly white". I was rather excited over the dissection, spoiled them and found nothing; The 20 August, 1895 [sic] — the anniversary of which I always call, "Mosquito Day" — was, I think, a cloudy, dull, hot day. I went to the hospital at 7:00 A.M., examined my patients, and attended to official correspondence; but was much annoyed because my men had failed to bring any more larvae of the dappled-winged mosquitoes, and still more because one of my three remaining Anopheles had died during the night, and had swelled up with decay. After a hurried breakfast at the Mess, I returned to dissect the cadaver (Mosquito 36), but found nothing new in it. . . . At about 1:00 P.M., I determined to sacrifice the seventh Anopheles of the

batch fed on the sixteenth, Mosquito 38 although my eyesight was already fatigued. Only one more of the batch remained. The dissection was excellent, and I went carefully through the tissues, now so familiar to me, searching every micron with the same passion and care as one would search some vast ruined palace for a little hidden treasure. Nothing. No, these new mosquitoes were also going to be a failure; there was something wrong with the theory. But the stomach tissue still remained to be examined lying there, empty and flaccid, before me on the glass slide, a great white expanse of cells like the courtyard of flagstones, each one of which must be scrutinized — half an hour's labor at least. I was tired, and what was the use? I must have examined the stomachs of a thousand mosquitoes by this time. But the Angel of Fate fortunately laid his hand on my head; and I had scarcely commenced the search again when I saw a clear and almost perfectly circular outline before me of about 12 microns in diameter. The outline was much too sharp, the cell too small to be an ordinary stomach cell of a mosquito. I looked a little further. Here was another, and another exactly similar cell. The afternoon was very hot and overcast; and I remember opening the diaphragm of the substage condenser of the microscope to admit more light and then changing the focus. In each of these cells there was a cluster of small granules, black as jet and exactly like the black pigment granules of the Plasmodium crescents. As with that pigment, the granules numbered about twelve to sixteen in each cell and became blacker and more visible when more light was admitted through the diaphragm. I laughed and shouted for the Hospital Assistant — he was away at his siesta. "No, No," I said, "Dame Nature, you are sorceress, but you don't trick me so easily. The malarial pigment cannot get into the walls of the mosquito's stomach; the flagella have no pigment; you are playing another trick upon me." I counted twelve of the cells, all of the same size and appearance and all containing exactly the same granules. Then I made rough drawings of

> nine of the cells on page 107 of my notebook, scribbled my notes, sealed my specimen, went home to tea (about 3:00 P.M.) and slept solidly for an hour. When I awoke with my mind refreshed my first thought was: Eureka, the problem is solved! I seemed to have solved in my sleep an explanation for the pigment. The flagellated spores grow in the gastric cells of the . . . mosquito just the young Plasmodia grow in the human blood cells and as they grow they absorb hemoglobin from the blood in the mosquito's stomach. I was wrong: my cells were in fact the female crescents themselves which had been fertilized by the male crescents and were now beginning to grow, still containing their original pigment in the gastric cells of the anopheles . . . one thing was really done . . . we had to discover two unknown quantities simultaneously — the kind of mosquito which carried the parasite, and the form and position of the parasite within it. We could not find the first without knowing the second, nor the second without knowing the first. By an extremely lucky observation, I had now discovered both the unknown quantities at the same moment. The mosquito was the Anopheles, and the parasite lives in or on its gastric wall.[55]

The great discovery led Ross to write the following poem, which he sent to his wife:

> This day relenting God
> Hath placed within my hand
> A wondrous thing; and God
> Be praised. At His command
> Seeking His secret deeds
> With tears and toiling breath,
> I find thy cunning seeds,
> O million-murdering Death
> I know this little Death
> I know this little thing
> A myriad men will save.
> O death, where is thy sting?
> Thy victory, O'Grave.[56]

Ronald Ross would eventually win the Nobel Prize for his discovery, but it got scant attention initially, although it was published in December, 1897. His army superiors either through ignorance of his work on malaria or possibly because they were jealous or vindictive, sent him to a isolated station in India where there was no malaria, and he was unable to carry on his studies for four months. But with many letters of protest, and pressure by Manson in London, he was finally transferred to Calcutta where he was given a laboratory with instructions to study both malaria and kala-azar. However, the army only gave him six months to accomplish these difficult tasks, and he was disgusted to find no medical library available. Additionally, it was winter and the cool period in Calcutta, the mosquitoes were not biting, and very few human cases were found. Consequently Ross, with encouragement from Manson, decided to work with birds — sparrows, crows and larks — which also had malarial-type parasites, and fortunately he quickly found that the number of oocytes in the stomach of mosquitoes fed on bird blood was proportional to the number of parasites in the blood of the bird. He then transmitted the organism from infected birds to uninfected ones showing the various stages of the parasite in addition to finding the parasite in the salivary glands of the mosquito. This, of course, showed that the parasite was transmitted to a new host through the bite of an infected mosquito.[57] Unfortunately, on his return to England, Ross was not received with the honors and acclaim he felt he deserved, and opportunities to continue his studies in tropical medicine were not offered to him. Many of the medical community refused to believe that mosquitoes were involved with malaria, and the biologists simply felt that a physician such as Ross "didn't know anything about biology." Ross was so bitter that he decided to devote his further endeavors to mathematics and literature saying that "the word, malaria, made me nearly as sick as the thing itself would have done." The problem was that discussed in Chapter IV, simply that the English government had no interest in supporting medical research, and those individuals who were interested in such studies were really expected to do so on their own initiative as a hobby, or in their spare time as soldiers or officials. To make the situation even worse, Ross, Bruce, and W.G. King, who were primarily considered soldiers, were often punished for their scientific endeavors by their superior officers. Instead of sending a commission of scientists to India to assist Ross and to help in combating malaria which killed more than a million individuals each year in India, the English government sent him one "expert" to evaluate his findings. This was only after the eminent men Patrick Manson and Lord Lister had pleaded his case before the highest authorities in England. To further infuriate Ross, several Italian scientists, particularly Giovanni Grassi, either minimized his work or simply tried to take credit for it.

Fortunately, Ross's work was finally recognized in Sweden when he was awarded the Nobel Prize in 1902, and, belatedly, was knighted by his government. But he never seemed to recover from his earlier lack of recognition, and later he was frustrated by the obstacles put up by others in his campaigns to reduce malaria in the English colonies.

African Trypanosomiasis

The saga of the connection of African sleeping sickness with the presence of blood trypanosomes took place over a period of more than 150 years. The first modern description of a disease of natives of Africa characterized by somnolence and eventually death was made by an English naval surgeon in 1834, although there are earlier writers as far back as the twelfth century that describe a disease that was probably sleeping sickness. However, the disease was a comparatively rare one and most likely occurred in epidemic proportions only in isolated communities near the mouth of the Congo River and perhaps other small localities.

It was probably the starting of the slave trade, with movements of populations from previously isolated tribes on the western coast, that upset the delicate balance between the hosts, the parasite, and the vectors of the trypanosomes and increased the incidence of sleeping sickness. There were slaves that died of the disease in the West Indies, but they did not transmit it to other individuals, which, in retrospect, was because there were no tsetse flies in those islands. However, with the numerous explorations of Europeans in Africa in the nineteenth century, particularly those in which large caravans such as those of Stanley that went from the Congo area east to the region of Lake Victoria, pandemics occurred among the population there. The new use of steamboats on the rivers in the area also dispersed not only infected individuals but also the tsetse flies. As a result, during the last decade of the century, it has been estimated that, in some parts of Uganda, 200,000 individuals out of a population of 300,000 died of sleeping sickness, and, during the first half of the twentieth century, millions were infected and died. At the present time the disease is under control, but, with the vast increase in populations that are increasingly more mobile due to faster means of transportation and almost uncontrollable deforestation of the vast jungles, the ecological balance can be so disturbed that sleeping sickness could become epidemic again. There is a particular danger during times of drought when both the tsetse fly and infected individuals concentrate around the diminishing water holes. Also, less funding is being allocated for disease control now than a few years ago, no vaccines have been devised, and the trypanosomes show great ability to become resistant to new chemotherapeutic agents.

The impetus to the study of sleeping sickness was basically that the English saw a threat to their commercial interests in Africa (although they were not interested in following up Ross's malaria work in India) especially in South Africa, which gave great promise of agricultural and mineral wealth. The problem was an age-old disease called "nagana," which is the Zulu term for "depressed spirit," and is deadly for camels, horses, and oxen and prevented first the Arabs and later the Portuguese in the fifteenth century from developing the eastern side of southern and central Africa. The only manner in which to make explorations and development in this area was by using humans for portage, because they were not affected by nagana, and certainly this was not efficient. Then in 1894, the English governor of Natal in South Africa met with David Bruce, who after his success work with Malta Fever was teaching bacteriology at the military medical school in England, and explained how nagana was preventing the development of cattle and horse herds in the region. The idea of going to Africa and studying nagana fascinated the adventurous Bruce, and, although the military authorities (as always) attempted to prevent his going, the governor of Natal was his ally, and was able to arrange his transfer. He, of course, took his wife assistant and, as always, paid her way with his own funds. From Natal, he went to Ubombo in Northern Zululand, where nagana was present in the lowlands but not in the hills where he set up a small laboratory. His skills as a bacteriologist very quickly enabled him to exclude those microorganisms as a cause of nagana, but his skill as a microscopist, especially with the new stains of Ehrlich, found him soon locating a trypanosome in the blood of animals dying of nagana. Trypanosomes had been described as early as the 1840s by the early microscopists Gabriel Valentin,[58] who found them in the blood of a trout, and David Grüby,[59] who saw them in frog blood, but it was not until almost forty years later that they were found in the blood of mammals. At that time in India, T. Lewis saw them in the blood of rats[60] and shortly after Griffith Evans, a veterinary officer, identified them in the blood of horses, mules, and camels suffering from a disease known as "surra."[61] But Bruce was the first to positively identify them in Africa, and he set about to determine if they were the etiological factor in nagana.

Bruce was aware of the fact that for many years the natives had described a "fly disease" that sometimes killed their domestic animals in the lowlands, and he also knew that some early explorers had described a "tsetse fly" that was supposed to kill horses and oxen and that was identified as a species of *Glossina* by a French naturalist. By taking two young, healthy oxen and some dogs with no evidence of trypanosomes in their blood down into the areas where the "fly disease" was severe, he was able to show that, shortly after, they were infected with the parasite and became ill. He then caught several tsetse flies in the same area, brought them up into the hills, and, with a contraption that he devised, attached it to healthy dogs thus allowing the flies to bite these animals. The dogs soon showed trypanosomes in their blood and became ill, proving not only that the "fly disease" and nagana were the same entity but that it was transmitted by the tsetse fly.[62] To avoid any criticism that the tsetse flies had an inherent ability to produce the disease, he allowed flies without any trypanosomes in their intestine to bite healthy dogs and showed that no disease resulted. The next question was how the tsetse fly became infected with the parasite, and again he listened to the local inhabitants who knew that "where there are no wild animals there is no nagana." Bruce therefore caught or shot several wild animals but found either no trypanosomes or very few in their blood. However, if he injected substantial amounts of blood from these animals into healthy dogs, he was able to produce the disease with resulting high numbers of parasites, which indicated that the game animals were the reservoir for the trypanosome but had a natural resistance to the disease and were asymptomatic. The trypanosome was named *T. brucei*, after its discoverer.

It is ironic that while the problem of nagana was being solved, thousands of people, including Europeans, were dying in Uganda from sleeping sickness, and the attempts to determine the etiology of this deadly disease was minimal. In fact it was in May of 1901 when an English captain of a government launch on the Gambia river became ill that an examination of his fresh, unstained blood showed an unidentified motile worm-like organism. He was sent back to England, no parasites were found, and he seemed to recover; but when he returned to Africa, he became ill again. However, this time his blood was examined by J.E. Dutton from the Liverpool School of Tropical Medicine, who not only identified an organism as a trypanosome but sent slides to Laveran in Paris who said it was a new species. It was given the name *T. gambiense*.[63] Dutton died a short time later in an African village in the Congo, but not before he found *T. gambiense* in a few asymptomatic natives and concluded that the native population was a reservoir for the parasite and that occasionally it was transmitted to a European with a resulting mild febrile illness. He did not associate it with the rampant sleeping sickness in Uganda at the time. Eventually, the danger to the commercial interests of the European countries in the area became so severe that King Leopold II of Belgium subsidized an expedition in 1902 from the Liverpool School of Tropical Medicine. These investigators examined the blood of a thousand natives in the Senegambia region, found the trypanosome in seven, and concluded, like Dutton, that the trypanosome was not related to the sleeping sickness.

However, in Uganda the epidemic still raged; finally, the Royal Society in England appointed a commission to go there to investigate. Unfortunately the three individuals selected were completely incompatible, — George Low, 30 years of age and supposedly the head of the group, got into a physical fight with Cuthbert Christy, an egotistical man who was supposedly more interested in collecting butterflies than tsetse flies, and Aldo Castellani, who was a student at the London School of Tropical Medicine and was selected on the basis of a competitive examination for the commission of bacteriologist, was secretive and ambitious. Low attempted to link sleeping sickness with a filarial parasite, Castellani thought initially it was due to a streptococcus, and Christy went off on a field trip for several months to obtain epidemiological information. By the time he returned, Low had returned to England and Christy followed suit but by crossing northern Africa and leaving from Cairo, collecting insects along the way but without any hint about the cause of sleeping sickness. Castellani stayed on in Uganda and was shortly joined by a second commission consisting of David Bruce, D. N. Nabarro, an army sergeant, and, unofficially, Mrs. Bruce.

In the meantime, Castellani was still pursuing his streptococcus theory, but he had noted a trypanosome in the cerebrospinal fluid of a sleeping sickness patient, although he did not know whether it was significant. However, he would not tell Bruce of this finding until the latter agreed that, if this organism proved to be the etiological factor in sleeping sickness, he would be able to publish the discovery under his name alone, and he persuaded Bruce to promise not to tell Nabarro of the finding. Then together, Bruce and Castellani found the trypanosome in the cerebrospinal fluid of 20 out of 34 cases of advanced sleeping sickness, while in 20 control patients there were none. When he returned to England, Castellani reported that the trypanosome was the cause of the disease but that streptococcus also played a part in producing the symptoms, and he took entire credit for the work. Bruce stayed on in Uganda, now interested in the means of transmission of the trypanosome from victim to victim. He found that sleeping sickness occurred only along rivers and on islands in the large lakes, and he therefore suspected that there was a blood sucking insect like that in nagana that was restricted to the localities where the disease occurred. Although he was assured that the tsetse was not present, the natives talked about a blood sucking insect they called Kivu. By going into the sleeping sickness areas, the commission soon realized that Kivu was the Ugandan name for the tsetse fly, and, taking a major chance that they could contract the fatal disease themselves, they collected tsetse flies, took them back to the laboratory, fed them on patients dying of sleeping sickness, and then allowed the flies to bite monkeys.

But while they waited for the monkeys to get sick, Bruce wasted no time. According to Paul de Kruif, who interviewed Bruce before his death, Bruce enlisted the help of Apolo Kagwa, the plumed and colorfully dressed Prime Minister of Uganda, to get his people to send him, in envelopes, samples of Kivu insects from the various villages in Uganda along with information about cases of sleeping sickness in those localities. Then as the specimens came in he put a red pin in the localities on a map where the tsetse fly was caught and a black pin where there was a newly identified case of sleeping sickness. Very shortly he found that where the disease occurred there were always tsetse flies and where there were no tsetses there was no sleeping sickness. In the meantime the monkeys that had been bitten by infected tsetse flies were sick and showed trypanosomes. The proof of the manner of transmission was complete. But Bruce was not finished. He persuaded the Prime Minister to evacuate the areas along the water for a period of time to stop the epidemic. His ideas were complied with and would have worked except that other animals in the area, both domestic and wild, remained constant hosts for the parasite, and the disease could not be eradicated in that manner. As brilliant as Bruce was, there was one major belief he had that he was reluctant to change — the idea that the trypanosome of nagana was the same one that produced sleeping sickness but was somehow modified for man in Central Africa. Therefore, when a young German scientist that wanted to prove him wrong inoculated himself with blood from an animal dying of nagana that contained millions of *T. brucei*, in addition to allowing infected tsetse flies to bite him, and still did not become ill, Bruce's reaction was not shock but disappointment. According to de Kruif, Bruce said, "It is a matter for some scientific regret that these experiments were not successful — though we can ill spare our bold and somewhat rash colleague — for then the question would have been answered . . . as it is, these negative experiments prove nothing. It may be that only one man in a thousand can be infected that way." David Bruce was not only tough minded, but he was correct. In a recent review of African trypanosomiasis, the author criticizes modern investigators because they work in Europe or the United States and rely on syringe passaged trypanosomes and laboratory animals and says they either do not know of Bruce's work, have forgotten it, or are ignoring it. In 1913 regarding the trypanosome that affects monkeys, Bruce stated that:

> The rapidity with which the virulence of T. simiae becomes modified is also remarkable. When a cage containing wild G. morsitans is placed on a monkey and a goat, both animals take the disease and the monkey in such an acute form that the average duration of life is only a few days. But if it is attempted to pass T. simiae from an infected goat to a healthy monkey by the inoculation of goat's blood the experiment usually fails, showing that a short sojourn in the blood of a goat has almost nullified the virulence of the parasite for the monkey . . . but it is interesting as showing the fallacy of judging from the action of laboratory strains as to what will occur in nature.[64]

In 1990, there appear to be only two trypanosomes that affect humans: *T. rhodesiense,* which has a more acute course and can kill the victim within nine months; and *T. gambiense*, which produces a more chronic and wasting pattern (if in either case no chemotherapy is undertaken). Usually, the tsetse fly in the case of *T. rhodesiense* is *Glossina morsitans,* and, for *T. gambiense*, the vector is more likely *G. palpalis*. There are at least eight trypanosomes that affect animals, and more than seven different species or subspecies of tsetse flies, with considerable overlap of hosts. It is very likely that this ecology of parasite, vector, and host has shifted and continues to shift since Bruce started in studies in 1894.

Bibliography

1. Mahmoud, A.A.F., Diseases Caused by Protozoa and Metazoa, p. 1775, in *Textbook of Medicine*, edited by J.B. Wyngaarden and K.H. Smith, Jr., W.B. Saunders Co., Philadelphia, 1985.
2. Redi, F., *Osservazioni* . . . intorno agli animali viventi che si trovano negli animali viventi. Matini, Florence, 1684.
3. Goeze, J.A.E., *Vers. ein. Naturgesch. d. Eingeweidewurmer*, 1782.
4. Rudolphi, K., *Entozoorum, sive verminum intestinalium, historia naturalis*. 2 vols. Amsterdam, 1808-10.
5. Steenstrup, J., *Om Fortplantning og Udvikling gjennem vexlende Generationsraekker,* Reitzel, Copenhagen, 1842.
6. Davaine, C.J., *Traité des entozoaires et des maladies vermineuses.* Baillière, Paris, 1860.
7. Cobbold, T.S. *Entozoa*. 2 kts. Groombridge and Sons, London, 1864-69.
8. Foster, W.D., *A History of Parasitology*, Livington, Edinburgh, 1965.
9. Leuckart, R., *Die menschlichen Parasiten und die von ihnen herrührenden Krankheiten*, 2 vols. Winter, Leipzig, 1863–76.
10. Küchenmeister, G. *Über Cestoden im allgemeinen und die des Menschen insbesondere*, Pahl, 1853.
11. Owen, R. Description of a microscopic entozooan (Trichina spiralis) infesting the muscles of the human body. *Lond. Med. Gas.*, **16**, p. 125, 1834-35.
12. Wood, H. *London Med. Jour.*, p. 190, 1835.
13. Leidy, J., Trichina spiralis in hogs. *Proc. Acad. Nat. Sci. Phila.*, **3**, p. 107, 1846.
14. Herbst, G., Beobacht über Trichina spiralis. *Göttinger Nachr.* p. 260, 1851.
15. Leuckart, R., *Untersuchungen über Trichina spiralis,* Winter. Leipzig, 1860.
16. Zenker, F.A., Ueber die Trichinen-Krankheit des Menschen. *Virchow's Archiv*. **18**, p. 561, 1860.
17. Virchow, R., *Die Lehre von den Trichinen*, Reimer, Berlin, 1866.
18. Zimmermann, W.J., Trichinosis, in *Diseases Transmitted from Animals to Man*, p. 545, Edited by W. Hubbert, and W. McCulloch, C. Thomas, Springfield, Illinois, 1975.
19. Bilharz, T.M., Ein Beitrag zur Helminthographia humana. *Zeitschr.f.*

wiss. *Zool.*, **4**, p. 53, 1852.
20. Ref. 7.
21. Brock G.S., *J. Path. Bact.*, **2**, p. 52, 1894.
22. Katsurada, F., Schistosomum japonicum, ein neuer menschl., *Annot. Zool. Japon*, **3**, p. 147, 1904.
23. Catto, J., *Brit. Med. J.*, p. 11, 1905.
24. Manson, P., *Tropical Diseases*, p. 661, Cassel and Co. London, 1907.
25. Miyairi, and Suzuki, On the Development of Schistosomum japonicum, *Tokyo Med. Journ.*, p. 1836, 1913.
26. Leiper, R.T., Observations on the Mode of Spread and Prevention of Vesical and Intestinal Bilharziosis in Egypt. *Proc. Roy. Soc. Med.*, **9**, No. 9, 1916.
26a. Barlow, C.H., *Amer. Jour. Trop. Med.*, **29** p. 79, 1949.
27. Dubini, A., Nuovo verme intestinale urmono (Agchylostoma duodenale), *Ann. univ. Med.* (Milano), **106**, p. 5, 1843.
28. Wucherer, O., Estudos sobre a hypoemia intertropical. *Gaz. med. Bahia*, **1**, p. 27, 1866.
29. Grassi, G.B., Intorno all'Anchilostoma duodenale. *Gazz. med. lombardia*, **5**, p. 193, 1878.
30. Loos, A., Ueber das Eindringen der Ankylostomalarven in die menschliche Haut. *Zbl. Bakt.*, **29**, p. 733, 1901.
31. Bentley, C.A., On the causal relationship beween "ground itch" or pani ghao and the presence of the ankylostoma duodenale in the soil, *Brit. Med Jour.*, p. 190, 1902.
32. Stiles, C.W., A new species of hookworm (Uncinaria americana) parasitic in man. *Amer. Med.*, **3**, p. 777, 1902.
33. Ashford, B.K., Ankylostomiasis in Puerto Rico. *N.Y. Med.* J., **71**, p. 552, 1900.
34. Rockefeller Foundation, *Bibliography of hookworm disease*, Rockefeller Foundation, New York, 1922.
35. Demarquay, J.N., Note sur une tumeur des bourses contenant un liquide laiteux et renfermant de petits etres vermiformes . . . *Gaz. med. Paris*, **18**, p. 665, 1863.
36. Wucherer, O., Noticiar preliminar sobre vermes de uma especie ainda não descripta, encontrados na urina de doentes de hematuria intertropical no Brazil. *Gas. med. Bahia*, **3**, p. 97, 1868.
37. Lewis, T.R., On a hematozooan inhabiting human blood. Its relation

to chyluria and other diseases. *Ann. Rep. sanit. comm. India*, **8**, p. 24dl, 1871.

38. Bancroft, J., Cases of filarious disease. *Trans. path. Soc. Lond.*, **29**, p. 406, 1878.
39. Manson-Bahr, P.H., and Alcock, A., *The Life and Work of Sir Patrick Manson*, p.45, Cassell and Co., London, 1927.
40. Ibid, p. 55.
41. Bancroft, T., *Journal and Proceedings of the Royal Society of New South Wales*, **32**, p. 62, 1899.
42. Lancisi, G., *De noxiis paludum effluviis, eorumque remediis.* Salvioni, Rome, 1717.
43. Meckel, H., Ueber schwarzes Pigment in der Milz und im Blute einer Geisteskranken. *Zeitschr. f. Psychiatric*, p. 198, 1847.
44. Virchow, R., *Cellular Pathology*, 1863, p. 256, Translated by F.Chance, Dover Publications, NY, 1971.
45. Klebs, E., and Tommasi-Crudeli, C., Studien über die Ursache des Wechselfiebers und uber die Natur der Malaria. *Archiv. fur. exper. Path. und Pharm.*, **11** p. 311, 1879.
46. Laveran, C.L., Note sur un nouveau parasite trouvé dans le sang de plusieurs malades atteints de fièvre palustre. Communiquée à I'Academie de Médicine, Bull., séance due 23 Nov. 1880.
47. Richard, E., *Communication à l'Academie des Sciences sur les parasites de l'impaludisme*, séance du 20 Fév., 1882.
48. Sternberg, G., *Malaria and Malarial Diseases*, p.75, William Wood, N.Y.1884.
49. Councilman, W., Certain Elements Found in the Blood in Cases of Malarial Fever. *Transactions Association of American Physicians*, First Session, June 17 and 18, 1886.
50. Osler, W., On the value of Laveran's organisms in the diagnosis of malaria. *Johns Hopkins Hosp. Bull.*, **1**, p. 11, 1889-90.
51. Osler, W., The Hematozoa of malaria. *Brit. Med. Jour.*, **1**, p. 556, 1887.
52. Osler,W., *The Principles and Practice of Medicine*, p. 144, D. Appleton, New York, 1892.
53. Ross, R., *Memoirs*, p. 127, John Murray, London, 1923.
54. Ibid, p. 220.
55. Ibid, p. 222.
56. Ibid, p. 226.

57. Ross, R., Report on the Cultivation of Proteosoma. Labbe, in Grey Mosquitoes, *Ind. Med. Gaz.*, Nov. and Dec. 1898.
58. Valentin, G., Ueber ein Entozooan im Blute von Salmo fario. *Arch. Anat. Physiol. wiss. Med.*, p. 435, 1841.
59. Grüby, D., Recherches et observations sur une nouvelle espèce d'hématozoaire. C.B. Acad. Sci. Paris, **17**, p. 1134, 1843.
60. Lewis, T.R., The microscopic organism found in the blood of man and animals and their relation to disease. *Ann. rep. sanit. Comm. India*, **14**, p. 157, 1878.
61. Evans, G., On a horse disease in India known as "surra", probably due to a hematozooan. *Vet. J.*, **13**, 1881, p. 1, p. 82, p. 180, p. 326.
62. Bruce, D., *Preliminary report on the tsetse fly disease or nagana, in Zululand.* Bennett and Davis, Durbin, 1895.
63. Dutton, J.E., Preliminary note upon a trypanosome occurring in the blood of man. *Thompson Yates Lab. Rep.*, **4**, p. 455, 1902.
64. Bruce, D., Harvey, D., Hamerton, A., and Bruce, M.E., Trypanosomes of the domestic animals in Nyasaland I., *Proc. R. Soc. Ser. B.*, **87**, p. 48, 1913.

CHAPTER XVI

I can see you (Metchnikoff) now at the Budapest Congress in 1894, disputing with your antagonist; with your fiery face, sparkling eyes, and dishevelled hair, you looked like the Demon of Science, but your words, your irresistible arguments raised the applause of your audience The new facts, which at first seemed to contradict the phagocyte theory, now entered into harmony with it.

— E. Roux

The Cellular and Humoral Immunity Debate

Just as the first important work on bacteria in the study of disease was implemented by the chemist Pasteur, some of the first experiments on the reaction of animal organisms to invasion by extrinsic sources were carried out by the zoologist Elie Metchnikoff, another colorful character in the history of pathology.

Metchnikoff was born in 1845 and studied biology at the University of Kharkoff, but the repressive atmosphere in Russia was too much for the hyperactive, imaginative, enthusiastic, revolutionary, idealistic, neurotic Russian, who, without planning well, dashed to Wurzburg, Germany, to study cells with Kölliker, who along with the rest of the university was on vacation. Rejected by fellow Russians in Wurzburg because he was not only eccentric but a Jew, he was overcome with homesickness and went back to Russia. He next read Darwin's *Origin of Species* and was so taken with this book that he became an ardent evolutionist, determined to solve problems related to living organisms fighting for survival. During the years 1868–1875, he went from one laboratory to the other, shouting and arguing, and usually ending up being either asked to leave or ostracized. He married a Russian girl, who had tuberculosis and had to be carried to the altar, and they traveled throughout Europe looking for a cure. She died in Madeira, and Metchnikoff, despondent, became addicted to morphine and attempted suicide but did not succeed because the overdose of morphine simply made him vomit. Two years later, in 1875, while a professor at the University of Odessa, he married a girl of 15 years, whose family was very wealthy. After getting into a dispute with the university authorities, he moved to Messina in Sicily with his wife and her small brothers and sisters. He set up a small private laboratory where he started to work on invertebrates from the nearby straits, studying the reaction of mesoderm cells to foreign bodies such as bacteria. He gives the background of these experiments as follows:

> I have never prosecuted any medical studies; but sometime before my departure for Messina, I listened to the reading of Cohnheim's treatise on General Pathology, and I was struck by the description of the facts and of his theory of inflammation. The former, especially his description of the diapedesis of the white blood corpuscles through the vessel wall, seemed to be of momentous interest. His theory, on the other hand, appeared to be extremely vague and nebulous. It occurred to me that a comparative study of inflammation in lower animals of simple organization would certainly throw light on the very complex pathological phenomena in the Vertebrate, even in the frog which had served as the starting point for Cohnheim's remarkable experiments. I knew quite well that, at the period when I made my researches [1882], pathologists regarded inflammation as the consequence, if not always, at least in the majority of cases, of the penetration of microorganisms. From this followed the conclusion that the diapedesis and accumulation of white corpuscles in inflammatory diseases must be regarded as modes of defence of the organism against microorganisms, the leukocytes in this struggle devouring and destroying the parasites. According to this hypothesis the significance of inflammation at once became simple and clear. With the object of verifying my hypothesis I began to make experiments on the lower animals, so abundant in the Straits of Messina, and to make myself acquainted with the results that had been obtained in general pathology and in pathological histology. . . . Sometime later I had the great pleasure of meeting the celebrated Professor Virchow at Messina. I imparted to him my ideas and he was kind enough to come with me to examine my preparations of Bipinnaria larvae and other lower animals in which I had set up the phenomena of inflammation without the assistance of nervous and vascular systems. This eminent observer greatly encouraged me to continue my in-

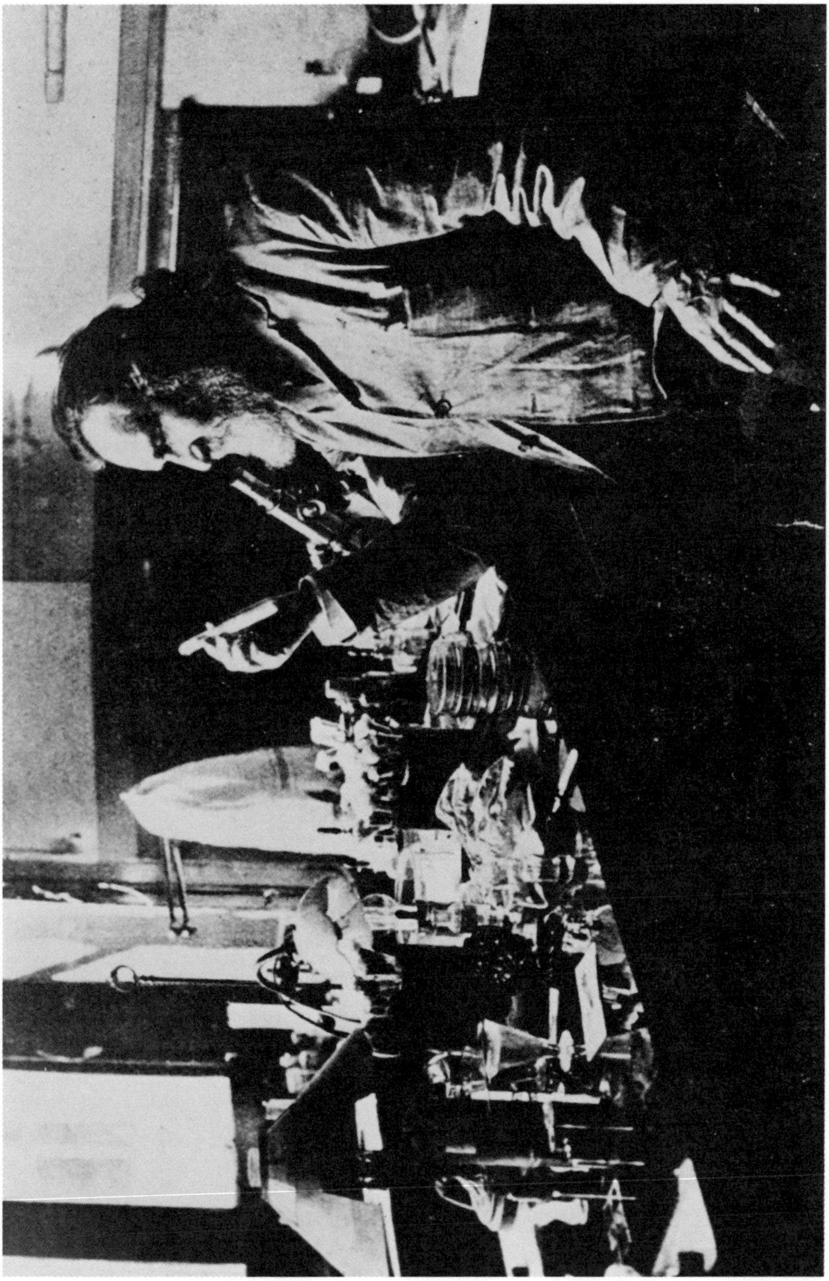

ELIE METCHNIKOFF

vestigations. When I explained to him my view that the inflammatory reaction on the part of the amoeboid cells could only be understood by accepting the hypothesis that the white corpuscles gave chase to the microorganisms and destroyed them, Virchow replied that in pathology just the opposite was invariably taught. The general opinion was that microorganisms were certainly found inside the leukocytes and that they made use of these cells as a means of transport and of dissemination through the body. Some time afterwards, I published in the same journal my work on the anthrax bacillus, in which I attempted to demonstrate that in the Vertebrata also, the invasion of pathogenic microorganisms sets up a desperate struggle between them and the amoeboid cells. In these works I made use of the term "phagocytes" to designate the amoeboid cells capable of seizing and digesting the microorganisms and other formed elements. To the theory based on this property of the defensive cells, I gave the name of "theory of phagocytes." I thought . . . that the observations on absorption and leukocytes, which had been accumulating for years in pathological histology, had sufficiently paved the way for a favorable reception to the idea that the amoeboid cells are defensive elements of the body capable of guaranteeing to it immunity and cure. In this I was mistaken. It was precisely the specialists in this branch of science who from the first manifested the most lively opposition to this theory. The publication . . . of bacterial anthrax, immediately roused severe criticism. Baumgarten [Paul], the well known pathologist . . . attempted to sap the basis of my theory, and not contented with a priori arguments, he set his pupils to make a series of researches on the fate of microorganisms in the refractory animal. Later Baumgarten published a long and above all admirably written analytical article in which, with much talent and wit, he attempted to demolish the bases and conclusions of the phagocyte theory. [His] example was followed by many other pathologists. Zeigler, the well known author of a textbook, vigorously attacked the theory of phagocytosis. . . . The intervention of these cells, according to him, must be purely accidental and their role in the defence of the body against microorganisms very insignificant. . . . The opposition emanating from Weigert, particularly impressed me, because this investigator is known not only to be an observer of great accuracy, but to possess a mind of great imagination and generaliz-

> ing power. . . . He would recognize neither the importance of phagocytosis in healing and immunity, nor the defensive function of the giant cells. It must be stated, however, that although there has been such opposition on the part of certain of our most eminent pathologists, others among them have, from the beginning expressed themselves in more favorable terms. Thus Virchow in an introductory article in the 101st volume of his Archive, continued his friendly attitude with regard to the works on phagocytic defence and spoke of them as opening up a new field of research.
>
> The attacks directed against the theory of phagocytosis by bacteriologists have been of a very different character. Not content with over turning this hypothesis, these observers have sought to build upon its ruins new theories capable of offering a better explanation of the phenomena of immunity. I must here confess at the onset that these attacks have been much more important than those coming from the pathologists and have led to discoveries of the greatest value.[1]

The first indication that there might be another manner, independent of phagocytes, in which to explain bodily defense against microorganisms came from the American George Nuttall (1862–1937). While working in Flugge's laboratory in 1888, Nuttall confirmed the phagocytosis of anthrax bacteria by leukocytes but also was able to follow, step by step under the microscope, the degeneration of anthrax by cell-free serum from immunized animals.[2] Metchnikoff's theory was also challenged by the work of Behring and Kitosato, who found that toxins produced by both diphtheria and tetanus organisms could be neutralized in cell-free serum of immunized animals by substances called antitoxins.[3] These studies opened a whole new field of humoral immunity.

In 1892, Richard Pfeiffer (1858–1945) extended the proof of humoral factors by immunizing guinea pigs with intraperitoneal injections of killed cholera bacteria. After periods of 6 days and 15 days, he injected intraperitoneally living cholera bacteria and then aspirated small amounts of peritoneal fluid at various intervals. He found that after 10-20 minutes, "before my eyes the cholera vibrios were lysed without participation of phagocytes." He also found that he could transfer living cholera bacteria mixed with some peritoneal fluid from an immune guinea pig to a non-immune pig, and that interval studies of peritoneal fluid showed the same type of lysis. However, when he placed the same mixture of immune fluid with bacteria in the incubator, he found that the bacteria were not used, but multiplied. He concluded that the peritoneal space was not simply a receptacle but "reacts to the stimulus of the vibrios under the influence of the immune substances in serum to elicit the bacteriocidal action."[4] (The existence and lability of complement was not known at this time.)

During this period, Max Gruber (1853–1927) and his English assistant H. Durham were studying bacteriolytic phenomena and had noted that, with cholera vibrios and anti-cholera immune sera, an agglutination reaction in vitro occurred. As discussed earlier (see Typhoid Fever discussion in Chapter XIII), this reaction allowed them to confirm the identity of colonies of pathogens on an agar plate.[5] Shiga then used this procedure to identify specific bacillary dysentery organisms at a time when biochemical differentiation was not satisfactory. In the meantime, Metchnikoff, whose "phagocyte theory" appealed to Louis Pasteur, was offered space in the new institute in Paris, where he stayed until his death in 1916. He idolized Pasteur, and in spite of his volatile nature, he was loved and respected by his French colleagues, spent his last days in Pasteur's apartment, and had his ashes placed in an urn in the Institute's Library.

Metchnikoff attracted many students, and one of his best was the young Belgian Jules Bordet (1870–1961), who was awarded the Nobel prize in 1919. Bordet investigated the "Pfeiffer phenomenon," and was the first to show the presence of the protein complement, which acts in conjunction with other immunological factors, in normal serum. (Bordet called the substance "alexin" but later Ehrlich called it "complement.") He demonstrated that there were two distinct substances necessary for lysis of bacteria in the immune reaction — the antibodies stimulated by the microorganism plus normal complement, which is destroyed by heating the sera to 60 degrees. Bordet concluded that antibodies can agglutinate bacteria, but complement is necessary for bacteriolysis. He also stated that normal serum was by itself very weakly bacteriocidal, but, when added to immune sera, together they became highly destructive to the specific bacteria.[6] But as a true scientist, although most likely very disappointing to Metchnikoff, Bordet also said this action was the same whether phagocytes were present in the normal serum or not. Then in 1898, Bordet worked with O. Gengou (1875–1959) to develop the complement fixation test, which has been used throughout the twentieth century when an antibody-antigen reaction cannot be detected visually, as can be done in agglutination, precipitation, or bacteriolysis. In this case an indicator system is added to determine if an invisible antigen-antibody reaction has occurred. The indicator system usually consists of sheep cells that have been added to rabbit serum previously sensitized to sheep cells and heated to 60 degrees to destroy complement. This indicator system is then added to a reaction mixture in which it is desired to determine if a soluble antigen has combined with a specific antibody (which could establish a diagnosis) but is invisible. Then a known amount of guinea pig serum containing active complement, which will only combine with an antigen-antibody complex, is added. If there has been no such complex formed, the guinea pig complement will combine with the sheep cells — sheep cell antibodies complex (which does not reveal itself under the microscope) and hemolysis will then result, which indicates a negative complement fixation test.[7] This test was the principle of the Wasserman test for syphilis.[8] In 1971 McFarlane Burnet wrote that:

> . . . In 1898 there came a major turning point in the history of immunology when Bordet found that rabbits could be immunized against red blood cells from another species, producing antibody which could specifically dissolve the red blood cells. Immunology became immediately a biological science in its own right instead of a mere approach to the understanding of infections.[9]

Metchnikoff continued to emphasize that his phagocyte theory was the dominant one in protecting the host from pathogenic organisms. He had the support of Virchow, who, in defending his Cellular Pathology, was also attempting to minimize the importance of the new humoral factors being discovered at the time and which they both thought threatened their pet concepts. In retrospect, modern information indicates that all parties were correct, although at the time the polemics of cellular versus humoral factors were very unfortunate and demeaning to those involved. It was a situation that has occurred so frequently simply because egos interfere with objectivity. Bertrand Russell gave a definition of the scientific spirit as

> the sweeping away of all other desires in the interest of the desire to know — it involves suppression of hopes and fears,

> loves and hates, and the whole subjective emotional life until we become subdued to the material, able to see it frankly, without preconceptions, without bias, without any wish to see it as it is, and without any belief that what it is must be determined by some relation, positive or negative, to what we should like it to be, or to what we can imagine it to be.[10]

This concept of course is ideal, and Russell, who emotionally embraced so many controversial beliefs during his life, realistically states that this spirit was not yet achieved at the time he wrote it (1917). And the question is whether it will ever be. Perhaps with advancements in computer science, artificial intelligence might approximate the ideal, if the human programmers can be trusted. On the other hand, it is most likely that without the passion and egos of such individuals as Metchnikoff, Virchow, Pasteur, Koch, Ehrlich, Bernard, and Magendie, there would be little progress in human knowledge about nature. And eventually, evaluations of the accomplishments and errors of such great men are made by later generations of scientists in the same fields who can give them historical perspective.

With regard to the problem of defense against extrinsic factors, if the old Russian zoologist and the Prussian pathologist were to come back to earth now and learn of modern immunology and inflammation, with the identification of so many different types of blood cells, and find that antibodies are produced by B lymphocytes they would undoubtedly say "We were right, the cells are the important factors!" But in the last decade of the twentieth century, the explanations of the response of the human body to pathogenic organisms are extremely complex, and are excellent examples of how explanations of biological phenomena simply become more detailed descriptions of what is occurring at lower and lower levels of physiology, until the matter is a discussion of the interaction of molecules, large and small. For example, whereas during the middle of the twentieth century there was essentially one type of lymphocyte, there are now B lymphocytes, which produce many types of immunoglobulins and antibodies, T lymphocytes, which are subdivided into helper and suppressor cells (each producing different substances that mediate immunity), null cells or killer cells, monocytes, which become macrophages in inflammation, and the various granulocyte cells (neutrophils, basophils, and eosinophils), each with their own complex response and actions to foreign material and microorganisms. Complement is found to be a group of at least 20 different plasma proteins, each with different functions and interrelationships with the other immune factors, both humoral and cellular. The discussion of immunity in a current textbook of pathology[11] is so complex and specialized that several authors are evidently necessary to cover the most up-to-date information, which continues to change very quickly. Knowledge in the field of immunology, which now encompasses biochemistry, molecular biology, and genetics, has become so vast that it is difficult to imagine a few colorful giants like the above mentioned men of the nineteenth century ever dominating the world stage in biology and medicine again.

Bibliography

1. Metchnikoff, E., *Immunity in Infective Diseases*, p. 518, Translated from the French by F.G. Binnie, Cambridge Univ. Press, Cambridge, 1907.
2. Nuttall, G., Experimente über die bacterienfeindlichen Einflüsse des thierischen Körpers. *Z. Hyg. Infekt Kr.* 4, p. 353, 1888.
3. Behring, E., and Kitosato,S., Ueber das Zustandekommen der Diphtherie-Immunität un der Tetanus-Immunitat bei Thieren. *Dtsch. med. Wschr.*, **16**, pp. 1113, 1890.
4. Pfeiffer, R., and Isayev, V., Ueber die specifische Bedeutung der Cholerimmunität (Bakteriolyse). *Z. Hyg.*, **17**, p. 355, 1894.
5. Gruber, M., and Durham, H., Eine neue Methode zur raschen Erkennung des Cholera vibrio und des Typhusbacillus. *Münch. med. Wschr.*, **43**, p. 285, 1896.
6. Robinson, V., Elie Metchnikoff, in *Pathfinders in Medicine*, p. 748, Medical Life Press, NY, 1929.
7. Bordet, J., Contribution à l'étude du sérum chez les animaux vaccinés. *Ann. Soc. Roy. Sci. Méd. Nat. Brux.*, 4, p. 455, 1895.
8. Wassermann, A., Eine serodiagnostische Reaktion bei Syphilis. *Dtsch. Med. Wschr., Berlin*, **32**. p. 745, 1906.
9. Burnet, M., and White. D.O., *Natural History of Infectious Disease*, p. 70, 4th Edition, Cambridge Univ. Press, Cambridge, 1972.
10. Russell, B., *Mysticism and Logic*, p.42, Doubleday Anchor Books, Garden City, N.Y., 1957.
11. Rubin, E., and Farber, J., *Pathology*. Saunders, Phil., 1988.

CHAPTER XVII

Blood is the life.

— Deuteronomy 12:23

The Pathology of the Blood

Normal Physiology of the Blood

The understanding of the nature of blood at the beginning of the nineteenth century had not progressed much over the prior thousands of years. This bodily fluid was accorded an almost magical vital quality that was expressed in Deuteronomy (12:23) as "blood is the life," most likely because primitive man as a hunter knew that a wounded animal would soon die if the flow of blood did not cease. This idea of the importance of the blood was intellectualized for thousands of years through the humoral theory and even in the early nineteenth century, manifested itself with the ideas of Rokitansky. Even Magendie, the great skeptic, thought the causes of many diseases would be found in the blood, and Virchow, who it will be remembered so severely castigated Rokitansky for his humoral ideas, early in his own career believed that cells arose from a "formless blastema" such as the blood plasma.[1] Another prominent but erroneous idea that continued through much of the nineteenth century was that the major oxidation and heat production occurred in the blood and its vessels. This belief was championed by two of the most prominent physiologists at that time, Claude Bernard[2] and Carl Ludwig.[3] Although Spallanzani in the eighteenth century performed experiments that indicated that oxidation occurred in the tissues themselves,[4] it was Eduard Pfluger during the years 1872–74 who showed conclusively that oxidation occurs intracellularly in all the tissues of the body.[5]

But by the end of the nineteenth century, the basic functions of the blood were established, although most of the details relating to these functions were determined after 1900. These functions were to (1) transport oxygen from the lungs to the cells of the body, through the mechanism of binding this gas to the hemoglobin of the erythrocytes, and carrying off the carbon dioxide from the cells back to the lungs; (2) transport nutrients from the intestinal tract to the cells; (3) transport metabolic waste products, primarily those containing nitrogen, to the kidneys, skin, and intestine for removal from the body; (4) maintain the water balance of the body; (5) transport substances (hormones) from their point of origin to their site of action; (6) regulate body temperature by distributing body heat; (7) maintain the normal acid–base balance of the body; (8) provide defense against microorganisms and foreign proteins through the action of leukocytes and the various soluble proteins such as antibodies and complement; (9) aid in the resolution of inflammation by providing clotting materials to stabilize lesions and promote healing.

With regard to function 5, in spite of the fact that it was not until 1905 that Ernest Starling used the term "hormones" to describe secretions of some of the ductless glands,[6] Berthold had already proved the existence of an internal secretion when he transferred the testes of a cock to another part of its body without a diminution in the male characteristics,[7] and Oliver and Sharpey-Schafer had extracted a pressor substance from the adrenal medulla.[8] Also Michael Foster in his 1895 textbook of physiology anticipated such substances in his discussion of the thyroid and adrenal organs.[9] Regarding function 7, clinicians who had been working with patients in diabetic coma[10-12] already knew about "acidosis," although the measurement of blood acidity and the nature of the buffer system of plasma was not accomplished until the twentieth century.[13-16]

Chemical Analysis of the Blood

As discussed in Chapter VII, Rokitansky, Andral, and Magendie thought that careful chemical analyses of blood in normal and abnormal conditions would throw light on the nature of disease when no anatomical lesions could be found, but this approach was premature. The result was that, except for semiquantitative determinations of glucose in blood by Claude Bernard in his studies on diabetes, glycogen function, and metabolism[17, 18] and uric acid determinations in gout by Garrod,[19] quantitative chemical blood analyses diminished in numbers in the mid nineteenth century. However, although separations and chemical characterization of metabolic substances were carried out in a limited way, it was not until Otto Folin (1867–1934),[20] Ivar Bang (1869–1918),[21] and Donald Van Slyke (1883–1971)[22] independently developed practical quantitative methods for determining such metabolites as urea, glucose, uric acid, creatinine, cholesterol, proteins, and carbon dioxide during the first two decades of the twentieth century that extensive studies of blood in pathological conditions became possible.

Studies of the Cellular Elements

With regard to the study of the cellular elements of the blood, the situation was quite different. As a result of the improvement of the compound microscope in 1830, the development of instruments for determining the numbers of the different blood cells per unit of volume, and the classification of the various leukocytes (made possible by the staining techniques of Paul Ehrlich), the field of hematology began during the last half of the nineteenth century.

In the early years of the century, anemia was basically a clinical term used for pallor of the skin and mucous membranes. Then Andral and Gavarret determined the relative weights of the clot, the fibrin, and the serum, and calculated each as a percentage of the whole sample. The problem, of course, was that a clot not only had all the cellular elements in it but also serum, so that gravimetric separations were only very imprecise. However, the procedure was able to distinguish severe anemia from normal blood,[23] but because it was so tedious to perform, it had only limited use. Also it seemed that Andral was more interested in the changes in fibrin content of the blood in various pathological conditions. By the beginning of the second half of the century, it became obvious that for the study of blood to become scientific, it would be necessary to have better methods of studying not only the chemical components of this vital fluid, but also the cellular elements. The compound microscope made it possible to make some preliminary studies of the cellular components, but the magnification of 300-400 × was simply not enough for careful studies of the red and white blood cells, and platelets were easily confused with granules, debris, or bacteria. The situation was best described in the medical textbook of Austin Flint in 1866:

> Of the manner in which the causes of anemia, exclusive of hemorrhage, occasion diminution of the red globules, all that can be said, with our present knowledge, is that they generally appear to act by impairing the liquor sanguinis. Further than

> this, the pathologist cannot go until the physiologist explains how and where the red globules are formed from the elements of the blood plasma in health. A pathological condition of much interest and importance has been heretofore, and is still called pyemia, or purulent infection of the blood, called also pyogenic fever, pus-blood and the pus crasis. The entrance of pus-corpuscles into the circulation by passing through the coats of the vessels, is . . . impossible. It can only enter into the circulation through an opening into a vein.[24]

Two years later Cohnheim conclusively proved that white blood cells move out into the tissue from the blood vessels, and it soon became clear that inflammation and suppuration in organs was primarily cellular exudate from the blood into the tissues and not vice versa. Cohnheim did not know the source of the white blood cells or their function in migrating through the walls of the small blood vessels; he simply determined the direction.[25] The cases in which there were very high amounts of white blood cells in the blood, in retrospect, were either cases of leukemia or leukocytosis, but it was difficult to differentiate these two conditions at the time. Neumann[26] and Bizzozero[27] in the same year discovered that the bone marrow was the source of blood cells, and Neumann first described myelogenous leukemia as differentiated from the lymphatic type in 1870;[28] thus, the mystery of the character and function of the white blood cells began to be solved. In the meantime, new instruments and methods were being developed independently to quantify the cellular elements.

The Development of the Blood Count

Starting with the work of Karl Vierordt (1818–1884) in 1852, there were many investigators who over the remainder of the century devised various types of equipment to determine accurately the numbers of the various blood cells and the amount of hemoglobin extracted from the erythrocytes in a given volume of blood. Vierordt's method[29] consisted of making a dilution of blood, drawing a small amount of the liquid up into a volumetrically calibrated capillary tube, expelling a known quantity onto a glass slide and counting the cells with the aid of a micrometer in the eyepiece. He determined that his own blood contained

5,010,000 cells per cubic millimeter, and he was able to duplicate this value with a small error. Two years later, his student, Welcher,[30] found an erythrocyte count of 3,300,000 in a patient with chlorosis. The problem with the technique was that it was tedious and impractical to be used routinely.

New devices were invented, most of which involved adding a diluted sample of blood to a calibrated chamber or capillary tube and counting the cells in an observed volume under the microscope. William Gowers, in 1877, was the first to have a chamber made that had rulings on the floor of the chamber, which eliminated the ocular micrometer.[31] Richard Thoma (1847–1923), in addition to devising the red cell pipette that still bears his name, improved the counting chamber of Gowers by having the gratings on a platform of ground glass surrounded by a moat. The counting area was one square millimeter and was divided into 400 square fields; when a cover slip was placed on the platform, a space of one millimeter remained.[32] The instrument was made by Carl Zeiss. Later Thoma made the leukocyte count simpler by devising a pipette that diluted the blood 20 times with dilute acetic acid to dissolve the erythrocytes.[33] The counting chamber over the many years was improved to make the cells easier to count, but the error was high, particularly for the erythrocyte calculation when one pipette and one chamber was used for a given blood determination. The error was evaluated in 1940 and it was calculated that if the true count were 5,000,000, any number between 4,210,000 and 5,790,000 could be expected. Therefore there was more diagnostic emphasis placed on the hemoglobin and packed-cell-volume determination until the electronic Coulter counters, which were able to give extremely accurate and precise counts,[34] came into existence in 1956.

Determination of the Hemoglobin and Packed Cell Volume

The method of determining the hemoglobin concentration of blood also went through several stages of development, and perhaps there has been no substance in the blood that has been so difficult to standardize and determine accurately. It became particularly important when Hoppe-Seyler showed that oxygen combined with hemoglobin to greatly improve the capacity of the blood to carry this gas to the body's cells.[35]

The first instruments were often ingenious but all relied on the comparison of blood or its dilutions with colored standards unrelated to hemoglobin. Sometimes these were dyes such as picrocarmine,[36] or colored glass with visual comparison[37] being made with white paper behind a standard tube. The blood was often treated with acid or alkali, which changed the nature of the hemoglobin before a comparison was made. There were four major problems with the early methods. The first was that the human eye was attempting to match two colors which were spectrally different. Second, even if the substances were identical, the concentration was assumed to be linearly proportional to the transmitted light. Third, there were no standard hemoglobin solutions that were stable for comparison purposes, and fourth, the assumption was made that hemoglobin in all bloods was homogeneous in composition. The errors were usually more than 20% and were to remain at this level into the 1940s, when the cyanmethemoglobin method[38] became the standard method used in the United States. This method, when used with a monochromatic spectrophotometer and compared with commercially available and reasonably stable standards that were based upon iron analyses and combination with carbon monoxide, can give accuracy and precision within three percent.

The measure of the packed cell volume, or hematocrit, was first used by Hedin,[39] who used a water-driven centrifuge to determine the percentage volume of the blood occupied by the blood cells after initial dilution. The problem was that the early solutions were not always isotonic and the swelling and shrinking of the erythrocytes gave variable results. Daland[40] used undiluted blood, but the centrifugal forces varied at that time, therefore results were inconsistent. It was not until many years later that the problem was corrected by using heparin or EDTA as the anticoagulant and new and standardized centrifuges, which gave consistent timing and centrifugal forces.

Thus the diagnosis of the type of anemia could not be determined accurately in terms of blood indices. The visual subjective evaluation of the peripheral blood and bone marrow smears was relied upon more for the differential diagnosis of the various types of erythrocyte dyscrasias until the quantitation of the concentration of the number of cells, the hemoglobin, and the packed cell volume was significantly improved.

Blood Cell Morphology

The morphologic evaluation of the blood cells also underwent a slow development. Swammerdam was the first to observe erythrocytes in 1658,[41] followed by Malpighi in 1661[42] in frogs, and then Leeuwenhoek in his own blood.[43]

With regard to the white blood cells, investigators reported seeing them in the eighteenth century, but the poor-quality microscopes made it difficult to differentiate them from various globules or air bubbles. However in 1777, William Hewson, using lenses especially ground for him and giving him a magnification of 400 ×, made careful observations on more than one hundred species of animals, drew pictures, and made measurements of the blood cells. Besides noting for the first time that the human red blood cell is "flat as a guinea," he made extensive studies of the lymphatic system and noted that the white corpuscles that are found in the lymph glands and thymus could be found in the peripheral blood. Hewson wrote that

> we have proved that vast numbers of central particles made by the thymus and lymphatic glands, are poured into the blood vessels through the thoracic duct, and if we examine the blood attentively we see them floating in it.[44]

Following Hewson's work, although others confirmed his findings, the study of the cellular components of the blood was neglected for almost seventy years. Then in 1846, T.W. Jones (1808–1891), the teacher of Thomas Huxley, made a substantial advance in the study of white blood cells by doing a comparative study of animals from the skate to man.[45] Without using stains, Jones differentiated the various cells in terms of granules and the lobes of the nuclei, but he believed that all of the white cells were stages in the development of the erythrocyte. William Addison also added knowledge about the white blood cells.[46] Then Max Schultze (1825–1874), who invented the term "protoplasm," in 1865 placed fresh blood mixed with ground carmine on a warm microscopic stage and observed the amoeboid movement of the white blood cells. He noted that the coarsely granular cells were less phagocytic of the carmine particles than were the finely granular ones and proposed a classification on this basis without considering the type of nucleus present in each cell.[47] The problem, of course, was that in spite of the great improvement in compound microscopes available during the years 1840–1877 and observations of such brilliant men as Virchow, Bennett, Schultze, Jones, Hayem, Cohnheim, Weigert, and others, the study of fresh unstained blood had its limitations. Besides the fact that there simply was not enough effective magnification, the contrast necessary to make intracellular differentiation of the various types of leukocytes was not available. In addition, although investigators knew that, with the new methods of counting blood cells, a low concentration of erythrocytes indicated an anemia and a high concentration of leukocytes could lead to a diagnosis of leukemia, the numerical values alone not only left the distinction between leukocytosis and leukemia indistinct, but also did not make possible a method of studying the pathogenesis of these conditions.

Paul Ehrlich (1854–1915)

But all this changed with the work of Paul Ehrlich, who early in his career developed methods of staining dried blood smears on cover slips or slides. The result was that the field of "hematology" was born.[48] The limits of the staining techniques pioneered by Ehrlich were only realized during the second half of the twentieth century with the discoveries of functionally different but morphologically similar lymphocytes.[49] Ehrlich was undoubtedly, as was Louis Pasteur, one of the greatest experimental geniuses in biology during the nineteenth century. In spite of their completely different backgrounds — Ehrlich being the product of a prosperous, German Jewish family and Pasteur being the son of poor, rural tanner in France — these two had much in common. Both were passionate, sentimental, colorful, humanistic, nonmaterialistic, and driven in their capacity for work. But the most remarkable similarity was that they both, very early in their careers, thought about biology in chemical terms. This alone placed them above the crowd working in biology and medicine and enabled them to become trailblazers in their respective fields of endeavor. While Pasteur's key to originality had its origins in the asymmetry of molecular structures of microbiological substrates, Ehrlich's primary idea was that certain chemical substances, synthetic or natural, act on tissue or living cells by combining selectively with specific cell components. This led to his first series of studies using aniline dyes to make heretofore almost invisible cell structures easily seen under the microscope.

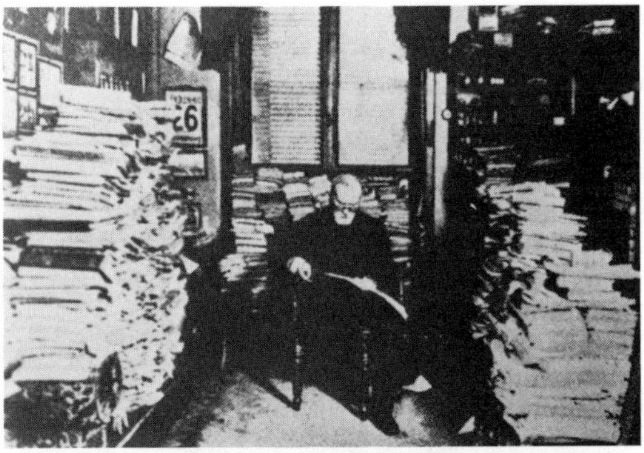

EHRLICH IN HIS OFFICE STUDY

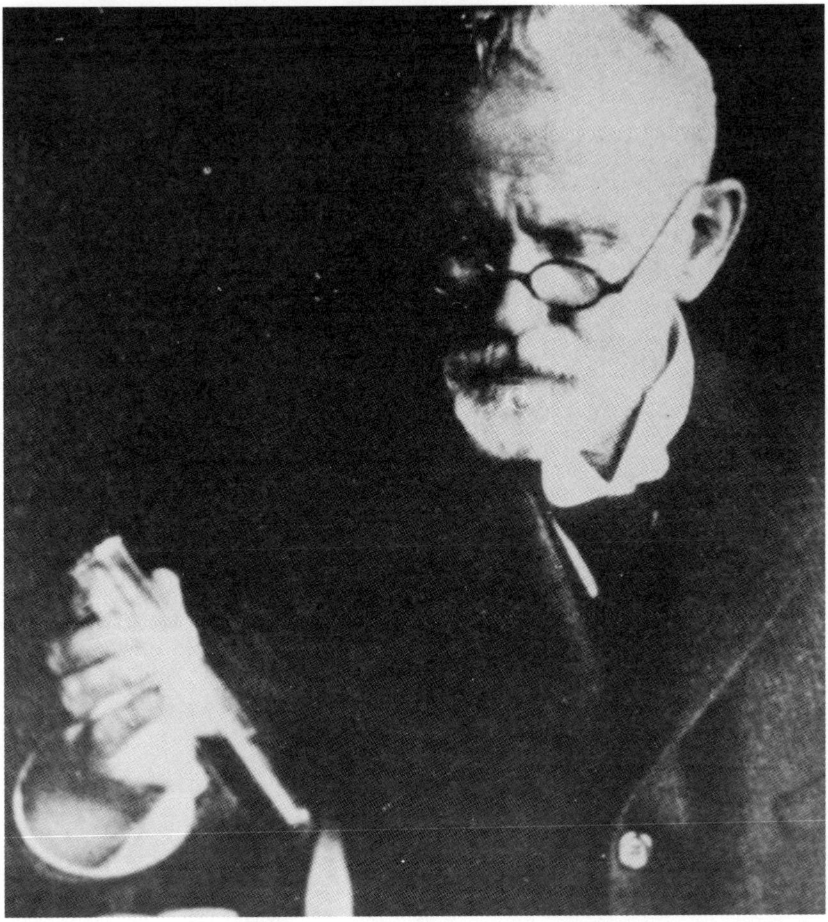

EHRLICH WITH HIS TEST-TUBE EXPERIMENTS

In the case of the white blood cells, which Ehrlich was the first to call "leukocytes," his staining techniques made it possible to study the origin and development of the blood cells in both health and disease. Although Ehrlich studied with the eminent histologists in Germany, Wilhelm Waldeyer (1836–1921), Rudolf Heidenhain (1834–1897), and his cousin, Carl Weigert (1845–1904), his approach to solving histological problems was always individual. The result was that early in his career, such outstanding investigators as Julius Cohnheim did not immediately recognize his brilliance and chided him for being a "master dyer" because of his enthusiasm for the new aniline dyes.[50] Ehrlich stated later in his career that:

> my talents lie in the field of chemistry; I can picture the chemical formula in my mental vision and I believe that this fact has been of greatest value to me in my studies. I had already foreseen many things in pure chemistry which only came to be known much later.[51]

Ehrlich received his medical degree in 1878 and went to work as an assistant to Friedrich Frerichs (1819–1885), Professor of Medicine at Berlin and one of Osler's "giants" in diagnostic medicine at the time.[52] Frerichs had studied with the chemist Wöhler early in his career, appreciated Ehrlich's chemical studies, and minimized his clinical responsibilities to give him time for his staining studies on blood cells. It was during the period 1878–1888 that Ehrlich did most of his work in hematology, although he published comparatively little during that time. But he was the first to show that certain cell structures have affinities for certain dyes based upon their acid or alkaline composition. In the case of leukocytes, he found that by mixing together both acid and basic dyes, he could produce neutral stains that differentially stained the nucleus, cytoplasm, and granules as a function of their pH. As a result, he made a classification of leukocytes that has essentially remained the same for the past one hundred years.

He identified six types of white blood cells, which he called (1) Lymphozyten, (2) Grossen mononuklearen leukozyten, (3) Ubergangsformen, (4) Polynuklearen, (5) Eosinophilen Zellen, and (6) Mastzellen. Ehrlich's descriptions of these cells were as follows:

> The lymphozyten are . . . small cells with a large round homogeneous nucleus, mostly reaction to alkaline dyes, possessing

> an unevenly staining protoplasm which is interpreted as a reticular structure rather than a granulation. The grossen mononuklearen are two to three times as large as erythrocytes, containing a large, oval, eccentric, weakly staining nucleus, and having a basophilic protoplasm. The ubergangsformen develop from the grossen mononuklearen of the blood, and are distinguished by a deep notching of the nucleus. . . . The ubergangsformen and gross mononuklearen together comprise 2-4% of the white blood corpuscles. The polynuklearen are described as having a polymorphous nucleus, irregularly bulged and indented, or even having the nucleus disintegrated into three or four distinct parts. . . . These cells compose about 70% of all white blood corpuscles . . . (and) derived from bone marrow, for the most part fully formed. . . . The eosinophilen are distinguished by a coarse, round granulation staining with acid dyes. The nucleus is similar to that of the polynuklearen though less deeply staining. These cells are . . . 2-4% of all white blood cells. The mastzellen composing 0.5% of all white blood cells in normal blood are described as intensely basophilic, containing basophilic granules of irregular size and uneven distribution.[53]

Essentially this is the modern classification except that the grossen mononuklearen and the ubergangsformen would be considered morphological variations of monocytes, the polynuklearen cells are called neutrophils, and the mastzellen are called basophils. Although Ernst Neumann (1834–1918)[54] and Giulio Bizzozero (1846–1901)[55] both discovered in 1868 that erythrocytes and granulocytes were formed in the bone marrow of adults, they did not use stains; therefore it was Ehrlich and his students who using variations of his aniline dye stains worked out many of the details of the development of these cells in the bone marrow. They showed that in the case of pernicious anemia there was in the bone marrow an abnormal megaloblast rather than an erythroblast that eventually led to the development of the pathological megalocyte. Ehrlich also showed that leukocytosis was produced by a greater activity of the precursor cells in the bone marrow, describing the presence of abnormal numbers of what he called “myelocytes,” which normally did not occur in the peripheral blood unless the stimulation of the marrow was extreme. He summarized his thoughts on the matter in 1892:

> The bone-marrow is a breeding place in which polynuclear cells are produced in large numbers from mononuclear pre-existing forms. These polynuclear cells possess above all other elements the power of emigration. . . . This readily explains the rapid and sudden appearance of large numbers of leukocytes, which so many substances bring about, and particularly the bacteria-proteins. . . . I regard leukocytosis therefore, . . . as a function of the bone-marrow.[56]

Ehrlich was the first to describe "aplastic anemia" in 1888 on the basis of the case of a postmortem on a patient with severe menorrhagia where the marrow was found to be fatty and devoid of erythocyte precursors.[57]

It is of interest, during these times of huge, well-equipped laboratories to relate how Ehrlich worked in a simple room during the early days of his career when his staining techniques attracted investigators from all over the world. According to his biographer, Marquardt:

> Visitors coming to see him there were kindly welcomed. Let us watch Ehrlich at work one day when, as so often happens, he has a visitor. Hardly looking up from his experiments over the Bunsen burner, he greets his visitor by holding out to him the little finger of his left hand. . . . The visitor looks inquiringly round the scantily equipped laboratory and remarks: "Well, Ehrlich, you know, the aspect of your laboratory is not at all imposing!" Ehrlich is busily engaged pouring the dye solution he has been heating in a test tube . . . onto a large sheet of white blotting paper which hangs from the big working bench, and is prevented from falling by bottles of dye used as weights along its upper edge. "As long as I have a water tap, a flame and some blotting paper, I can work just as well in a barn."[58]

Although no historian has commented on the significance of this portrayal of Ehrlich, it certainly indicated that this amazing man used paper chromatography to evaluate the components of the aniline dyes long before anyone else published this method of separation.

After Ehrlich left the Charité Hospital in Berlin following Frerichs's suicide, he no longer did any original work in hematology, leaving this field to his old colleagues, especially A. Lazarus with whom he published a book "Die Anemia" in 1898. This book presented to the medical public a summary of all the work done by himself and others in hematology up to that time.[59] In 1891 Ehrlich's triacid stain was replaced by the Romanovsky eosin methylene blue stain, which essentially used the principles of Ehrlich (combining an acid with a basic stain).[60] All such blood stains (such as the Wright[61] and Giemsa[62]) were modifications of the eosin methylene blue combination. The improvements gave better differentiation of the various blood cells but also allowed the staining of malarial and filarial parasites and made it unnecessary to fix the blood slide by heat because this was done by the alcohol in the stain itself.

Ehrlich joined Koch and worked on the staining of bacteria, particularly that for tuberculosis.[63] But stains and the morphology of blood cells and bacteria did not hold his interest, and he did pioneer work in immunology and later chemotherapy for syphilis, always using his concept of specific attachments to cellular components of various chemicals, for stains, immunity, and poisoning of spirochetes.

The Platelets

The platelets were the last of the cellular elements to be discovered, even though several investigators had reported seeing the small bodies.[64, 65] Max Schultze was the first to give convincing evidence for their existence[66] and along with Reiss[67] regarded them as remnants of disintegrated white blood cells. Osler[68] was not sure they were not related to bacteria and referred to them as "organisms." In 1878, Hayem referred to them as hematoblasts and thought they were the precursors of red blood cells.[69] Then in 1882 Bizzozero called them platelets and suggested that they may play a part in the formation of blood clots.[70] Homer Wright, in 1906, was the first to study the platelets with his new stain and correctly concluded that they were formed by budding of megakaryocytes in the bone marrow.[71]

Clinical Applications of the New Knowledge and Techniques

In comparison with Austin Flint's textbook of 1866, William Osler's textbook[72] published in 1892 reflected all of the above advances in the study of the blood cells. This information allowed him to attempt a classification of anemia into two categories — primary and secondary. Primary Anemia included the following: (1) chlorosis, an iron deficiency anemia in young women with characteristic low hemoglobin and erythrocytes that show hypochromia and poikilocytosis; (2) progressive pernicious anemia, with no obvious blood loss, no iron deficiency, no purpura, no malignancy, or any recognizable chronic disease. The hemoglobin is often very low, but the erythrocytes are larger than normal and nucleated forms are often present in the peripheral blood. Osler also places in this category the following anemias ("not to be distinguished from Addison's idiopathic form"): (a) pregnancy, (b) atrophy of the stomach, and (c) parasites such as hookworm. The Secondary Anemias were listed as due to: (1) hemorrhage; (2) chronic drain on the albuminous materials of the blood as in chronic suppuration, Bright's disease, or malignancy; (3) inanition brought about by poor nutrition; (4) toxins such as the action of lead, mercury, or arsenic or infections such as syphilis or malaria. No mention was made of the hemolytic anemias, which were not known at the time except clinically as liver disease. With regard to the white blood cells, by 1892, three forms of leukemia were recognized at that time — lymphatic, myelogenous, and splenic — although clinically and pathologically there sometimes appeared to be overlap of these three forms. Also leukocytosis was recognized as a response to inflammation and other pathological and physiological conditions, and eosinophilia was usually found in asthmas and parasite infections. However, during the 1890s the differentiation of leukemia and leukocytosis was not completely clear. It was thought by some that leukemia was likely to be an extreme and irreversible leukocytosis and that unexplained leukocytosis could be a benign and temporary leukemia. Only by careful investigations were many of the new blood morphologists able to prove that leukemia and leukocytosis represented entirely different pathological entities.

Toward the end of the century and the beginning of the twentieth the field of hematology was becoming a specialty, and several textbooks were devoted entirely to this subject.[73-75] The emphasis was almost entirely on morphological characteristics of the cellular elements and this focus would remain dominant throughout most of the century, although Wintrobe believes that the Modern Age of Hematology started with the discovery of the treatment of pernicious anemia by Minot and Murphy,[76] because it was the beginning of systematic experimental studies in this field.[77]

Bibliography

1. Virchow, R., Über die Reform der Pathologische und Therapeutischen Anschaungen durch die Mikroskopischen Untersuchungen. *Virchow's Arch.* **1**, p. 207, 1847.
2. Bernard, C., *Lecons sur les propriétés physiologiques et les altérations pathologiques des liquides de l'organisme.* Vol. 1, Baillière, Paris, 1859.
3. Müller, J.W. (in Ludwig's laboratory), Über die Spannung des Sauerstoffs der Blutscheiben. *Ber. Sächs Ges. (Akad) Wiss*, **22**, p. 351, 1870.
4. Senebier, J., *Rapports de l'air avec les etres organisés, tirés des journaux d'observations et d'expériences de Lazare Spallanzani, avec quelques mémoires de l'editeur sur ces matières.* Vol. II, J.J. Paschoud, Geneva, 1807.
5. Pflüger, E., Beiträge zur Lehre von der Respiration. *Pflüg. Arch. ges. Physiol.*, **10**, pp. 251, and 641, 1875.
6. Starling, E.H., The chemical correlation of the functions of the body. *Lancet* **2**, pp. 339, 423, 501 and 579.
7. Berthold, A., Transplantation der Hoden. *Arch. Anat. Physiol. wiss. Med.* p. 42, 1849.
8. Oliver, G., and Sharpey-Schafer, E.A., The physiological action of extract of the suprarenal capsules. *J. Physiol.*, **18**, p. 230, 1895.
9. Foster, M., *A Textbook of Physiology*, 6th American Edition, p. 466. Lea Brothers and Co., Philadelphia, 1895.
10. Stadelmann, E., Ueber die Ursachen der pathologische Ammoniakausscheidung beim Diabetes Mellitus und des Coma diabeticum. *Arch. Exp. Path. Pharm.*, **17**, p. 419, 1883.
11. Minkowski, O., Ueber das Vorkommen von Oxybuttersaüre im Harn bei Diabetes mellitus. Ein Beitrag sur Lehre von coma diabeticum. *Arch. Exp. Path. Pharm.*, **18**, p. 35, 1884.
12. Magnus-Levy, A., Die Oxybuttersaüre und ihre Beziehungen zum Coma diabeticum. *Arch. Exp. Path. Pharm.*, **42**, p. 149, 1899.
13. Henderson, L.J., The theory of neutrality regulation in the animal organism. *Amer. J. Physiol.*, **21**, p. 427, 1908.
14. Henderson, L.J., On the neutrality equilibrium in blood and protoplasm. *J. Biol. Chem.* **7**, p. 29, 1909.
15. Hasselbach, K.A., Elektrometrische Reaktionbestimmung

Kohlensaürehaltiger Flüssigkeiten. *Biochem. Z.*, **30**, p. 317, 1910.
16. Van Slyke, D.D., and Cullen, G.E., Studies of acidosis. 1. The bicarbonate concentration of the blood plasma; its significance, and its determination as a method of acidosis. *J. Biol. Chem.*, **30**, p.289, 1917.
17. Bernard, C., *Lecons sur le diabète et la glycogènese animale.* Baillière, Paris, 1877.
18. Bernard, C., *Lecons de physiologie expérimentale appliquée à la médicine,* Baillière, Paris, 1855.
19. Garrod, A.B., Observations on certain pathological conditions of the blood in gout, rheumatism, and Bright's disease. *Med.-chir. Trans.*, **31**, p. 83, 1848, and **37**, p. 49, 1854.
20. Folin, O., and Wu, H., A system of blood analyses. *J. Biol. Chem.*, **38**, p. 81, 1919.
21. Bang, I., Ein Verfahren zur Mikrobestimmung von Blutbestandteilen. *Biochem. Z.*, **49**, p. 19, 1913.
22. Peters, J.P., and Van Slyke, D.D., *Quantitative Clinical Chemistry.* Vol. II, William and Wilkins, Baltimore, 1932.
23. Andral, G., Essai d'hématologie pathologique, p. 48, Fortin, Masson et Cie, Paris, 1843.
24. Flint, A., *A Treatise on the Principles and Practice of Medicine*, 2nd Edition, p. 65, p. 88, Henry C. Lea, Philadelphia, 1867.
25. Cohnheim, L., Ueber Entzündung und Eiterung. *Virchow's Arch.* **40**, p. 1, 1867.
26. Neumann, E., Ueber die Bedeutung des Knochenmarkes für die Blutbildung. *Zbl. Med.* Wiss., **6**, p. 689, 1868.
27. Bizzozero, G., Sulla funzione ematopoietica del midollo delle ossa., R.C.R. 1st. *Lomb. Sci. Lett.*, **1**, 2 ser., p. 815, 1868.
28. Neumann, E., Ein Fall von Leukämie mit Erkrankung des Knochenmarkes. *Arch Heilk. (Lpz)*, **11**, p. 1, 1870.
29. Vierordt, K., Neue Method der quantitativen Mikroskopischen Analyse des Blutes. *Arch. Physiol. Heilk.*, 11, p. 26, 1852.
30. Welcher, H., *Blutkörperchenzählung und farbeprüfende Methode.* Vierteljahrschrift für die Praktische Heilkunde (Prague), **44**, p. 12, 1854.
31. Gowers, W.R., On the numeration of blood corpuscles. *Lancet*, **ii**, p. 797, 1877.
32. Lyon, J.F., and Thoma, R., Über die Methode der

Blutkorperzählung. *Virchow's Archiv*. **84**, p. 131, 1881.
33 . Thoma, R., Die Zählung der weissen Zellen des Blutes. *Virchow's Archiv.*, **87**, p. 201, 1882.
34. Brecher, G., Schneiderman, M., and Williams, G.Z., Evolution of an electronic blood cell counter. *Am. J. Clin. Path.*, **26**, p. 1439, 1956.
35. Hoppe-Seyler, F., Ueber den chemischen und optischen Eigenschaften des Blutfarbstoffs. *Virchow's Archiv.*, **29**, pp. 233 and 597, 1864.
36 . Limbeck, R., *The Clinical Pathology of the Blood.* Translated by A. Latham and J. Nachbar, p. 30., The New Sydenham Society, London, 1901.
37. Ibid, p. 37.
38. Crosby, W.H., Munn, J.J., and Furth, F.W., Standardizing a Method for Clinical Hemoglobinometry., US. Armed Forces Med. Jour., **5**, 693, 1954.
39. Hedin, S.G., Der Hämatokrit, ein neuer Apparat zur Untersuchung des Blutes. *Skand. Arch. Physiol.*, **2**, p. 134, 1890-91.
40. Daland, J., Über das Volumen der rothen und weissen Blutkorperchen im Blute des gesunden und kranken Menschen. *Fortschr. d. Med., Berlin*, **8**, p. 867, 1891.
41. Swammerdam, J., *Book of Nature or the History of Insects*, p. 121, London, 1658.
42. Malpighi, M., *Opera omnia*, p. 35, Leyden, 1687.
43. Leeuwenhoek, A., Philosophical Transactions of the Royal Society of London, p. 22, 1674.
44. Hewson, W., *The Works of William Hewson*, Sydenham Society, London, 1846.
45. Jones, T.W., The blood corpuscles considered in its different phases of development in the Animal Series. *Phil. Trans.*, p. 65, 136, 1846.
46. Addison W., *Experimental and Practical Researches on Inflammation and on the Origin and Nature of Tubercles of the Lungs*. J. Churchill, London, 1848.
47. Schultze, M., Ein heizharer Objekttisch und Seine Verwendung bei untersuchungen des Blutes. *Arch. Mikr. Anat.*, **1**, p. 35, 1865.
48. Ehrlich, P., and Lazarus, A., *Histology of the Blood, Normal and Pathological.* Translated by W. Myers, Univ. Press, Cambridge, 1900.
49. Ford, W.L., The Lymphocyte — Its Transformation from a Frustrat-

ing Enigma to A Model of Cellular Function. p. 457, in M. Wintrobe's *Blood*, Pure McGraw Hill, 1980.

50. Salomonsen, C.L., Reminiscences of the Summer Semester, 1877, at Breslau. Translated by C.L. Temkin. *Bull. Hist. Med.* **24**, p. 333, 1950.
51. Marquardt, M., *Paul Ehrlich*, p. 15, Henry Schuman, N.Y., 1951.
52. Osler, W., Allgemeines Krankenhaus. *Can. Med. Surg. Jour.*, **11**, p. 451, 1873.
53. Ref. 48, p. 69.
54. Neumann, E., Ueber die Bedeutung des Knochenmarkes für die Blutbildung. *Zentralbl. Med. Wissensch.*, **6**, p. 689, 1868.
55. Bizzozero, G., Sulla funzione ematopoetica del midollo delle ossa. *Zentralbl. Med. Wissensch.* **6**, p. 885, 1868.
56. Ref. 48, p. 147.
57. Ehrlich, P., Ueber einen Fall von Anämie mit Bemerkungen ueber regenerative Veraenderungen des Knochenmarks. *Charité Ann.*, **13** p. 300, 1888.
58. Ref. 51, p. 134.
59. Ehrlich, P., and Lazarus, A., *Anemia.* Second Edition, Translated by W.W. Armit, Rebman Limited, London, 1910.
60. Romanovsky, D., Zur Frage der Parasitologie und Therapie der Malaria. *St. Petersburg Med. Wehnschr.* **16**, p. 297, 1891.
61. Wright, J.H., A rapid method for the differential staining of blood films and malarial parasites. *J. Med. Res.*, **7**, p. 138, 1902.
62. Giemsa, G., Färbemethoden für Malariaparasiten. *Centrbl. Bakt., I Abt.*, **31**, p. 429 and **32**, p. 307, 1902.
63. Koch, R., The Etiology of Tuberculosis, in *Microparasites in Disease*, Translated by Stanley Boyd, p. 74, New Sydenham Society, London, 1886.
64. Donné, A., *Cours de Microscopie.* Bailliere, Paris, 1844.
65. Zimmermann, G., Ueber die Formgebilde des menschlichen Blutes in ihrem naehren Verhaeltniss zum Prozesse der Entzuendung und Eiterung. *Rust's Mag. für d. ges. Heilk.* **66**, p. 171, 1846.
66. Ref. 47.
67. Reiss, L., Zur pathologischen Anatomie des Blutes. *Arch. f. Anat. Phys. u. Wissensch. Med.*, p. 237, 1872.
68. Osler, W., An Account of Certain Organisms occurring in the liquor sanguinis. *Monthly. Micro. Jour.*, **12**, p. 141, 1874.

69. Hayem, G., Recherches sur l'évolution des hématies dans le sang de l'homme et des vertébrés. *Arch. Physiol. Norm. Path.*, **5**, p. 692, 1878.
70. Bizzozero, G., Über einen neuen Formbestandteil des Blutes und dessen Rolle bei der Thrombose und der Blutgerinnung. *Virchow's Archiv.*, **90**, p. 261, 1882.
71. Wright, J.H., The origin and nature of blood plates. *Boston Med. and Surg. Jour.*, **154**, p. 643, 1906.
72. Osler, W., *The Principles and Practice of Medicine.* Appleton and Co., N.Y., 1892.
73. Hayem, G., *Du Sang et ses altérations anatomiques.* G. Masson, Paris, 1889.
74. Ref. 36.
75. Cabot, R.C., *A Guide to the Clinical Examination of the Blood.* William Wood and Company, New York, 1897.
76. Minot, G.R., and Murphy, W.P., Treatment of pernicious anemia by a special diet. *J.A.M.A.*, **87**, p. 470, 1926.
77. Wintrobe, M., *Blood, Pure, and Eloquent*, McGraw-Hill Book Co., 1980.

Chapter XVIII

Tumors

The nature and etiology of tumors has been a challenge for the medical community since antiquity. Although significant progress in understanding them has been made during the past two centuries, using reductionist techniques that have been so successful in gaining knowledge about cell metabolism and genetics, there is still a great deal of mystery surrounding tumors. And until investigators determine the precise mechanism by which genetic codes manifest themselves through the various nucleic acids and proteins that relate to normal growth, development, aging, and internal and external influences on the immune system, the ultimate mechanism by which tumors arise and grow will probably remain an enigma. This is said in spite of the ingenious and imaginative studies on oncogenes and their relationships to viruses,[1] and that some therapeutic progress against some specific neoplasms has been made.

Antiquity to 1800

Medical writings since ancient times have addressed the problem of tumors and cancers. Both the Edwin Smith Papyrus[2] and the Ebers Papyrus,[3] written in approximately 1500 B.C., mentioned these lesions. Later Hippocrates recognized cancers of the skin, breast, uterus, stomach, and mouth and attempted to treat some of them with ointments or cauterization.[4] Galen classified tumors into three general categories: natural ones such as the enlargement of the uterus in pregnancy, those formed by healing such as bone callus and skin keloids, and tumors that we would call true neoplasms but that undoubtedly included, at the time, such lesions as chronic inflammation and cysts.[5] Hippocrates and Galen both considered the origin of the third group to be due to an imbalance of the four humors (black bile, yellow bile, blood, and phlegm). They thought that malignant cancers were due to an accumulation of black bile, a theory that persisted until the fiery protests of Paracelsus in the sixteenth century. Paracelsus, however, used some alchemical ideas to formulate a different type of humoralism, which added no lasting knowledge to understanding disease processes.[6] Antonio Benivieni (1443–

1502),[7] Gabriele Falloppio (1523–1562),[8] and other medical men described tumors, but there was still confusion about malignant neoplasms because in descriptions not only were benign neoplasms included but sometimes also ulcers, chancres, gangrene, carbuncles, erysipelas, leprosy, scabies, buboes, and aneurysms. Morgagni, during his 700 autopsies, encountered cancers of the breast, stomach, rectum, and pancreas and sometimes noted accompanying lesions in the lymph nodes, lungs, and liver, which were undoubtedly metastatic lesions from a primary cancer, but he did not speculate on the relationship.[9] Charles Deshais Gentron (1663–1700), a French physician, published a small book on cancer in 1700 and was the first to suggest that a cancer starts as a local lesion that represents a transformed part of the affected organ that continues to grow, destroying the surrounding tissue and is refractive to any type of medication.[10] But Gendron's ideas were also unproven speculation and the humoral concept or its modifications continued to be the more popular theory. Certainly the more astute clinicians through the hundreds of years since Hippocrates were able to recognize and differentiate various tumors on the basis of location, appearance, degree of hardness, and the symptoms of the patient and to make accurate prognoses. However, with regard to therapy, the applied poultices and remedies were for the most part useless, although it is possible that some of the later barber surgeons could have achieved some degree of success with excision if the resulting infection did not kill the patient.

With regard to experimental work on tumors, perhaps the first individual to take this approach was Jean Astruc (1684–1766) who took pieces of cancerous breast and an equivalent amount of beefsteak and, after distilling them both using a retort in a sand bath, examined both the residues and the distillates.[11] He concluded that there was no significant difference, either qualitatively or quantitatively, in the composition of cancers or normal tissue. He used the extremely crude methods of assaying — using precipitation techniques, treatment with acids, solubility in alcohol, testing for changes in color of indicators made by extracts of flowers, and finally tasting the fractions. He then stated " I conclude that for all that has been said about an acrid, corrosive humour in cancers, it is a false assumption, and consequently it is necessary to look for some other explanation regarding the generation of these tumors." Although this experiment would not be considered a positive proof for his conclusion by modern scientific standards, certainly the spirit of Francis Bacon, William Harvey, and Robert Boyle was there, and the concept of cancers being caused by an accumulation of black bile lost much of its credibility.

There were other astute and specific observations regarding cancers made by other medical men whose validity have stood the test of time. The English physician John Hill in 1761 reported six cases of polyps in the nose when the individuals were snuff users, and in one case he stated that one swelling that was hard, black, and painless at first developed "all the frightful symptoms of an open cancer. He warned against the immoderate use of snuff, saying "no man should venture upon snuff, who is not sure that he is not so far liable to cancer; and no man can be sure of that."[12] In 1795, Samuel von Soemmerring, practicing in Mainz, found that "carcinoma of the lips occurs most frequently where men indulge in pipe smoking; the lower lip is particularly affected by cancer when it is compressed between the tobacco pipe and the teeth."[13] In 1775, Percivall Pott called the attention of the medical profession to the correlation of scrotal cancer to the occupation of chimney sweep, although the members of this occupation had already recognized "sootwart" as one of the hazards of their trade.[14]

1800–1839

It is of interest that in 1802 a committee in England, represented by some of the most eminent medical men in England, assembled a group of questions regarding cancer, questions that were extremely astute in that they were the ones specifically answered during the nineteenth and twentieth centuries.[15] The questions proposed were the following: (1) What are the diagnostic signs of cancer? (2) Does any alteration take place in the structure of a part, preceding that more obvious change which is called cancer? If there does, what is the nature of that alteration? (3) Is cancer always an original and primary disease, or may other diseases degenerate into cancer? (4) Are there any proofs of cancer being a hereditary disease? (5) Are there any proofs of cancer being a contagious disease? (6) Is there any well-marked relation between cancer and any other diseases? If there is, what are those diseases to which it bears the nearest resemblance in its origin, progress, and termination? (7) May cancer be regarded at any period, or under any circumstances, merely as a local disease? Or, does the existence of cancer in one part, afford a presumption that there is a tendency to a similar morbid alteration in other parts of the animal system? (8) Has climate, or local situation, any influence in rendering the human constitution more or less liable to cancer, under any form, or in any part? (9) Is there a particular temperament of body more liable to be affected with cancer than others? (10) Are brute-creatures subject to any disease resembling cancer in the human subject? (11) Is there any period of life absolutely exempt from the attack of the disease? (12) Are the lymphatic glands ever affected primarily in cancer? (13) Is cancer under any circumstances susceptible to a natural cure?

Although the brilliant Bichat at the beginning of the nineteenth century recognized that organs were made up of various types of tissues, which could be specifically affected by inflammation, he could not determine with any degree of accuracy whether a growth was primarily inflammation or a benign or malignant lesion.

In 1813 in the monumental sixty volumes entitled *Dictionaire Des Sciences Medicales*, Gaspard Bayle and Jean Cayol wrote 142 pages about cancer, discussing the diagnosis, prognosis, and therapy (when possible) on 15 different cancers. However, with regard to their etiology and pathogenesis, they were only to say a few words:

> We have nothing to say regarding the immediate cause of cancer . . . (but) with regard to the more distant causes, these (can be) divided into general and local. The first (would include) sadness, prolonged grief, sexual abuse, celibacy, sterility, suppression of natural evacuations as menstruation, hemorrhoids, or (lesions) produced by cautery or other such procedures. Local causes are blows, bruises, acute or chronic phlegmases, engorgements or ulcers, syphilitic, scrofulous or other such afflictions, constant or intermittent stimulations such as that on the stomach by alcoholic beverages. There is no doubt that all these causes, individually or together . . . are able to provoke the formation of cancer . . . this is a fact confirmed by all the previous centuries. But it is also certain that cancer can develop without these causes. . . . Cancer of the liver, the brain, and other internal organs prove incontestably that cancer can be produced without a local cause. On the other hand we often see all the above mentioned causes present, but nevertheless, a cancer is never produced. . . . A rigorous conclusion of the above facts . . . is that there exists an internal disposition without which the above external factors cannot produce cancer. . . . Without trying to define this disposition, which will perhaps always remain unknown as to its nature, we can call it

> a cancer diathesis. It is this disposition that is a true and unique cause of the recurrence of cancer after extirpation and is responsible for the simultaneous cancers produced in diverse organs that are often very far from each other. . . . The diathesis does not exist equally in the different parts of the body . . . certain individuals seem to be especially disposed towards cancer of the skin, (and) others cancer of the glands or other organs. . . . Cancer is not a local disease . . . because there is a cancerous cachexia. . . . This cachexia exists in various ways . . . it alters nutrition and other body functions to produce a general depravation of the body. . . . Is cancer contagious? It is not at all likely that cancer is contagious (in spite of various anecdote cited).[16]

From this quotation, it is obvious that the questions posed in 1802 were far from being answered. The major problem was that during the first quarter of the century, as much as anatomical pathology had advanced, particularly in France, the observations made on both the living and dead were entirely macroscopic, and it was often impossible to determine with the naked eye the difference between a swelling due to inflammation or cancer early in the development of the lesion, especially if there was ulceration and necrosis, which can occur in both types of lesions.

The result was that the pathogenesis of tumors was expressed by early nineteenth century pathologists, who did not believe the older ideas such as imbalances of acids and bases, salts, and minerals as proposed by the sixteenth- and seventeenth-century iatrochemists such as Paraselsus, Sylvius, and van Helmont. Rather they did espouse almost equally simplistic ideas such as the "coagulated lymph" of John Hunter, a cancer diathesis, and finally the concept of blastema, which was supposed to be part of the blood plasma and would appear in literature discussions of cancers until the middle of the century. The pathologists of that period, J.F. Lobstein, Julius Vogel, Gabriele Andral, Robert Carswell, Thomas Hodgkin, and John Abernethy, all believed in some aspect of humoralism. Perhaps the "last hurrah" for the humoral idea was expressed in Karl Rokitansky's 1839 *Handbook of Pathology*, who proposed an elaborate system that used his concepts of crases and dyscrases, which were generalized states of the body that were predisposed to the production of normal and abnormal blastemas to produce different diseases. Thus he used such terms as typhus crasis, tubercle crasis, croupous crasis, exanthematous crasis, and cancer dyscrasis to explain the pathogenesis of these conditions and diseases (see Chapter VI).

But as discussed in earlier chapters, a major breakthrough in the study of the pathology was the great improvement in the optics of the compound microscope in 1830. The first great advancement in biology that used the newly almost-perfected instrument and that soon influenced the opinions of the early pathologists was the development of the Cell Theory as proposed by Schwann in 1839. This theory essentially stated that the cell was the basic unit of living matter and was one of the first steps in the successful method of reductionism in biology and medicine. When Johannes Müller started to study tumors in 1836, he did not recognize the importance of cells, and his observations had no significant value. But in 1838, when he became aware of his student Schwann's work, he revised his earlier studies, noted the cellular composition of tumors, and described such cells, pointing out their variation in size and shape, but also stated that he did not believe that microscopical analysis could be used as a practical means to diagnose cancers.[17]

1839–1855

Although the Cell Theory was quickly accepted, Müller, like his students Schwann, Virchow, and Kölliker, had difficulty accepting the fact that cells can only arise from other cells by division. They still had faith in the validity of the blastema concept, in which a liquid component of the blood plasma or the intercellular fluid could give rise to new cells by a method of accretion around granules. Kölliker wrote in 1853:

> Among the few hypotheses which have . . . been proposed, . . . that of Schwann, who compares it with the formation of crystals, is certainly the most attractive. . . . In a fluid containing organic matters dissolved in considerable proportions, a granule, the nucleolus, is precipitated. Once formed, this attracts nutriment from the cytoblastema, and thus becomes the nucleus, which Schwann considers to be solid. This still goes on attracting to itself a substance, which, becoming more and more condensed, at last forms a membrane; which, allowing for the passage of fluid cytoblastema through its pores, becomes detached from the nucleus, and we have a cell.[18]

But by 1860, Kölliker changed his mind:

> With regard to the formation of cells, a distinction has hitherto been made between the free origin of them, and their production through the intervention of other cells. The farther, however, investigation is prosecuted, the occurrence of a free cell-formation becomes more and more doubtful; and it appears that all animal cells only arise, as in plants, in dependence upon other pre-existing cells.[19]

The individual who actually established this fact was Robert Remak, another student of Müller, who while studying embryological development recognized that all of the cells of an early embryo come from cleavage of the zygote and discovered the germ layers; he also observed dividing blood cells in the later stages of an embryo.[20] But it was Virchow, who in 1855 finally admitting the validity of Remak's conclusions and enunciated his famous "omnis cellula e cellula." This fact, in addition to the establishment of the Cell Theory, then provided an excellent basis for the study of not only all aspects of biology but also pathology. Only with the later findings of Oscar Hertwig,[21] Eduard Strasburger,[22] and Walther Flemming[23] in the late 1870s, using the new methods of fixing and staining for the study of mitosis and cell division, was it possible to extend Virchow's axiom to "omnis cellula e cellula, omnis nucleus e nucleo," and in this manner provide the foundation for evolution studies and modern genetics.[24]

The Problem of Metastatic Cancer

The term metastasis, although presently used exclusively to denote the process of the spread of a primary cancer through blood or lymphatic vessels to other parts of the body where secondary growths are established, was until the middle of the nineteenth century used to describe the displacement of any disease from one part of the body to another. In 1829, J.C.A. Récamier, Professor of Medicine at the College de France, reported local infiltration and invasion of veins and brain lesions in patients who had died of breast cancer.[25] However, the mechanism by which this occurred remained a mystery until many years later. Johannes Müller first suggested that a fluid blastema promoted such secondary growths, but after the establishment of the Cell Theory, he expressed the possibility that a cancer could spread by cells or "germ-nuclei" through the circulation. Then in 1840, a young physician in Göttingen, Bernard Langenbeck, found in autopsies on two patients with uterine cancer that there were "cancer cells" in the pelvic veins, right heart, and pulmonary arteries. Although Cruveilhier had seen similar situations, this pathologist believed that cancers had their origins in the blood vessels. On the other hand, Langenbeck noted that the cancer cells were not attached to the vein wall, appeared as well developed as in the primary lesion, did not always appear in the veins around the organ where the primary cancer was located, were never seen in arteries around the cancers, and therefore it was very unlikely that these lesions could form from a cancerous degeneration of vessel walls. He therefore concluded that in secondary growths of cancers:

> Cell-nuclei, young cells, or particles of the carcinoma enter veins or lymphatics vessels laid open by (carcinomatous) ulceration and reach the circulation by virtue of the movements of fluids in these vessels from the branches to the main trunks and the right heart. Here they seat themselves firmly either in some or one of the greater vessels, e.g. the thoracic duct, or in the right heart and develop into a carcinoma or — as appears to be most frequently the case — because their diameter is far greater than that of the finest capillary vessels, they lodge in the capillary vascular system of the lungs (or the hepatic portal vessels when the primary carcinoma is situated in the gut) and there grow into cancerous tumors in complete accordance with the known laws of cell growth, i.e. by the development and multiplication of young cells within (by) already formed older cells.[26]

However, Langenbeck's conclusions were not generally accepted, one of the major reasons being that Rudolf Virchow, who at that time still thought that cells arose from a humoral cytoplastema, had stated that metastatic cancers were more likely to have arisen as a result of an acellular cancerous blastema. In 1858 Virchow said in a series of lectures:

> The lungs, as is well known, are much more rarely invaded by cancerous disease than the liver, not only after gastric and uterine, but also after mammary cancer which would necessar-

> ily rather produce cancer in the lungs, if it were anything corpuscular which was conveyed away, became stagnant and gave rise to a new eruption of the disease. The manner in which the metastatic diffusion takes place seems, on the contrary, to render it probable that the transference takes place by means of certain fluids, and these possess the power of producing an infection which disposes different parts to a reproduction of a mass of the same nature as the one which originally existed . . . in the course of heteroplastic (cancerous) processes dyscrasiae occur which do not burst out afresh at points, which, according to the direction of the current of blood or lymph, would be most directly exposed to them, but at remote spots.[27]

This statement at this time is remarkable since Virchow had not only become an advocate for the Cell Theory and had enunciated his "omnis cellula e cellula" but also had so severely criticized Rokitansky several years before for use of the concept of crases and dyscrases, which he called neohumoralism. Then in 1865, Carl Thiersch carried out careful observations on epithelial cancers of the skin, in which he found cells similar to those in skin carcinomas in distant lymph nodes.[28] He argued that because there was no epithelium in lymph nodes it was most likely that they arrived there through an embolic process from the primary skin lesion. In 1889, Stephen Paget published studies on 735 cases of carcinoma of the breast and noted that 241 had metastases of the liver and 66 cases of metastases of the spleen and compared these results with 340 cases of pyemia, which resulted in 66 cases of abscesses in the liver and 39 in the spleen.[29] He explained the discrepancy by assuming that the liver and spleen possessed different properties that made them differ in susceptibility to cancers on the one hand and pyemic infections on the other. These ideas were finally accepted by most pathologists at that time.

The Question of the Origin of Cancer and the Specificity of the Cancer Cell

After the general acceptance of both the Cell Theory and the fact that cells are only derived from other cells, Virchow wrote during the 1860s that not only cancers but also inflammatory lesions such as tubercles arise from undifferentiated cells in the connective tissue cells in response to different stimuli that can produce either cancers, pus, or tubercle cells. However, his old rival and nemesis Robert Remak, who had come to the conclusion that "omnis cellula e cellula" while Virchow still believed in the cytoblastema, also was the first to suggest in 1854 that epithelial cancers typically arose from normal epithelium.[30] Remak had quietly over the years pioneered the field of embryology and had discovered the three germ layers and that epithelial surfaces arise, except in the possible case of parts of the urogenital system, from ectoderm and entoderm, whereas connective tissue arises from the mesoderm. However, Remak was primarily a biologist and, because he was only peripherally interested in pathology, he did not propose complex theories such as those of Virchow, who by that time was considered the czar of German pathology. For some reason Virchow, although acknowledging the importance of Remak's work on the germ layers, chose to ignore an embryological basis for epithelial cancers and therefore stated even ten years later that epithelial cancers arose from connective tissue cells. However, it was Thiersch's observations that eventually proved Virchow in error.

During his study of cancers of the skin, Thiersch, using fixation by alcohol or chromic acid, sectioning with a hand blade, and staining with carmine, was able to show a transition of obvious cancer cells from the basal layer cells of the skin and not with any connective tissue cells.

Inflammatory Tumors

Until the last half of the nineteenth century, the nature of tumors or "swellings" were differentiated by their clinical evaluation and gross observations, and often the visual distinction between true neoplasms and inflammatory granulomas such as tubercles was confused. With the microscope, the basic differences became clearer. Using this instrument, Julius Cohnheim in 1868 described inflammation at the cellular level and proved that the swelling character of some inflammations was in great part due to the migration of leukocytes from the small vessels into an irritated area to produce "pus." Although it was not until the 1880s that Pasteur and Koch (Chapter XIII) discovered the inciting action of microorganisms to produce infection and that Metchnikoff (Chapter XVI) recognized the phagocytic actions of leukocytes on such organisms, the German pathologist, in spite of the lack of this knowledge at the time, called such lesions "infective tumors," particularly those associated with tuberculosis, leprosy, glanders, actinomycoses, and syphilis. He also recognized that such tumors as the leukocytomata of Klebs was characterized by many leukocytes, epithelioid giant cells, and other such inflammatory elements not typically found in true neoplasms, whether benign or malignant.[31]

The Definitive Studies of Wilhelm Waldeyer

Although the microscope was beginning to resolve histologically the various types of tumors, there was still a clear-cut disagreement with regard to the cellular derivation of malignant tumors. Wilhelm Waldeyer (1836–1921), a student of both Jacob Henle and Karl Reichert and one of the outstanding histologists of the nineteenth century, was early in his career in charge of pathology at Breslau. There he carried out careful studies of breast cancers, using large sections and carmine stain, and published his work during the years 1870–1872.[32] He showed that early breast cancer is characterized by multiplication of cells in the glandular acini, with some proliferation of supporting connective tissue. Next, the epithelial cells become very atypical and soon rupture the basal membranes of the acini, after which they spread to the surrounding interlobular connective tissue. A soft or medullary cancer has a large number of carcinomatous epithelial cells, whereas a scirrhous tumor has very few but more connective tissue present. In carcinoma of the stomach, a similar situation occurs, and Waldeyer was able to show in sections that the malignant mucosal cells often showed continuity through all the layers of the stomach wall, which was strong, though static evidence that the origin of epithelial cancer of the stomach originated in the mucosal cells, and that this invasion was local and primarily by cell division. These studies also offered strong evidence that epithelial cancer growing in more distant organs or tissues arrived there by an embolic process and not as a result of an independent growth stimulated by a type of acellular factor in the blood or lymph, as was proposed by Virchow. Waldeyer also could find no evidence anywhere of a transformation of any connective tissue elements to epithelial cancer cells, although he stressed that various amounts and forms of supporting connective tissue could be stimulated to grow by these cancer cells. But, on the other hand, he did believe that connective tissue cells or other cells and other types of tissue whose original derivation was the embryonic mesoderm could give rise to sarcomas that did not possess epithelial characteristics. The ideas and circumstantial evidence of cancer origin by Waldeyer have continued to be accepted to the present time and have essentially not been seriously challenged by modern anatomic pathologists. Leland Rather (1913–1990), the eminent historian of pathology, summarized the consequences of Waldeyer's studies:

> What did happen was that the assumptions so clearly articulated and skillfully employed by Waldeyer in 1867 continued to suffice, as the nineteenth century wore on, to more or less satisfactorily explain all additional histological data garnered by students of the tumor problem. Histological techniques, with the introduction of the rotary microtome and aniline cell and tissue stains, became increasingly refined in the 1870s and 1880s, and apochromatic objectives and substage condensers sharpened the microscopic image. The perfection of these techniques was a powerful stimulant to convert pathologists into histopathologists and to stunt the growth of other procedures in the study of tumors. As Virchow pointed out in 1898, pathologists were becoming captive interpreters of static images, "readers of glass slides". Meanwhile no decisive evidence in favor of any alternatives to Waldeyer's set of assumptions appeared: those hypotheses gradually lost credibility because they were unnecessary rather than because they were refuted by further observation . . . then as now, a slice of tumor tissue—growing ever thinner—available to the microscopist, tumor histogenesis was still interpretative, whereas tumor histology was descriptive. . . . Leaving aside the near certainty that the initial step in the transformation of a normal cell into a cancer cell is not visible under the light microscope, it was still necessary for histopathologists to infer temporal developmental sequences from static spatial arrangements. And in most instances tumors became available for microscopic study only after they were well past their initial states of development and growth.[33]

Nineteenth Century Ideas on the Etiology of Cancer

Until 1850, most concepts on the origin of cancers related to the influence of some unknown humors, or pathological blastemas. But with the acceptance of the Cell Theory and Remak's truth that cells can only arise from other cells, newer theories were proposed. Virchow, who placed much faith in the developmental ability of connective tissue cells, not only stated that all inflammatory cells arose from division of cells in that tissue, but cancers by a process of "metaplasia," a term he invented to describe cells under the influence of some factor in the blood. Then his student, Julius Cohnheim, not only experimentally demolished Virchow's idea on the origin of inflammatory cells (see Chapter XII), but also proposed that cancers arose from embryonic cells that had not developed in the fetus, and persisted in the newborn and adult, that became reactivated to produce neoplasms. In his famous *Lectures on General Pathology* published in 1877, Cohnheim, after eliminating trauma and infection as etiological agents, wrote the following:

> The simplest view appears to me undoubtedly to be that in an early stage of embryonic development more cells are produced than are required for building up the part concerned, so that there remains unappropriated a quantity of cells — it may be a very few in number — which, owing to their embryonic character, are endowed with a marked capacity for proliferation.[31]

As indirect evidence to support his idea, Cohnheim sites the fact that cancers often originate around specific orifices of the body such as the lips, tongue, eyelids, rectum, esophagus, cervix, and he gives these reasons:

> The above named localities are most of them the seat, at some stage or other of embryonic development, of a certain complication. There occurs at the various orifices either a prolongation of the epiblast inwards or a conjunction between it and another epithelial tube . . . ; and during the process some slight irregularity may, I think, easily happen, which would give rise to a group of superfluous epithelial cells — that is, to the rudiment of a tumor . . . the almost constant localization of epithelioma of the esophagus . . . is due to the fact that the esophagus and bronchus were originally here united. In the rectum, too, it is noted on the orifice itself, the anus, that a [cancer] develops, but at the spot where the epithelial tube formed by the hinder portion of the gut unites with the anal invagination of the epiblast. . . . In the female . . . the favorite seat of cancer, [is] the region in which the pavement epithe-

> lium of the sinus urogenitalis coalesces with the cylindrical epithelium of Müller ducts.[31]

Cohnheim also cited as evidence for his embryonic rest theory the nature of dermoid tumors and teratomas, both benign and malignant. However, the embryonic rest theory lost its popularity as more information was developed about tumors, particularly the realization that Cohnheim's theory did not explain why all embryonic rest cells did not produce tumors. The visualization of a transition of normal epithelium to precancerous to frankly malignant cells in multiple sites as in the skin cancer, the production of cancers in animals by viruses and chemical carcinogens, and the influence of heredity on cancer production also contributed to the demise of Cohnheim's theory. In addition, as more knowledge was gained about the internal functions of the cell, particularly as related to the cell nucleus and chromosomes and finally nucleic acid and gene action, it became clear that tumor productions clearly have as their etiology many different factors that probably act in complex sequences and that each tumor is very likely different in its pathogenesis. This has been an expanding recognition since Cohnheim's ideas more than one hundred years ago.[34]

Bibliography

1. Bishop, J.M., Cellular oncogenes and retroviruses. *Annu. Rev. Biochem.*, **54**, p. 302, 1983.
2. Breasted, J.H., *The Edwin Smith Surgical Papyrus*. Univ. Chicago Press, Chicago, 1930.
3. Effell, B., *The Papyrus Ebers: The Greatest Egyptian Medical Document*. Levin and Munksgaard, Copenhagen, 1937.
4. Adams, F., *The Genuine Works of Hippocrates*. Sydenham Society, London, 1849.
5. Galen, De tumoribus praeter naturum. In his *Opera*, Vol. 7, p. 705, Ed. C.G. Kuhn, Leipzig, 1824.
6. Major, R., *A History of Medicine*. Vol. 1, p. 384, C. Thomas, Springfield, Id. 1954.
7. Benivieni, A., De abditis nonnullis ac mirandis morborum et sanationum causis, 1507. Translated by C. Singer, C. Thomas, Springfield, Ill., 1954.
8. Falloppio, G., *Omnia quaeadhuc extant opera . . .* Andreae Wecheli, 1584.
9. Morgagni, J.B., *De sedibus, et causis morborum per anatomen indagatis libri quinque, Remondiniana*. Venice, 1761, English Translation by B. Alexander, London, 1769.
10. Gendron, D., *Enquiries into the Nature, Knowledge and Cure of Cancers*. J. Taylor, London, 1701.
11. Astruc, J., *Traité des tumeurs et des ulceres*. 2 Vols. P. Guillaume Cavelier, Paris, 1769.
12. Redmond, D.E., Tobacco and cancer: the first clinical report. *New Engl. J. Med.*, **282**, p. 18, 1970.
13. Soemmerring, S., *De morbis vasorum abserventium corporis humani*, Frankfurt, 1795.
14. Pott, P., Percivall Pott's contribution to cancer research. *N.C.I.* Monograph No. 10, p. 1, 1963.
15. Medical Committee, Institution for Investigating the Nature and Cure of Cancer. *Edinburgh Med. Surg. Journ.*, **2**, p. 382, 1802.
16. Bayle, G., and Cayol, J., Cancer, Vol.3, p. 537, in *Dictionaire Des Sciences Médicales*. C.L.F. Panckoucke, Paris, 1812.
17. Müller, J., *On the Nature and Structural Characteristics of Cancer*. Trans. by Charles West, Sherwood, Gilbert, and Piper, London, 1840.

18. Kölliker, A., *Manual of Human Histology,* Vol.1, p. 31, Translated by G. Busk, and T. Huxley, The Sydenham Society, London, 1853.
19. Kölliker, A., *A Manual of Human Microscopic Anatomy*. p. 16, John W. Parker and Son, London, 1860.
20. Remak, R., Sur le developpement des animaux vertebres. *Comptes rendus.*, **35**, p. 341, 1852.
21. Hertwig, O., Berträge zur Kenntnis der Bildung, Befruchtung und Theilung des thierischen Eies., *Morph. J.*, **1**, p. 347, 1876.
22. Strasburger, E., *Über Zellbildung und Zelltheilung*. 3rd Edition, G. Fischer, Jena, 1880.
23. Flemming,W., Beiträge zur Kenntniss der Zelle und ihrer Lebenserscheinungen., *Arch. Mikr. Anat.*, **16**, p. 302, 1879 and 18, p. 151, 1880.
24. Hertwig, 0., *Textbook of the Embryology of Man and Mammals*. p. 71, Translated by E. Mark, The Macmillan Co., New York, 1901.
25. Récamier, J.C.A., *Recherches sur le Traitement du Cancer, parla Compression Méthodique Simple ou Combinée et sur I'Histoire Generale de la Meme Maladie*. Gabon, Paris, 1829.
26. Langenbeck, B., Ueber die Entstehung des Venenkrebses und die Moeglichkeit, Carcinoma vom Menschen auf Thiere zu übertragen. *Jahr. in-und Auslaend. Gesem. Med.*, **25**, p. 99, 1840.
27. Virchow, R., *Cellular Pathology, 1858*. Translated by Frank Chance, Dover Publications, Inc., New York, 1971.
28. Thiersch, C., *Der Epitheliakrebs, Namentlich der Haut*. Engelmann, Leipzig, 1865.
29. Paget, S., The Distribution of Secondary Growths in Cancer of the Breast. *Lancet*, **1**, p. 571, 1889.
30. Remak, R., Ein Beitrag zur Entwickelungsgeschichte der krebshaften Geschwuelste. *Deutsche Klinik*, p. 170, 1854.
31. Cohnheim, J., *Lectures on General Pathology*. Vol. 11, Translated by A. McKee, New Sydenham Society, London, pp. 760 768, 1889
32. Waldeyer, W., Die Entwickelung der Carcinome. *Arch. Path. Anat. Phys. Klin.* Med., **41**, p. 470, 1867, and **55**, p. 67, 1872.
33. Rather, L., *The Genesis of Cancer*. p. 155, Johns Hopkins University Press, Baltimore, 1978.
34. Rubin, E., and Farber, J.L., Neoplasia. In *Pathology*. Lippincott, Philadelphia, Chapter 5, 1988.

CHAPTER XIX

> I was often asked in Germany how it is that no scientific work in medicine is done in this country, how it is that many good men who do well in Germany and show evident talent there are never heard of and never do any good work when they come back here. The answer is that there is no opportunity for, no appreciation of, no demand for that kind of work here.
>
> — William Henry Welch (1878)

The Beginnings of the Study of Pathology in the United States

In the preceding chapters, there is a paucity of American names and institutions with regard to the study of pathology. The reason is that before the beginning of the twentieth century, scientific medicine in the United States was almost nonexistent. There were four major factors responsible for this dismal performance. The first was that as a basically commercial people, the philosophy of Adam Smith permeated almost every part of American society. It is interesting that in 1776, the year of the Declaration of Independence, Smith wrote that:

> Every individual is continually exerting himself to find out the most advantageous employment for whatever capital he can command. It is his own advantage, indeed, and not that of society, which he has in view. But the study of his own advantage naturally, or rather necessarily, leads him to prefer that employment which is most advantageous to society. . . . By pursuing his own interest, he frequently promotes that of the society more effectively than when he really intends to promote it.[1]

After the Civil War, the protagonists of this philosophy created great amounts of wealth in the United States. The West was opened up with private capital, and new corporations were formed that developed coal mines and oil fields in Pennsylvania and Ohio while gold and silver mines were established in the western mountains. The steel industry grew dramatically, which provided the materials for the building of the transcontinental railroads. These were all accomplished with the help or blessing of the politicians in federal and state governments and large corporations such as Standard Oil Company established by John T. Rockefeller, United States Steel organized by Andrew Carnegie, banks by J.P. Morgan, and steamships and railroads by Cornelius Vanderbilt, all of which became dominant factors in the economic life of the United States. Inventions became commonplace: the rotary press for printing, the telegraph for providing immediate communication through the vast territories, the steel plough, the reaper, the cash register, the stock ticker, and, later in the century, the telephone of Alexander Graham Bell, and the incandescent electric light of Thomas Edison. Although these inventions changed and improved the standard of living for many segments of American society, it should be pointed out that most of these developments were technological and contributed very little to basic scientific knowledge compared with the type of developments being carried out in Europe. Research in biology and medicine was almost completely neglected because American society could see no immediate monetary profit from such activities, and no laboratories or funds were provided for this purpose. Americans as a people have never had great respect for and indeed are often contemptuous of theoretical or abstract ideas — individuals who profess them are often dismissed as impractical dreamers. Although there were great epidemics of such diseases as typhoid fever and yellow fever in the United States, it was not until the work of Louis Pasteur on the prevention of anthrax and rabies, which showed for the first time that Man can control disease through research, that there was a change in American philosophy. This was manifested in the work at the end of the nineteenth century by Walter Reed and his coworkers, work that was sponsored by the Federal Government and showed that yellow fever could be eradicated by mosquito control. But even in this case, it was the outrage of the American population regarding the deaths of its soldiers due to disease not battle during the Spanish American War in 1898 that demanded governmental action. It was certainly not an interest in the new science of microbiology and pathology as intellectual disciplines.

The second factor inhibiting basic studies in biology in the advancement of medicine was the influence of the church hierarchies. These institutions were not only condemning the striving for material wealth by American society, but they were also fighting the new dominant theme in biology — Evolution — which came about with the publication of Charles Darwin's *Origin of Species*. The concept was regarded as blasphemous because it appeared to attack the literal meaning of the Bible. It is difficult for a modern person to appreciate the conflict, but it was so fundamental that the three pioneer pathologists in North America, William Osler,[2] William Henry Welch,[3] and T. Mitchell Prudden,[4] all of whom were raised in orthodox Christian environments where the Bible was considered infallible, had unhappy breaks with their church or misunderstandings with members of their families. Their study of the new biology and medicine required of them a skepticism of any theory or dogma and encouraged proofs by observation or experimentation. But since many of the new colleges in the United States at that time were established by churches, religion took priority over science and thus the modern teaching of biology was stifled. Nondenominational colleges and universities sprouted forth after the Civil War in large numbers as a result of the Federal Government giving large land grants to the states for education. In addition, large sums of money were beginning to be donated to them by large corporations and newly wealthy citizens. On the other hand, although American families wanted their children to obtain "practical" education to prepare them for material success with its accompanying prestige and were willing to sacrifice the classical education copied from their English ancestors at Oxford and Cambridge, many balked at having their children exposed to ideas such as evolution. In some instances more liberal professors who were skeptical of religious dogma were discharged. Experimental science was almost non-existant. As a result, the more progressive students in biology and medicine went to Europe to study and perform experiments in the commodious laboratories, particularly in Germany. However, they were usually disappointed and disenchanted when they returned to the United States to teach and do research, because not only was there prejudice against the ideas of Darwin, which became the foundation for modern biology, but laboratory facilities were almost non-existent.

The third factor was the recognition by political leaders that to become elected and remain in office, it was necessary to be proponents of only those ideas and activities that were popular with the general population. Suggesting such activities as the study and possible control of such diseases as yellow fever, which ravaged the cities along the eastern coast and the Mississippi River, but would require the expenditure of money and would necessarily ultimately require increased taxation of the citizenry was then, and still is, unpopular.

The fourth factor was that medical training in the United States during the nineteenth century was appalling. An individual usually became a physician in the United States by becoming an apprentice to another physician for as much time as agreed to by the two individuals. The medical schools — except for the University of Pennsylvania, Harvard, Yale, Jefferson Medical College, and the College of Physicians and Surgeons in New York — were essentially commercial ventures; it was possible to get a diploma simply by paying a fee and taking a few lectures on medical subjects. In some cases, it was unnecessary to be able to read or write. During the last half of the nineteenth century, there were as many as 150 such schools, most of them essentially diploma mills, with the object being to turn out the most doctors in the shortest time to produce the most profit for the owners of the school. However, in the United States during the period between 1800 and 1825, there were a few anatomist clinicians associated with the better medical schools who recognized the importance of pathological anatomy. Usually they were trained in England under John Hunter, in Edinburgh under one of the Munro anatomists, or in Paris with Bichat, and they taught anatomy and performed autopsies on occasion. At the University of Pennsylvania there were Philip Syng Physick (1768–1837) and Samuel Jackson, in New York there were David Hosak (1769–1835) and Valentine Mott (1785–1865), and at Harvard there were Benjamin Waterhouse (1754–1846) and later James Jackson (1777–1868), all of whom performed autopsies and taught rudimentary pathology. But these efforts were sporadic and not as systematized as those in France or Great Britain. Pathological museums were established, but for the most part they consisted of curiosities such as monsters, large stones, or tumors.

During the second quarter of the century, more specific efforts were made to emphasize pathological anatomy in the few better medical schools, and two books devoted to the subject were written by Americans. The first was by William E. Horner (1793–1853), Professor of Anatomy at Pennsylvania, and contained good descriptions of lesions of the major organs, but the general pathology was permeated by the erroneous theories of Broussais, rather than Bichat or Laennec, and thus was of little value.[5] The second book was *Elements of Pathology,* published in 1839 and written by Samuel Gross, the eminent Professor of Surgery at Jefferson. It is of value to quote from Gross's book because it gives the perspective of an outstanding medical man on pathology and medicine at that time:

> It is certainly an anomaly in the history of our profession, that a science which admits of such extensive application as the present, and which may be regarded as constituting the very foundation of the grand edifice of medicine should still be so neglected as a branch of elementary study in the United States. The utility of an extended knowledge of this science, cannot, indeed, be anymore a matter of doubt or dispute. Without the light which it furnishes, our views of disease must necessarily be limited and confused; whilst by its help, the nature and seat of every lesion is comparatively easily comprehended.[6]

However, Gross reflected the Fundamentalist philosophy in his pessimism regarding the possibility of pathology ever truly understanding the nature of disease by stating that:

> Of the essence of disease, very little is known; indeed, nothing at all; nor can the utmost ingenuity hope to remove the veil which still envelopes the subject, until the physiology and pathology of the muscular and nervous system shall be better understood. The proximate cause of morbid action, and the immediate cause of life in the healthy state, are as inscrutable to the human mind as the cause of gravitation, of attraction, and repulsion. All we can boast of is, that we know something of their effects; beyond this, it is extremely problematical whether we shall ever be able to penetrate. With this, indeed, every philosophical inquirer after truth should be contented, remembering that the secrets of nature are not easily detected, and that to God alone belongs the knowledge of the intrinsic property of things.[7]

But the American character has always emphasized pragmatism and action, and as a result of the Civil War there were produced, in spite of their poor training, many daring and proficient surgeons. The terrible war wounds provided great opportunities for imaginative and resourceful surgeons, and the result was that many American surgeons during the last half of the nineteenth century were as skilled as many of those in the best hospitals in Europe. But for those physicians who wanted to understand disease processes, it was necessary to go to Europe for postgraduate training. They first went to Edinburgh, but in the first half of the nineteenth century, they studied in France where most came under the influence of Louis.[8] These were James Jackson, Jr. (1810–1834), H.I.

Bowditch (1808–1892), Oliver Wendell Holmes (1809–1894), W.W. Gerhard (1809–1872), Alfred Stillé (1813–1900), J. Mason Warren (1811–1867), and Alonzo Clark (1807–1887), among others. These men learned the value of careful history taking, physical examination, and the importance of good record keeping, but with regard to systematic correlations of their clinical findings with postmortem examinations, the emphasis was not there. The study of pathology was considered not important enough to be a separate part of medicine, but was looked upon in the same way as therapy or prognosis. Consequently, it was given a separate paragraph or two in the discussion of each clinical entity in the textbooks, but this was primarily for teaching purposes.

In the United States, the realization that pathological anatomy and the other basic sciences of physiology and biochemistry were the foundation on which scientific medicine was based did not occur until the last quarter of the nineteenth century. It was at this time that a few medical men from North America, who went to Europe to train under such outstanding individuals as Virchow, Cohnheim, Koch, and Ludwig, established in the major medical centers of New York, Boston, Baltimore, and Philadelphia institutions and departments that either directly or through their students resulted in bringing to prominence laboratory medicine in the United States during the twentieth century. But it was primarily at the new Johns Hopkins Hospital and Medical School during the last twenty years of the century that a renaissance in medicine occurred. In retrospect, this renaissance was equivalent to that which occurred in Italy with Vesalius and Harvey; in Holland with Boerhaave; in France with Bichat, Laennec, Corvisart, and Louis; in England's Guy's Hospital with John Hunter, Astley Cooper, Richard Bright, Thomas Addison, and Thomas Hodgkin; in Vienna with Rokitansky, Skoda, and Hebra; and finally in Germany with Müller, Virchow, Traube, Frerichs, Ludwig, and Ehrlich. The next chapter discusses this American renaissance in medicine that occurred at the Johns Hopkins, the factors that were responsible, the men involved, and its ultimate influence on the field of medicine in the twentieth century.

Bibliography

1. Smith, A., Wealth of Nations, Book IV, Chapter 11, quoted in *Encylopedia Brittanica*, Vol. 20, p. 691, W. Benton, Chicago, 1973.
2. Wyn, N., The Early Life of Sir William Osler, in *Appreciations and Reminiscences of Sir William Osler*, p. 149, Bulletin IX , Internal. Assoc. Med. Museums, Edited by Maude E. Abbott, Montreal, 1926.
3. Flexner, S., and Flexner, J., *William Henry Welch and the Heroic Age of American Medicine*, p. 87, Dover Publications, N.Y., 1966.
4. Prudden, T. M., *Biographical Sketches and Letters of T. Mitchell Prudden*, M.D., Yale Univ. Press, New Haven, 1927.
5. Horner, W.E., *Treatise on Pathological Anatomy*, Lea and Blanchard, Philadelphia, 1829.
6. Gross, S., *Pathological Anatomy*, Marsh, Capen, Lyon and Webb, Boston, 1839.
7. Ibid, Vol. 1, p. 23.
8. Osler, W., *Influence of Louis on American medicine*, Johns Hopkins Hosp. Bull., **8**, p. 161, 1897.

CHAPTER XX

> The generations past and the generations to come form with those alive one single whole; all live eternally, though it is only some that happen at any moment to live upon earth
> — Osler (quoting a Chinese)

Renaissance in Medicine in Baltimore at Johns Hopkins Hospital and Medical School

In the William Henry Welch Memorial Library at Johns Hopkins University in Baltimore there hangs a portrait by Sir John Singer Sargent called "The Four Physicians," which represents Sir William Osler, William Henry Welch, William S. Halsted, and Howard A. Kelly. It was these individuals and others who, during the heroic years of 1876–1905 at the Johns Hopkins University and later the Hospital and Medical School, were primarily responsible for bringing American medicine to the forefront of the world in the twentieth century. These times were best described by contemporary and colleague Bertram Bernheim:

> All four physicians were present at the birth of the Hopkins (1889, capacity 220 beds) and a new era in American Medical Education dawned. Pathologist, physician, surgeon, gynecologist, the Four took the new infant to themselves and literally swept it to maturity and first rank without so much as a gesture to the usual childhood years. Working as a team, but individualistic just the same, they plotted new courses and followed through with a judgment and a verve and an enthusiasm that made them preeminent in American medicine almost overnight. They had spirit, they had humanity, they had knowledge and deep understanding of illness, disease, and people. Especially did they understand people, and their sympathy knew no bounds. Yet they didn't stand around and wring their hands and cry their eyes out over the suffering they saw and the woe they had to deal with. It was by fortuitous circumstances that they came to the Hopkins at one and the same time, at the psychological moment. A break; a quirk of

> fate. Any one of them would have brought renown, but together they brought fame. For they were the spirit and they were inspired, and theirs was a God-given quality that you see once in a great while when the need is great and the time is ripe. Welch, Osler, Halsted, Kelly were naturals for the Hopkins Medical Department. They were more than doctors; they were men; they were teachers; they were executives, organizers, compilers, lecturers, research workers, writers, advisers — even actors and propagandists though they probably didn't realize that. Did you say I am being extravagant? Of course I am. They were extravagant men. They'd have done well in any walk of life — industry, finance, politics. They'd have taken over because they had what it takes — individually and collectively. I haven't the slightest doubt they'd have made a night club of Alcatraz if by some strange fate they had been sent there and had wanted to. Men just naturally flocked to them — doctors, students, the sick, the lowly, the rich, gamblers, men, women, and children. All gave them their confidence; all hung on their words; all took their advice; all went their ways happy and believing. They comprised the most extraordinary group the world of medicine ever saw or probably ever will see. And that in a nutshell spells the fame of the Johns Hopkins Hospital and Medical School.[1]

Of course, it was actually more complicated than that, although Bernheim, who knew them well but was still in awe of his colleagues, certainly expressed the most important and necessary spirit of those days.

As the twenty-first century is approaching, it can be stated that there was indeed a medical renaissance in Baltimore between the years 1876 when Johns Hopkins University was established and 1905 when Osler left to go to Oxford. At that time it is clear that Osler himself did not recognize this renaissance in which he played such an important part. He was too close to the time and the situation, and certainly too modest a man to ever make such a claim, even if he were aware. Certainly his letter from Vienna in 1907 (Ref. 25 in Introduction) indicates that he did not have that perspective, because he wrote that he did not believe that Minerva Medica had yet decided to move to the New World. In retrospect, she had certainly already moved to Baltimore, although Osler and probably the other participants were completely unaware of her presence. Her "chief temples" were not only the university, but also the new

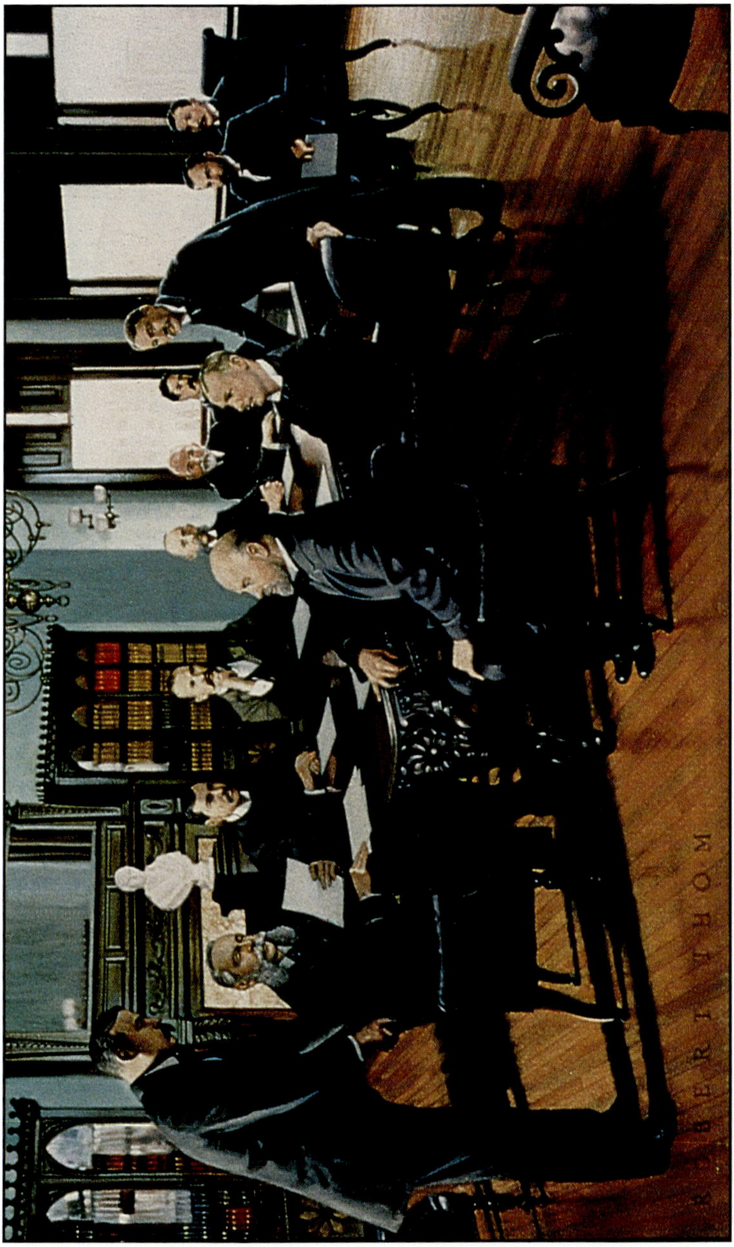

John Shaw Billings Daniel Coit Gilman Howard A. Kelly William Osler Henry M. Hurd Ira Remsen J. Whitridge Williams
William H. Welch William S. Halsted Franklin P. Mall John J. Abel William H. Howell

THE HOPKINS: A REVOLUTION IN MEDICAL EDUCATION

temples that were soon built in the form of the Johns Hopkins Hospital and then the Medical School. And whether they realized it or not, Welch, Osler, Halsted, Kelly, and earlier Martin and Councilman, were the new "high priests" of medicine who had come to "teach, practice, and worship the old Hippocratic service" and "to whom from all quarters the young disciples flocked." By 1914 Osler, writing from Oxford at the time of the twenty-fifth anniversary of the John Hopkins Hospital was beginning to recognize the significance of the Hopkins program. He wrote the following:

> It was not the men, though success could not have come without them, so much as the method, the organization, and the collective new outlook on old problems. They were gathered here from all parts to do one thing, to show that the primary function of a university was to contribute to the general sum of human knowledge. . . . Individuals here and there for generations had in this country those ideals but never before a studium generate, a whole body of men gathered in one place to form a university. That part of the university which, with the hospital, forms the medical school has only had twenty-five years of existence, not a generation, a mere fraction of time in the long history of the growth of science, so that it seems presumptuous to claim any powerful influence on the profession at large. The feeling, however, is strong, too strong to be passed over, that the year 1889 did mean something in the history of medicine in this country.[2]

In retrospect it might have been expected that if there were to be a renaissance in American medicine it would have occurred in Boston, New York, or Philadelphia, which already had important medical schools and hospitals of long standing with cultural traditions. Baltimore, on the other hand, in the 1870s was a small Southern commercial center dealing primarily in cotton, flour, and tobacco and had changed very little since the Civil War a decade before. The streets were lined with miles of little brick residences with Georgian entrances and there were essentially no large buildings. But it was in Padua, not Rome, where the first renaissance in medicine occurred with the work of Vesalius and Harvey, and later in Leyden, not Amsterdam, where Boerhaave and his disciples produced a second renaissance. So why was it unreasonable that Baltimore could become the site for the significant rebirth in Western medicine and that the brilliant men who came there from afar and would become the new "high priests" would make with their students comparable discoveries as those by such men as Vesalius, Harvey, Hunter, Virchow, Cohnheim, Pasteur, Koch, and Ehrlich?

It all started in 1873 when a successful Baltimore merchant, Johns Hopkins, left half of his entire seven million dollar fortune for the establishment of a high-quality university and the other half for the building of a hospital in association with a new medical school. Hopkins appointed an astute group of trustees to carry out his wishes. This group in turn selected Daniel Coit Gilman, originally a Yale librarian and later the president of the new University of California, to find and hire the best possible faculty. Within a few years the graduate school at Johns Hopkins University began attracting the brightest young men who wanted the best education in such diverse fields as the classics, political science, and the natural sciences. There were no rah-rah activities such as secret societies or organized athletics, or even such goals as producing "good Christian citizens," which was so specified in many schools such as Harvard, Yale, or Princeton. Scholarship and not family background or "connections" determined success in Baltimore. After the university was launched, Gilman turned to the development of the hospital and medical school. But instead of following the traditional custom of recruiting local, financially successful physicians as faculty members, he enlisted the help of John S. Billings, who was the librarian of the Surgeon General's Library and one of the first medical scholars in the United States. Billings was sent to Europe with Gilman's plans and was soon persuaded by the eminent medical men there to base the new medical school on the field of pathology and the basic sciences. Taking their advice, Billings and Gilman with the help of Ira Remsen, the outstanding chemist, then proceeded to establish not only the first graduate program in experimental biology and physiology in the new university in 1876 under the leadership of Henry Newell Martin, but also for the first and last time in United States formed in 1885 a pathology department in the university, which was four years before the opening of the hospital and eight years before opening of the medical school.

William Henry Welch

The man selected not only to head this important new department but also to organize the hospital and medical school was William Henry Welch. Julius Cohnheim, the new star in pathology in Germany, had worked with Welch in 1877 and recommended him as the man who could accomplish the task. Thus in 1884, Gilman went to New York to offer Welch the first position in the United States that included not only the first full-time professorship in pathology with laboratory facilities but also the deanship of the new school. This was perhaps the most important and astute appointment ever made in American medicine and, considering that Welch not only had not achieved an international reputation as a pathologist but also had essentially no experience as an organizer and administrator, it was an extremely risky selection. But Welch was no ordinary man, and he soon began a new career of leadership that lasted until his death in 1934 at the age of 84. During this long career there were approximately seventy individuals who worked with him at some time or claimed him as their mentor. Many of these medical people went on to distinguish themselves in departments of pathology, bacteriology, medicine, surgery, or anatomy throughout the United States. Some of his more notable disciples were: in pathology, W.C. MacCallum of Johns Hopkins and Columbia, Milton Winternitz at Yale, Eugene Opie of Washington University and then the Rockefeller Institute, W.T. Howard of Western Reserve, George Blumer at Albany, Simon Flexner at the Rockefeller Institute, and George Whipple at Rochester; in bacteriology, Stanhope Bayne-Jones at Johns Hopkins, Alexander Abbott at Pennsylvania, and George Nuttall at Cambridge in England; in medicine, Lewellys Barker, who took Osler's place in 1905, William Sidney Thayer, also a professor of medicine at Johns Hopkins, and Rufus Cole, who was also at the Rockefeller Institute and Hospital; in gynecology, Thomas Cullen, who would eventually take Kelly's place as head of gynecology and worked for several years in pathology under Welch, and John Whitridge Williams, who would later head the obstetric department; and in pediatrics, William D. Booker, who was the first head of this department at Johns Hopkins and had worked in Welch's department studying the bacteria of the stools of children with summer diarrhea.

It was not that Welch was an active director of the work in his department but rather that he created an atmosphere in his department that stimulated excellent men to do outstanding work and also to help each other to do so. Collaborative work between different individuals with diverse talents and training (as in the case of Halsted and Mall described below) contributed significantly to the advancement of medicine. But always it was the emphasis on the field of pathology that was the foundation of the practice of medicine at Johns Hopkins. Simon Flexner described Welch's department in this manner:

> (Welch) never devoted his laboratory to the investigation of a single subject. . . . And he never set a student to work on a concrete problem . . . Welch's success as a teacher depended on that illusive thing, atmosphere. He rarely interfered in what went on around him, yet example, his intelligence, and his comprehensive knowledge formed the keystone of the arch of scientific medicine in America. MacCallum tells us that although Welch never gave him a problem to study, he never undertook a problem without asking himself: "What will Dr. Welch think of it?" The desire to be like Dr. Welch, the desire to win his approval, these were the principal incentives of the eager young men who crowded his laboratory.[3]

Welch was born in 1850, in Norfolk, Connecticut, the son of a physician, and attended Yale University where he graduated with honors in the classics in 1870. This was a time when Yale patterned itself after Oxford and Cambridge, essentially offering no science courses because this subject was not considered intellectual but rather utilitarian and not a proper part of a college education. There was, of course, the newly formed and pioneer Sheffield Scientific School, but this institution at that time was separate from the main college and there was no necessity to take any courses there for earning a bachelor's degree. Welch, therefore had basically no exposure to science during his undergraduate years.

Following his graduation he had hoped to obtain a faculty position teaching Greek and the classics, but there were no positions open at the college level and he was forced to take a position for a year at a private school for boys where he tutored them for university examinations. The next year he returned home to become an apprentice physician to his father, but he quickly saw that this was a poor manner in which to learn medicine. Therefore, after a short time, he enrolled at the College of Physicians and Surgeons in New York City, but again recognized that he was too weak in his knowledge of science to take good advantage of this training. Welch was never one to settle for mediocrity, and he swallowed his pride and returned to Yale where he attended the Sheffield School and learned chemistry and worked in the laboratory for a year. (Welch said in his later years when he was asked to give a public lecture on "The Relation of Yale to Medicine" during the nineteenth century that it was such a barren subject that he wished the sponsors would have asked him to discuss Yale and Calvinism, or perhaps Yale and Football since then he would have had something to say.) After his year in chemistry, he again returned to the College of Physicians and Surgeons where he studied for three years, after which time he obtained an internship at Bellevue Hospital. It was there that he was introduced and learned pathology from Francis Delafield, who was at that time the most renowned pathologist in the United States. But Delafield did not teach him the use of the microscope because when Welch won an award for descriptions of gross pathology of the thyroid gland, the prize was a microscope, and he complained that he had no knowledge of how to use it!

Welch's ability was recognized by Abraham Jacobi, the father of pediatrics in the United States, who encouraged him to go to Germany for further training. Consequently, he first went to Strasbourg where he learned histology under the famous Waldeyer and worked with Hoppe-Seyler in chemistry. He had hoped to finalize his training with Virchow in Berlin. However, he was to change his mind in Leipzig where he studied under anatomic pathologist Ernst Wagner preparing pathological specimens for microscopic examination, especially neoplasms, with the latest staining techniques. At Leipzig, Welch also was exposed to the great Carl Ludwig, and the famous physiologist assigned him a project where he could use his newly learned techniques in studying the nerves and ganglions of the heart. With Ludwig, he also learned some of the newest methods of studying physiology, and his perspective in pathology started to change. At the end of his stay in Leipzig, Ludwig discouraged him from going to Berlin to study with Virchow, because he felt that this pathologist was too morphologically oriented, and he encouraged Welch to go to Breslau where Julius Cohnheim was approaching the study of disease from a physiological perspective. Convinced by Ludwig, he worked under Cohnheim for a year where he studied the factors involved in the production of pulmonary edema.

However, when he returned to New York, he did not find any medical school that was interested in supplying him facilities and a salary for the development of pathology on a full-time basis. He took a position at Bellevue Medical School where he taught pathology to a small group of students who paid him minimal fees for the course. It was expected by his friends that he would develop a consulting practice as his primary economic resource. However, both he and his friend T. Mitchell Prudden, another aspiring pathologist who worked at the College of Physicians and Surgeons, were frustrated by the lack of interest of the medical faculty in developing research facilities. Welch wrote in a letter:

> I was often asked in Germany how it is that no scientific work in medicine is done in this country, how is it that many good men who do well in Germany and show evident talent there are never heard of and never do any good work when they come back here. The answer is that there is no opportunity for, no appreciation of, no demand for that kind of work here. In Germany, on the other hand, every encouragement is held out to young men with taste for science. . . . I do think that the condition of medical education here is terrible.[4]

However, after six years of struggling in New York, teaching pathology, performing autopsies, and writing a section on pathology for the latest edition of Austin Flint's popular textbook in medicine, Welch was approached by John Billings in 1884 offering him the position at the Johns Hopkins,[3] as related in the last chapter. With his acceptance, Welch requested that he be allowed another year in Germany to learn the new bacteriology, which he knew would be very important to him as a leader at Johns Hopkins and which had developed dramatically since his last visit in 1877. Koch's laboratory was deluged with individuals from all over the world, and Welch had to go to Munich where he worked with Wilhelm Frobenius, a Koch student. He also worked with Max von Pettenkorfer, the director of the first hygienic institute in the world and was later to influence Welch in his endeavors on behalf of public health in America. After Munich, he went again to Leipzig to study with Carl Ludwig, stating that with the death of his former mentor, Julius Cohnheim, there was no longer an experimental pathologist in Germany. He eventually spent some time with Koch, but it is interesting that he made no effort to work with Virchow, perhaps because he felt that by

1885, this great pathologist was past his prime and not able to offer him any new knowledge. Then in October 1885, Welch went to Baltimore to assume his new duties and quickly showed his greatest talent, not knowledge of pathology, which was certainly important as background for his decisions, but his ability to evaluate the talent of other medical men and to stimulate and enhance the careers of promising students by exemplary teaching and by giving them advice and facilities for research work. Like Virchow in Germany, he was a politician academic, but his personality was quite different. He was not intimidating, arrogant, or pugnacious like the German but was able to achieve his goals by gentle but persistent persuasion. He never showed anger, used sarcasm, or attempted to belittle his opponents. These characteristics, together with altruism, left a legacy of great accomplishments in American medicine. At the same time he also achieved, like his colleague Osler, the affection and admiration of the entire profession, which was conveyed by his nickname of "Popsy."

His first task of organizing the hospital, the pathology department, and later the medical school at Johns Hopkins could have been overwhelming, but he had the support of both the older and more experienced President Gilman and John Billings. They not only had the same ideals and goals as Welch but also had actually prepared the groundwork with the selection of one of the almost-forgotten figures in biology, who was already on the scene in Baltimore when Welch arrived. This man was Henry Newell Martin. In addition to training many outstanding physiologists, Martin had selected as an assistant, perhaps as luck would have it, William Councilman, a well-trained pathologist who, when Councilman arrived three years later, became the right-hand man of Welch.

Henry Newell Martin

One of the best decisions of Gilman was to select the 28-year-old Irishman, Henry Newell Martin, to head the new department of biology at the new university in 1876, seventeen years before the beginning of the medical school. Martin had worked with both Michael Foster and Thomas Huxley, and, although his scientific publications were sparse, they both heartily recommended him. Gilman provided him with funds for equipment and research and a modest building for his exclusive use. The uniqueness of the program, in comparison with that in New York or

Bowditch's laboratory at Harvard, was the emphasis on offering young graduate students the opportunity to perform original experiments. In doing so, Martin recruited for the first time in the United States young graduates from universities throughout the country, some with bachelor's degrees and others who had graduated from medical schools but had little or no experience in physiological experimentation. As a result of this program, Martin developed several disciples in biology who had distinguished careers and in most cases established excellent departments in other universities. Among his most notable students were Henry Sewell, who obtained his Ph.D. under Martin in 1879 and became Professor of Physiology at the University of Michigan Medical School; Frederic Schiller Lee, who received his Ph.D. in 1882 and eventually headed the physiology department at Columbia; William Thompson Sedgwick, who after his Ph.D. went to MIT; H.H. Donaldson, who became professor at the University of Chicago and later the Wistar Institute; and finally William Henry Howell, who became head of the physiology department of the Johns Hopkins Medical School when it opened in 1893. Ross Harrison, the famous anatomist at Yale, and the geneticist Thomas Hunt Morgan were both students of Martin.

It is also significant that when the American Physiological Society was established in 1888, approximately half of the original 28 members were or had been affiliated with Johns Hopkins. Unfortunately, in spite of all of the success of Martin at Johns Hopkins, he became frustrated by being unable to keep his associates who were enticed by the more attractive salaries offered by other universities to head their departments. In fairness to the administration of the Johns Hopkins, their reluctance to increase the salaries of the associates was related to the recession during the late 1880s and particularly to the university's considerable investment in the Baltimore and Ohio Railroad, which did not give dividends for several years. But this did not help Martin. Overburdened with having to do his own teaching and research, attacked by anti-vivisectionists, and perhaps unable to keep abreast of new trends in physiology when his best students left, he succumbed to alcoholism, resigned his position at the university in 1893, and returned to England where he died three years later. He was indeed a tragic figure but certainly one that contributed greatly to scientific development of human physiology and medicine in the United States and was recognized as such by his many disciples.[4a]

William Councilman

A medical graduate of the University of Maryland in 1878, William Councilman was also a student of Martin and learned to use the microscope from the physiologist. He then went to Europe where he studied with Hans Chiari, then with Cohnheim and Weigert, and finally with von Recklinghausen in Strasbourg. In 1882, he returned to Johns Hopkins, became Martin's assistant, worked with George Sternberg and A.C. Abbott in some early bacteriology experiments in the biology department, taught at the University of Maryland Medical School, and performed most of the postmortem examinations in Baltimore. In October 1885, when Welch arrived in Baltimore to develop plans for the new hospital and later the medical school, Councilman became his assistant. It is of interest that although Councilman would be called upon to become the Shattuck Professor of Pathology at Harvard in 1892, a position he filled in a distinguished manner and during which time he organized the pathological departments of both Massachusetts General Hospital and later Peter Bent Brigham Hospital, he clearly was not regarded by Gilman and Billings as the person to head the new pathology department in the new Johns Hopkins Hospital. Councilman had a speech impediment and was also a man who was very frank to a point that he was sometimes perceived by those who did know him well as very undiplomatic. Nevertheless, Welch, as the new man in Baltimore, was able to develop a close and mutually respectful relationship with Councilman because he recognized the latter's equal if not superior knowledge of pathological anatomy, and he needed Councilman for performing the routine pathology in the hospital while Welch spent much of his time in the unacademic and often tedious tasks of administration. The relationship of the two men in those early days was aptly described by Welch at a dinner in honor of Councilman in 1913:

> The truth is that when I came to Baltimore I found pathology already represented in such a way that it might really be a surprise to anyone as to why they should have looked elsewhere for the incumbent of the chair . . . the hospital was building (at that time). One of my chief occupations, after having mastered the complicated system of heating and ventilation, was to serve as guide to many visitors. Councilman consistently refused to learn how the hospital was heated and

> ventilated, and declined to show anybody over those miles and miles of corridors and those ladders to be climbed. . . . Councilman, was however, tremendously absorbed in picking out the room he was going to occupy in the hospital. He would take me from the top to the bottom of the administration building . . . to get my opinion as to the relative advantages of this or that corner room. The association with Councilman is a matter to me so intimate and one of such a personal character that these memories are very dear to me. It is hardly necessary to say that . . . when he left, I felt as if my right hand had been taken off. It did not seem at that time as if it would ever be possible to fill his place. He was a very inspiring teacher, but there was one quality which in a measure disturbed me for a while. Dr. Councilman has probably never known that I was responsible for him becoming an editor of a medical dictionary. I had not then become so accustomed to the congenitally bad speller as I have since then, and the embarrassment of strangers visiting the museum occasionally and looking at the labels on the specimens was so great, I thought it would do Councilman good if I threw in his way, the opportunity of serving as the editor of a medical dictionary. I doubt if many here know that he worked hard on the spelling and derivation of medical terms, not only in English, but in Latin, French, German, and Italian, in that famous medical dictionary with which his name will always be associated.[5]

The Later Major Figures

William Osler

Perhaps Welch's major coup was the recruiting of William Osler to come to Johns Hopkins as Chief of Medicine in 1885. This man, born in a rural area of Canada in 1849, was already a medical legend when he died in 1919. Like Welch, he had not accomplished any outstanding research such as that of Pasteur, Koch, or Ehrlich, but his personality was much like the pathologist in that he was a natural leader with great capacity for work, vitality, ambition, unusual psychological understanding of himself and other human beings, combined with the best in Victorian concepts of good character, contagious optimism, historical understanding and perspective in the field of medicine, and brilliant ways of communicating clearly his ideas orally and in writing. The difference between the two men was that, although he was an expert pathologist, his

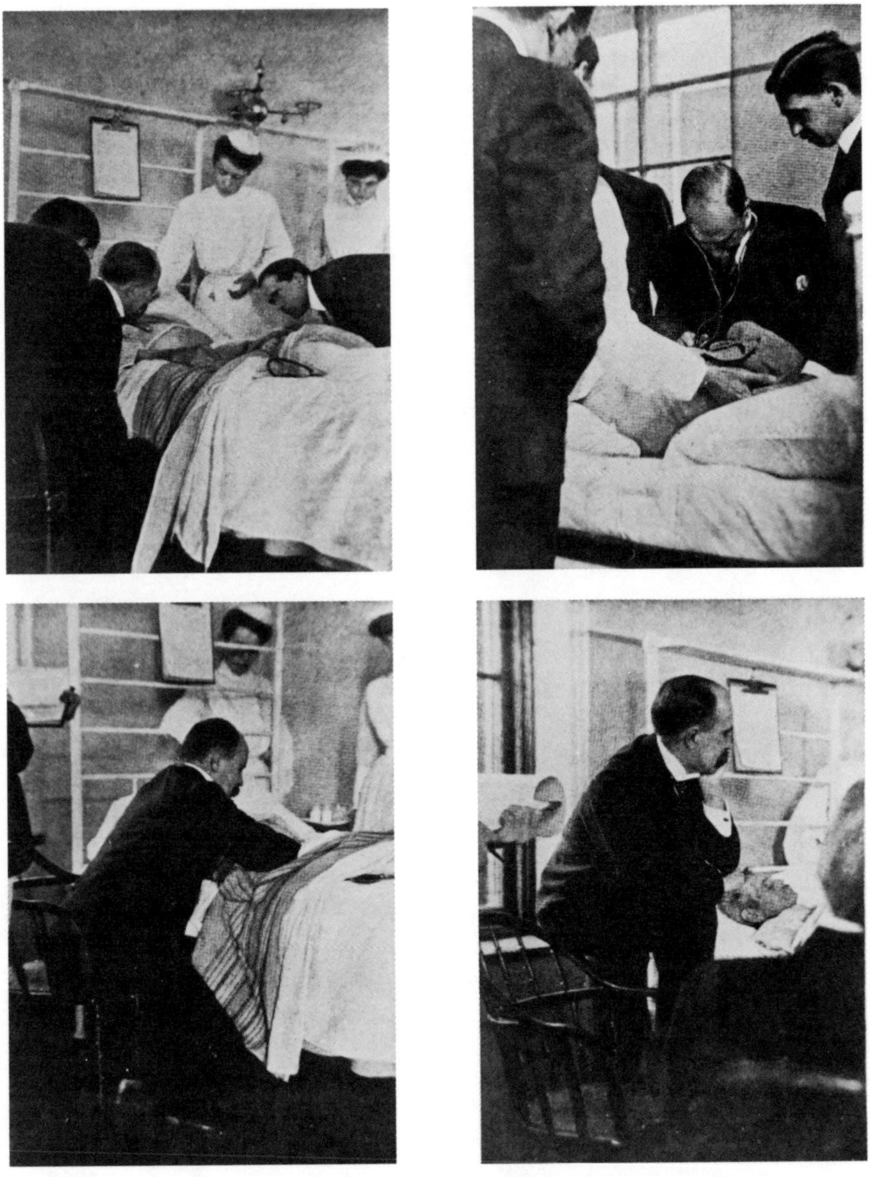

"OBSERVATION, PALPATION, PERCUSSION, AUSCULTATION"
WILLIAM OSLER: THE MASTER OF THE PHYSICAL EXAMINATION

scientific training was not as great as that of Welch, but for the last quarter of the nineteenth century his knowledge enabled him to advance clinical medicine in North America more than any other individual. It was at that time that the ability to correlate signs and symptoms of the patient with gross and microscopic findings was the most important first step in placing the practice of medicine on a scientific basis; no one in North America was Osler's superior. His appearance on the medical scene was at a time when medical America consisted mostly of physicians who were trained by apprenticeship, or had medical degrees from diploma mills, and hospitals were of extremely poor quality. First-class medical centers and research facilities were almost non-existent. In 1872 Osler graduated from McGill Medical School, which was the best in Canada, but like Welch, he was not satisfied with his training and on graduation went to England and then Germany for further study. Unlike Welch, however, Osler was already an expert microscopist, having learned the use of that instrument as a youngster from a schoolmaster who was a naturalist and encouraged Osler to study diatoms from the lakes near his home outside Toronto. In fact, in his biography of Osler, Harvey Cushing wrote that:

> It was apparent that at this time he looked upon his medical work more or less from the standpoint of a naturalist, with the microscope always at hand. . . . There can be little doubt that had William Osler at this time (1870) come under the influence of Leidy or Agassiz or possibly Huxley, he would have gone on with his biological studies and abandoned medicine.[6]

In England, Osler worked with the physiologist Burton Sanderson for 17 months on leukocytes and platelets and confirmed the observations of both Donné and Schultze with regard to platelets before Hayem and Bizzozero came to the conclusion that these bodies were normal particles in blood. Osler, on the other hand, had stated that he was not sure that these bodies were not related to bacteria and therefore his observations have historically been discounted, but his research was done before Ehrlich developed his so-important blood stains. After his work in England, Osler went to Germany where he was impressed by Virchow, Traube, and Frerichs.[7] When he returned to McGill in charge of teaching the institutes of medicine, which were essentially the basic sciences in those days, he was determined to make changes in the curriculum. He insisted that every student learn how to use the microscope and perform some laboratory work. In his introductory remarks to his students in 1874, he said that:

> In the spirit [of reforms in medical teaching] the course you are about to begin has been inaugurated. An opportunity will henceforth be afforded to the students attending this school of becoming practically acquainted with the use of the microscope in physiology and pathology; and I may venture to congratulate McGill College as the first in this country to offer such a course. The first essential in a course like this is proper supply of good microscopes; every student must be furnished with one to enable him to follow out the demonstrations with any degree of satisfaction. These have been obtained from Dr. Harnack of Paris and Potsdam and are the same as are in use in the chief laboratories in Europe.[8]

What Osler didn't say was that the 12 microscopes that he ordered were paid for by a small salary of $600 he received for volunteering to work in the smallpox wards, a task which was very dangerous, and ultimately led to his contracting a mild case himself, although he had been repeatedly vaccinated. Of that course, George Armstrong, who was a student at that time, wrote in later years:

> This first class in histology was held Saturday afternoon in the student cloakroom in the basement of the building. We were given bits of tissue which we embedded in little paper boxes of wax, and the sections were cut with razors.[9]

By 1881 Osler was giving four separate courses at McGill, Practical Physiology, Normal Histology, Morbid Anatomy, and his favorite course Clinical Microscopy, "especially designed to meet the requirements of a practitioner." In addition to his teaching responsibilities, Osler was actively engaged in research and writing. Related to the study of blood, he published an article on the development of blood cells in the bone marrow and discussed at length a case of progressive pernicious anemia with postmortem findings, giving detailed description of the various blood types in the bone marrow, many observations being quite original. This was most remarkable because they were made without any stains whatsoever. In gross pathology, Osler performed almost 800 autopsies on his return to McGill, obtaining 150 carefully dissected and prepared gross specimens that were preserved in the pathological museum at McGill, as were his careful and complete handwritten notes of many of his autopsies, several of which were published in the Montreal General Hospital Pathology Reports during the years 1877–1878. Osler, however, began to show a greater interest in practicing medicine and an opportunity to take over ward work at the University of Pennsylvania induced him to accept an appointment there. He again emphasized the importance of using autopsies as the method of evaluating premortem diagnoses and prognoses and the value of making laboratory examinations of blood and urine with the microscope to differentiate various illnesses from each other.

With regard to Osler's move to Johns Hopkins, Welch said many years later that he met Osler at a meeting at Delmonico's restaurant in New York in the late 1870s and was captivated by the thin, olive-skinned man with the huge moustache. Then, with Osler's reputation at McGill and Pennsylvania increasing by leaps and bounds, he immediately thought about asking him to join the faculty at Johns Hopkins shortly after his own appointment. However, Billings as a consultant wanted to appoint an older, more experienced clinician from England, but Welch was not dissuaded, and as a result, according to Osler, Billings came to his lodgings in Philadelphia early in 1889 and without sitting down asked, "Will you take charge of the Medical Department of the Johns Hopkins Hospital," to which Osler replied affirmatively. Billings then said as he was leaving "see Welch about the details" and left within a few minutes. The prime reason for Osler's decision to go to Baltimore was the opportunity and freedom it would give him to bring in new ideas without having to accommodate senior faculty men who were less inclined to change.

In May of 1889, Osler was at work in Baltimore organizing the medical clinic at the new Johns Hopkins Hospital. His new chief resident H.A. Lafleur, who later became professor of medicine at McGill, described the first days of the opening of the hospital:

> There was a feeling of elation — one might even say of exaltation that the structure which had taken twenty years to evolve, absorbing the energies and thought of so many able minds, had at last become a fait accompli. And to none other than to Dr. Osler was this a red letter day. To blaze perfectly new roads, untrammeled by tradition, vested interests or medi-

> cal "deadwood". The days that followed were filled with the many details of organization. There were records, forms and charts of various sorts to be devised, instruments of precision and appliances for diagnosis to be purchased, diet lists to be drawn up, and not the least, a clinical laboratory to be furnished and equipped — the latter a temporary affair, as those who had planned the magnificent pile of buildings had omitted to make provision for this essential feature of a medical clinic. . . . Dr. Osler appreciated very highly the laboratory side of medicine. He was well trained in pathology and clinical microscopy and urged his assistants to study biochemistry in all its relations to medicine. When he visited the laboratories of his department, and he did this quite regularly, he always came as a student, asking what we had to show him.[10]

As a physician-in-chief, Osler organized his department patterned after the best hospitals in Germany with a hierarchy of long-term residents. This was in contrast to the usual house staff of short-term interns, which was the practice in America at that time. Osler took young doctors, first as interns then as assistant residents usually for a specified number of years, but the individual who had the honor of becoming the chief resident stayed on indefinitely. The philosophy was that it was better to train one individual well than many in a mediocre manner, although assistant residents from Johns Hopkins were often recruited for other medical school faculties. Although these residencies did not pay a significant salary, such men as William Sidney Thayer, who was Osler's chief resident for nine years, were able to develop an outside medical practice that enabled them to live comfortably. Osler was also the first to bring medical students into the wards as part of their training under the guidance of the interns and residents. Thus the traditional hierarchy that became almost part of every medical school by the middle of the twentieth century had its origin in Osler's program at Johns Hopkins. Osler left Baltimore in 1905 to become the Regius Professor of Medicine at Oxford, and clinical medicine at the Hopkins was never the same without him. He left primarily because he had become the doctor's doctor, and he was overworked with consultations that he found himself unable to refuse. He resigned in spite of great pressure for him to stay, but his fragile health and his longing for more time for contemplation and the study of the history of medicine promised by the new position in England was too much for him to decline. Welch said this of Osler's accomplishments in Baltimore:

> Osler introduced three great reforms. (1) the creation of an upper resident staff, corresponding to assistants in a laboratory; . . . (2) the introduction of the British system of clinical clerks and surgical dressers . . . and (3) the establishment of laboratories as an integral part of the clinic where students were taught laboratory methods of diagnosis and of examination of excreta, secretions, blood . . . .[11]

But a considerable part of his accomplishments at Johns Hopkins were more nebulous. Bernheim said many years later, "the Hopkins was never the same without Osler. He was the soul of the Hopkins and will remain so till the end of time."[12]

In retrospect, it probably would have been a greater disaster if Welch had left during those heroic years at Johns Hopkins, since he had more scientific training and was better able to chart the course necessary for the school and American medicine over the next quarter of a century. But at the same time, seventy years after his death, Osler is remembered more than Welch. This was primarily because Osler was more colorful and dramatic and in a romantic manner seemed to exude the most humane qualities associated with the historic physicians throughout the ages. In addition, his speeches and essays had a poetic quality, and, in spite of having a Victorian quaintness when read today, they still convey an idealism and wisdom of the ages that can strike a responsive chord in many young doctors and medical students.

William Stewart Halsted

William Halsted (1852–1922) was the distinguished general surgeon and first experimental surgeon in America. A shy, polite, learned, introverted man, he was uninterested in fame or money and his passion was laboratory work on his animals. He disliked performing surgery on important personalities that came to Baltimore because of his outstanding reputation, rarely attended medical meetings, and never headed a surgical society. Although the more intellectual surgeons appreciated that his surgeries were like works of art, many others, who took pride in their speed and dexterity, found him exasperatingly slow. Bernheim, who was in his surgery department, many years later, wrote that

> [Halsted's] surgery was a poetry of sorts that few men understood. Halsted taught respect for tissues and control of bleeding. He taught the ultimate good for his patient; and the time

> element was not a consideration. No patient of his ever left the operating room in shock, nor ever had a bungled, messy operation . . . and to this day no surgeon has ever gotten better results, and few have equaled his.[13]

Halsted's accomplishments were new techniques for blood vessel and thyroid surgery and he designed the first rubber gloves to be used in the operating room. But some of his experiments led to personal tragedy. Before he came to Baltimore at Welch's request, he attempted, along with three other surgeons in New York, to use cocaine as a local anesthetic, and all the young doctors used it on themselves. Unfortunately all became addicted, and only Halsted continued to carry on his career. Welch befriended him and persuaded him to go to various sanatoriums which gave him only temporary results. But knowing of his surgical skills, Welch brought Halsted to Baltimore with him in 1889 where initially he was an assistant in the pathology laboratory. When it became clear that Halsted had his habit under control, he was made an Associate Professor of Surgery and a year later made head of the department. There is some question as to whether Halsted ever completely conquered his addiction before he died in 1922 and his only confidants in the matter were Osler and Welch, who never really knew or revealed the truth about him, since Halsted always remained reclusive and guarded.

Nevertheless, honors were bestowed upon him, and his disciples were many. Halsted recognized that with increasing surgical knowledge it would be necessary for subspecialties to develop. He was responsible for developing the first men in the following specialties in the United States: Hugh Young in urology; Samuel Crowe in ear, nose, and throat; Joseph Bloodgood in surgical pathology; F. H. Baetjer in radiology; William Baer in orthopedics; Willis Gatch in anesthesiology; and his most famous disciple, Harvey Cushing in neurological surgery. With regard to the latter, brain surgery at the beginning of the twentieth century had such a high mortality rate, that surgeons hated to take the cases. But knowing of Cushing's surgical skills as his chief surgical resident at the time, Halsted encouraged Cushing to take the brain cases, especially after he had spent some time in Europe working with the neurophysiologists Sir Charles Sherrington and Victor Horsley, England's famous neurosurgeon whose techniques horrified Cushing who, like his mentor Halsted, was a perfectionist. Thus the specialty of neurosurgery was pioneered by Cushing during the early years at the Hopkins, and his procedures attracted patients from all over the United States. The mortality rate dropped slightly but it was still so high that Halsted was heard to say privately that he "didn't know whether to say Cushing's poor patients, or poor Cushing's patients."[14]

The secret of Halsted's leadership was mysterious. His residents over the years were always in demand in other medical schools, and many became heads of surgery departments. Perhaps he led by example or that he recognized in the men he selected an ability that would manifest itself without verbal exhortation. He was never close to any of his residents. His only friends at Johns Hopkins were Welch and Franklin Mall of the anatomy department, and he trusted Osler as his personal physician. On his death, Harvey Cushing wrote that

> he . . . was one of the few American surgeons who may be considered to have established a school of surgery comparable, in a sense, to the school of Billroth in Vienna . . . many of his contributions, not only to his craft but to the science of medicine in general, were fundamental in character and of enduring importance.[15]

Howard A. Kelly

Howard Kelly was born in Camden, New Jersey, in 1858 and was educated at the University of Pennsylvania where he received his medical degree in 1882. He was an excellent anatomist, and, after taking some surgery training at the Episcopal Hospital in Philadelphia, he started a gynecological practice in the poor Kensington district of Philadelphia. He had significant success in treating cases that were considered inoperable by other surgeons. In 1886, he visited many of the gynecological and surgical centers in Europe and Great Britain and in 1888 went back to Berlin where he persuaded Virchow to allow him to work on cadavers with the objective of determining the best manner of catheterizing the ureters. On his return to Pennsylvania he was appointed an associate professor of gynecology, but his friend Osler, who called him the "Kensington colt" and recognized his outstanding surgical ability, persuaded Welch to ask Kelly to come to the new Johns Hopkins as the head of the gynecology department, although he was only 31 years old at the time.

Aside from Kelly being a prolific writer, producing during his career almost 500 papers relating to medical matters and aside from writing the definitive biography of Walter Reed,[16] he also published a book on botany, was a collector and expert on poisonous snakes, and like Osler and Welch, was a devotee of medical history. But his fame came from the fact that he was one of the most skilled and innovative gynecological and abdominal surgeons in the history of medicine, and his two-volume *Operative Gynecology*[17] and *Medical Gynecology*[18] of almost 700 pages were textbooks of world-wide acclaim. Kelly developed not only operative procedures for abnormalities of the female reproductive system but also those for the bladder, ureter, kidneys, and the intestinal tract. He was the first to make it possible to visualize the bladder and the orifices of the ureters with instruments of his own design. The speed with which he operated became legendary. The following is a description of a visit to his operating room by a Chicago surgeon in 1895:

> It was my good fortune to be placed in a desirable front seat, next to Dr. Nicholas Senn. At least two hundred surgeons and near surgeons were crowded into the horseshoe of the large operating amphitheater. A patient was wheeled in, anesthetized and prepared for the preliminary procedure — catheterization of the ureters. The nurses gowned in spotless white arranged the instruments . . . and several internes stood by, ready to serve their chief . . . as Professor Kelly appeared there was prolonged applause. Modestly he assumed his place on a stool at the end of the table. . . . The frontal mirror was slipped into place on the operator's forehead, as he picked up a ureteral speculum with one hand and his trusted bougie with the other — both instruments which he himself had devised. Then he turned and asked one of the spectators to time him. "We will not risk our patient by haste, but I do wish to demonstrate the simplicity of the procedure". In little more time than is necessary to tell about it, both ureters were catheterized with the stiff bougies, the patient's legs were extended, the abdominal incision was made, the diseased uterus explored, and the distended ureters identified — for they must not be injured; then the uterus . . . as it lay in the operator's hand, the broad ligaments were clamped on either side, cut separately, and the body of the uterus freed. The cervix was then severed, the stump ligated and the organ held high as the operator turned and called for "time". "Eight minutes" was the reply. Practically every man in the room was ready to testify to the miracle. The patient was wheeled to the side . . . and Dr.

> Clark proceeded to tie off the broad ligaments, to ligate the bleeding points, to suture the wound, to remove the ureteral bougies and to apply the dressings. Though there were dozens of our most eminent surgeons in the audience, probably not one of them could have completed the delicate procedure of placing those bougies in less than fifteen minutes, to say nothing of the real operation that followed. Someone said to me afterwards: "I was sitting watching Professor Nicholas Senn during Kelly's operation. Do you know what his expression reminded me of? The surprise that might have been seen on the face of an American Indian at the approach of civilization."[19]

Although his surgical style was completely different from Halsted's, the two men respected and admired each other for their respective contributions to surgery. They both insisted on perfect aseptic techniques and at a time when surgeons usually operated in street clothes with sleeves rolled up, Kelly and Halsted both insisted upon fresh cotton gowns, shirts and trousers, which were always sterilized after each procedure, thereby establishing a precedent that was soon copied throughout the United States. Kelly had no experience in pathological histology, but by his contact with his other three colleagues, quickly recognized its importance, and sent one of his early residents, Thomas Cullen, to work with Johannes Orth in Germany (a disciple of Virchow). When Cullen returned to Baltimore, Kelly had already selected another man, William Russell, to be his resident, but he encouraged Cullen to work under Welch's direction until a residency was open. At first Cullen was greatly disappointed but in later years when he became head of the department he wrote that:

> It was perfectly square. Billy was senior to me and entitled to it and as it turned out, it was the luckiest thing that could have happened. I went into the Pathological, was given charge of gynecological pathology, and stayed there three years. I didn't get any pay to speak of but I got my board and room and laundry, and experience that was priceless. It must have looked from the outside as though I was in a backwater, but those three years made all the difference. I had a chance to study all the material from Dr. Kelly's clinic and I had Dr. Welch and Simon Flexner as my laboratory seniors. When I came back to surgery I knew my way around the human belly and could

> recognize things I found there. I remember, years after, Dr. Kelly saying to me that he would give fifty thousand dollars to have had my experience in pathology. I told him I owed him the money then, because he gave me the experience. It was perfectly true. The place was made for me at Kelly's request and I stayed there doing Kelly's work and it was the time of my life.[20]

Howard Kelly's only aberration that might have detracted from his surgery accomplishments was his religious fervor in which he not only gave substantial funds to fundamentalist programs but also took part personally in crusades against prostitution (he tried to "save" them) and in anti-saloon activities. At times it concerned his colleagues, who were worried that he might give up surgery and become a missionary, especially when he would call them "Brother," and gently attempt to convert them to his causes at times. But they all loved him and accepted his fundamentalist ideas regarding the Bible and Jesus Christ as simply part of his complex personality, and they understood that these deep-seated beliefs very likely contributed to his compassion for patients and his desire to help mankind with his surgical inventiveness.

The Basic Scientists

Franklin Paine Mall

Another almost forgotten individual, besides Henry Newell Martin, who played a major part in the Baltimore renaissance was Franklin Paine Mall, the first Professor of Anatomy. Born in 1862 in the farming community of Belle Plaine, Iowa, he graduated in medicine from the University of Michigan in 1883. Then in spite of the fact that Henry Sewell, fresh from Martin's department in Baltimore and the new professor of physiology at Michigan, was said to have predicted that Mall (along with William Mayo) would not succeed in either science or medicine, Mall went to Germany and studied with both William His and Carl Ludwig. Both of these eminent scientists were greatly impressed with Mall's research and recommended him to Welch in 1885. Welch was organizing his pathology department, before the opening of the hospital, and selected him for one of the twenty fellowships given to the new department by the university. Mall worked with Welch during the years 1886–1889, and during those years developed a close relationship with

William Halsted, who had also come to Welch's department after temporarily giving up his surgical career in New York as a result of his cocaine addiction. The two men collaborated at the time Halsted was interested in anastomoses of sections of intestine as a result of injuries or cancers. Mall, having worked on the anatomy and physiology of the intestine in Germany, knew more about that subject than any other person in North America.

This fortuitous association certainly had a significant impact on Halsted, who was soon to become one of the most renowned surgeons in the United States, because the knowledge gained from Mall in terms of understanding the nature of the histology of the body, and the nature of wound healing undoubtedly influenced his method of surgery and all of his students and disciples. Halsted always stated that his "Halsted suture" which involved the submucosa layer in the intestine was inspired by his work with Mall, and, until the latter's death in 1917, Halsted would frequently go to the anatomy department to consult with Mall about his problems in surgery. Also, with regard to political problems such as that of "full-time clinicians," except perhaps for Welch, the influential Mall was the mentor for the shy and introverted Halsted.

Mall's primary interest was embryology, and he was instrumental in establishing the Carnegie Institution of Embryology. He also published 104 papers during his life. He made no monumental discoveries as did Pasteur, Koch, or Ehrlich, but with his precise ways he contributed valuable information and data in anatomy and embryology.

As a teacher, Mall was very controversial, disliked traditional lecturing, and encouraged his associates and medical students to search for information on their own. He believed in learning by doing, and in his course on gross anatomy, he would tell the students to obtain a good atlas and start dissecting, never telling them how to start, what to look for, nor how much they were expected to do and learn in a given period of time. His emphasis was on independence and not to "spoon" information to be memorized. When the first medical class started in 1893, Mall had not performed a human dissection since he was a beginning student himself, and therefore his specific knowledge of gross anatomy was not much greater than that of his new students. But he worked with the students, which he called "elbow training," and he learned with them. The result was that after a few years when he knew his human anatomy, he continued to make the students learn without initial demonstrations by an expert prosector. When the author was a medical student almost 60 years later, the stories about Mall teaching gross anatomy were legend. The most famous one was related by his assistant during those early years:

> One day he found a student standing around doing nothing and he asked him what was the matter. When the student said that he did not know what to do (next), Mall said nothing at all, went out into the hall, but soon returned and without a word put the janitor's broom into his hand.[21]

Needless to say, he was not loved by all of his students, and his teaching was criticized by some of the clinical surgeons, but there were those who eventually appreciated his teaching method, often later in their careers when they had to make a difficult decision in perhaps a life or death situation without anyone else to give advice. In any case, Mall was part of the renaissance, and about twenty five of his students went on to become heads of anatomy departments in medical schools throughout the United States, which was perhaps his greatest contribution.

John Jacob Abel

Born in 1857, John Jacob Abel graduated from Michigan, worked with Martin in Baltimore in 1884, went to Europe where he studied with Ludwig, His, von Frey, Kussmaul, von Recklinghausen and later Naunyn, Hoppe-Seyler, Schmiedeberg, and von Nencki. He returned to the University of Michigan in 1891 but he was not satisfied with the research facilities there and Osler recruited him to be Professor of Pharmacology at the Johns Hopkins, where he remained until he retired in 1932. During those years he isolated epinephrine from the adrenal medulla and showed its effect on blood pressure, purified insulin for the first time, studied pituitary extracts and the use of phenolsulfonephthalein, and developed a primitive but working artificial kidney. His more important students or associates were Leonard G. Rowntree, who became professor of medicine at the University of Minnesota, and Paul D. Lamson, Eugene M. Geiling, and Helen T. Graham, who became professors of pharmacology at Vanderbilt, the University of Chicago, and Washington University in St. Louis, respectively.

William Henry Howell

When Henry Newell Martin resigned from Johns Hopkins University, William Henry Howell, who was born in 1860 and had received his Ph. D. under Martin in 1884, was called back from his position as associate to H.P. Bowditch at Harvard to head the new department of physiology at the new medical school in 1893. He worked actively in the physiology department until 1918 when he became director of the School of Public Health. His research involved studies of erythrocytes (Howell-Jolly bodies), the pituitary gland, and the factors in blood coagulation, particularly as related to hemophilia. He was very active in academic matters; he was dean of the medical school for several years, was president of the American Physiological Society during the years 1905–1910, and was greatly involved in his popular textbook *Textbook of Physiology for Medical Students and Physicians,* which was one of the most used textbooks in American medical schools for more than a half century. Some of his students who later had distinguished careers were two Nobel prize winners: George Minot, who later became Professor of Medicine at Harvard and discovered the use of liver to treat pernicious anemia; and Joseph Erlanger, professor at Washington University in St. Louis who received the prize for his work on the neurophysiology of the heart. Other outstanding students of Howell were Arnold Rich, who later became professor of pathology, and E. Cowles Andrus, professor of medicine, both at Johns Hopkins, and L. Emmett Holt, professor of pediatrics at the New York College of Medicine.

Harvey Cushing

It is not possible to discuss the principal individuals responsible for the renaissance of medicine at Johns Hopkins without mentioning Harvey Cushing. This remarkable physician was actually a second-generation member of the original group, since he graduated in 1895 from Harvard and in 1912 returned there to become the first full professor of neurosurgery where, until 1932, he developed this field to the extent that there were few eminent neurosurgeons before 1950 who had not studied directly with him or one of his students. However, from the time he first arrived in Baltimore, his brilliance was recognized not only by Halsted, but also by Welch and Osler, with whom he developed a very close relationship. Personally, Cushing was described by one who knew and admired him as "a thin, medium sized man with snapping eyes, quick-thinking, quick-acting, short-tempered, nervous, charming, sarcastic, inconsiderate, impatient, ruthless (depending upon changing moods), jealous, lovable, selfish, domineering, demanding — he had a penetrating mind, stupendous ability, and there was nothing he couldn't do and do well once he decided to have a go at it."[22]

When he first came from his training at Harvard and Massachusetts General Hospital, where the emphasis was on operative techniques, Cushing was surprised that his new chief (Halsted) was so slow in his surgery and seemed to be interested not only in taking care not to injure every cell but, if it was a malignancy, in studying microscopically various areas of the removed neoplasm. However, Cushing soon recognized the merits of Halsted's method of surgery and incorporated them into his own procedures. In addition, there was a great interest in the bacteriological study of lesions, a subject about which he knew very little. Then in spite of the fact that he was very active in the surgery department as a general surgeon, he began to work with Welch in bacteriology, publishing papers on typhoid organisms in intestinal lesions and the gonococcus bacterium in peritonitis. Also, he had brought from Boston the first X-ray unit in Baltimore. As a medical student, he devised the method for charting the vital signs during anesthesia, which later included systolic blood pressure readings with the new sphygmomanometer. Almost alone, he championed the use of this method in the United States in 1903. This instrument, of course, was necessary in studying not only the new entity of hypertension, but also that of surgical shock.

In 1900, Cushing went to Europe where he was introduced to the study of physiology, working in Bern with Hugo Kronecker and Leon Asher, while he also performed surgery with Theodore Kocher. It was this experience that stimulated Cushing's life-long interest in physiology and prompted him to become an early member of the American Physiological Society. When Cushing returned to Baltimore, he developed a unique institution, the Hunterian Laboratory, which started as a bare room in which he taught operative surgery to third-year students. However, in 1904, the Hunterian was relocated in a modest building constructed in conjunction with the pathology department. It was there that experimental surgery and physiology were carried out. It was a huge success, especially with the early experiments on the pituitary, with Cushing and Samuel Crowe performing one of the first successful hypophysectomies. They used Halsted's principle of transplantation of organs suspected of having an internal secretion, and showed that pituitary transplantation into the cerebral cortex prolonged the life of animals compared to those who did not receive the transplantation. By 1912 when Cushing wrote his monumental *The Pituitary Body and Its Disorders*,[23] it was clear that the nature of hypo- and hyperactivity of this organ had been elucidated. Also the pathological processes leading to dys-

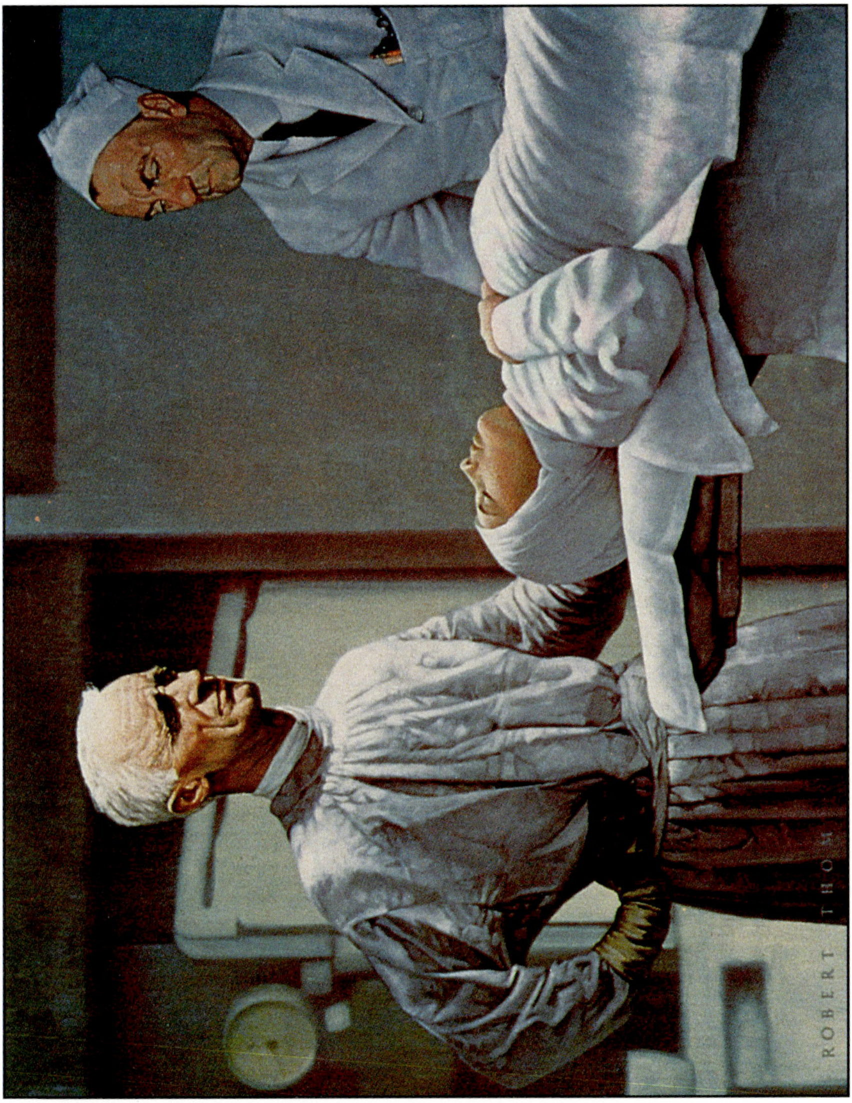

HARVEY CUSHING AND NEUROSURGERY

function of the pituitary, such as tumors, hyperplasia, infections, or congenital defects, were studied and this work certainly led to surgical improvements in the therapy of such lesions. The influence of this work culminated in the isolation of the adrenocorticotrophic and interstitial cell hormones of the pituitary by one of Cushing's early associates at the Hunterian, Herbert M. Evans, and his group at the University of California in the 1940s.

Inspiration for the Establishment of The Rockefeller Institute for Research

One of the great creations of William Osler was his writing of the *Principles and Practice of Medicine*, first published in 1892. This textbook, which was written in a clear, modern style, was the most popular book on internal medicine ever written, certainly until the middle of the twentieth century, and was translated into many languages and underwent several editions even after Osler's death in 1919. But, as important as the textbook was in educating medical students, it was also greatly responsible for the establishment of the first private center for medical research in the United States. In 1897, Osler's book was read by Frederick T. Gates, a former minister and advisor on philanthropic ventures for John D. Rockefeller. The following is taken from his memoirs:

> I read the whole book without skipping any of it. I speak of this, not to commemorate my industry or intelligence, but to testify to Osler's charm, for it is one of the very few scientific books that are possessed of high literary quality. But . . . besides its style that attracted and intensified my interest . . . to the layman student, like me, demanding cures, and specifics, he had no word of comfort whatever . . . medicine had — with few exceptions, no cures and that about all the medicine up to 1897 could do was to suggest some measure of relief, how to nurse the sick . . . . Beyond this, medicine as a cure had not progressed. . . . When I laid down this book I had begun to realize how woefully neglected in all civilized countries and perhaps most of all in this country, had been the scientific study of medicine. . . . It became clear to me that medicine could hardly hope to become a science until it should be endowed, and qualified men could give themselves to uninterrupted study and investigation, on ample salary, entirely inde-

> pendent of practice. . . . Here was an opportunity for Mr. Rockefeller to become a pioneer. This idea took possession of me. . . . I did not realize its enormous difficulty; the only thing I saw was the overwhelming and universal need. . . . I brought my Osler into the office . . . and there I dictated for Mr. Rockefeller's eye a memorandum in which I aimed to show to him the actual condition of medicine in the United States . . . I enumerated the infectious diseases and pointed out how few of the germs had yet been discovered and how great the field of discovery. . . . I pointed to the Koch [sic] Institute in Paris. . . . I remember insisting . . . that even if the proposed institute should fail to discover anything, the mere fact that he, Mr. Rockefeller, had established such an institute of research, . . . would result in other institutes of a similar kind, . . . until research in this country would be conducted on a great scale; and that out of the multitudes of workers we might be sure in the end of abundant rewards, even though those rewards did not come directly from the institute which he might found.[24]

The result was that in 1901, the Rockefeller Institute for Medical Research was founded, and the laboratories were opened in 1906. And Frederick Gates was correct in that one year later the Memorial Institute for Infectious Diseases was founded in Chicago by Mr. and Mrs. Harold F. McCormick, the same year The Carnegie Institution in Washington was established and two years later the Institute for the Study, Treatment and Prevention of Tuberculosis was established by Henry Phipps.

But the most dramatic and pragmatic result of the renaissance at Johns Hopkins in terms of the numbers of human lives saved in the New World and the illustration of how medical and scientific experimentation can lead to knowledge that allows Man to control disease, Nature, and to a great extent, his own destiny is the subject of the next chapter.

Bibliography

1. Bernheim, B.M., *The Story of Johns Hopkins*, p. 8, McGraw-Hill Book Co., New York, 1948.
2. Osler, W., Communication from Osler on the Twenty-Fifth Anniversary of the Johns Hopkins Hospital, 1889-1914. *Bull. Johns Hopkins Hosp.*, 25, p. 354, 1914.
3. Flexner, S.F., and Flexner, J.T, *William Henry Welch and the Heroic Age of American Medicine*, p. 163, The Viking Press, New York, 1941.
4. Ibid, p. 1 12.

4a. Fye, W.B., *The Development of American Physiology, Scientific Medicine in the Nineteenth Century*. Johns Hopkins Univ. Press 1987

5. Welch, W.H., *Papers and Addresses by William Henry Welch*. Vol. III, p. 424, Johns Hopkins Press, 1920.
6. Cushing, H., *The Life of Sir William Osler*. Vol.I, p.61, Clarendon Press, Oxford, 1925.
7. Osler, W., Berlin Correspondence, Canadian. *Med. and Surg. Jour.*, 11, p. 308, 1873-74.
8. Osler, W., Introductory remarks to, and synopsis at, practical course on institutes of medicine. *Canadian Med. and Surg. Jour.*, 4, p. 202, 1875-76.
9. Armstrong, G., *Student Reminiscences, Montreal Period.* International Association of Medical Museums, Sir William Osler Memorial Number, p. 177, Murray Printing Co., 1926.
10. LaFleur, H.A., *Early Days at the Johns Hopkins Hospital with Dr. Osler.*, International Assocation Medical Museums, Sir William Osler Memorial Number, Toronto, Murray Printing Co., p. 270, 1926.
11. Ref. 3, p. 500.
12. Ref. 1, p. 79.
13. Ref. 1, p. 21.
14. Ref. 1, p. 87.
15. Fulton, J.H., *Harvey Cushing, A Biography*, p. 120, Charles C. Thomas Springfield, Illinois, 1946.
16. Kelly, H.A., *Walter Reed and Yellow Fever*, McClure, Phillips and Co., 1906.
17. Kelly, H.A., *Operative Gynecology*. D. Appleton and Co, N.Y.,

1898.
18. Kelly, H.A., *Medical Gynecology*. D. Appleton and Co., N.Y., 1908.
19. Martin, F.H., *Fifty Years of Medicine and Surgery*. p. 233, Surg. Pub. Co., Chicago, 1934.
20. Robinson, J., *Tom Cullen of Baltimore*. p. 113, Oxford Univ. Press, Toronto, 1949.
21. Sabin, F., *Franklin Paine Mall, Anatomist*. Johns Hopkins Press, Baltimore, 1934.
22. Ref. 1, p. 25.
23. Cushing, H.W., *The Pituitary Body and Its Disorders*. Lippincott, Philadelphia, 1912.
24. Ref. 6, Vol. 1, p. 454.

General References

On the History of Johns Hopkins Hospital and Medical School

A. Harvey, A. McGehee, Adventures in Medical Research, Johns Hopkins Univ. Press, Baltimore, 1976.
B. Harvey, A. McGehee, *Research and Discovery in Medicine*. Johns Hopkins Univ. Press, Baltimore, 1981
C. Harvey, A. McGehee, et.al., *A Model of Its Kind*, Vols I & II., *A pictorial History of Medicine at Johns Hopkins*. Johns Hopkins Univ. Press, Baltimore, 1989.

CHAPTER XXI

The Conquest of Yellow Fever and the Influence of the Johns Hopkins

Yellow fever was the major scourge of the New World since 1692, when it was first recognized as a distinct disease in Guadeloupe in the Caribbean. It has been estimated that between the years 1793, when there was a major epidemic in Philadelphia, and 1878, when there was a severe epidemic in Memphis and other cities along the Mississippi River, there were approximately 500,000 cases of yellow fever with 100,000 deaths.[1] It decimated armies of the European countries that came to occupy the Caribbean islands, and, in the case of Haiti, it was the major factor in the defeat of Napoleon's armies that came from France to quell the rebellion of former slaves of the island.[2]

From the time it was first recognized until the last few years of the nineteenth century, its etiology remained a mystery. The only valid facts about the disease that seemed to be established were that it only occurred in sea ports or along river communities that could communicate with the Caribbean, that it disappeared as soon as the first frost occurred, and that individuals who recovered from the disease were immune. Thus the cities along the eastern and southern coast of North America (such as Charleston, Philadelphia, Norfolk, New York, Boston, Baltimore, Mobile, Pensacola, and St. Augustine) together with communities along the Mississippi River (New Orleans, Baton Rouge, Natchez, and Memphis) were the only ones affected during the summer and fall months. Cadiz, Malaga, and Xeres, which are along the southern coast of Spain and were the chief ports of the Spanish Main during the seventeenth, eighteenth, and early nineteenth century, and the island of Gibraltar also suffered severe epidemics that essentially decimated the populations.[3] None of the eminent medical men who went to investigate could ever agree whether the disease was contagious or not. The problem was that the bodies of the sick and dead did not always communicate the disease to non-immune members of the family who were taking care of the patient.

Even more mysterious was that individuals who visited an infected community could contract the disease even though there were no longer sick individuals present, and often by simply walking along deserted streets. In 1881 Hirsch wrote that:

> It is highly probable . . . that the development . . . of the yellow fever poison stands in a certain causal connection with the processes of decomposition in organic materials. Hypotheses as to the nature of the yellow fever poison . . . have exhausted the ingenuity of the profession without advancing our knowledge by a single step.[4]

Because of the development of microbiology as a result of the work of Pasteur and Koch, it was natural that investigators would attempt to identify a bacteria that causes yellow fever. In 1879 George Sternberg,[5] an army physician and the United States' first (and self-taught) bacteriologist, was sent to Cuba to investigate the cause and spread of yellow fever. He worked for several months and although at times thought he had isolated an organism that caused the disease, he finally admitted that he could not offer any unequivocal proof. After pleading unsuccessfully with the Army for several years, he was finally allowed to become a temporary fellow at the new Johns Hopkins University, where, instead of learning about bacteriology, he taught others. This was because the following year William Henry Welch went to Europe (after his appointment as the new Professor of Pathology in Baltimore) to learn from Koch and the other Germans. Alexander Abbott, another pioneer in bacteriology who worked with Welch for several years, wrote in 1916 that:

> it was my happy privilege to have been associated with Dr. Sternberg in the fall and winter of 1884–1885 — when his rank was that of major. He was then holding, by courtesy, a Fellowship in the Johns Hopkins University. . . . I became his assistant and it was from him that I received my first instruction in bacteriology. . . . At that time the accurate, simple, and logical methods of Koch were not available to workers in American laboratories. In fact, there were no workers at all in pure bacteriology in this country, Sternberg, to my knowledge, being the only one.[6]

However, the Army did not allow Sternberg to continue his studies at the Hopkins, and he was sent to confirm or refute the claims of two South American scientists that they had isolated a bacterium that caused yellow fever. Although he did not have faith in the work of these men, he attempted to repeat their work with negative results, and he was able to state in a report to the Surgeon General that "If I have not succeeded in making a positive demonstration which will satisfy the exactions of science, I have at least been able to exclude in a definite manner a majority of the microorganisms which I have encountered in my culture experiments, as well as those which various other investigators have supposed to be the specific cause of the disease."[7]

Following this work, he returned to Baltimore where he again worked at Johns Hopkins and had as his colleagues Welch, Councilman, and Abbott. By this time the problem of yellow fever was a paramount one in Sternberg's mind, and in 1889 he requested assignment back to Cuba to perform more experiments during an epidemic. Although he was again unsuccessful in isolating an etiological bacteria, he was convinced that the disease was produced by an infective agent, and he made an analogy to Pasteur's experiments on rabies. (Viruses, although suspected, had not been isolated at that time). In 1893, Sternberg was promoted to Surgeon General, the highest position in the Army Medical Department, but he did not forget yellow fever, the disease that almost killed him many years before. In an attempt to minimize the disease in Army soldiers during the occupation of Cuba after the war with Spain in 1898, he sent Aristides Agramonte (1868–1931) from the New York Health Department to investigate another bacteria, proposed by Giuseppe Sanarelli, a highly reputable Italian bacteriologist working in South America.[8] The studies were made during the summer of 1898, and, although other investigators confirmed Sanarelli's work, Agramonte could not. Frustrated and aware that important Americans had recently succumbed to the disease, Sternberg appointed an army board made up of Captain Walter Reed, James Carroll, Jesse Lazear, and Agramonte to go to Cuba to again attempt to solve the problem.

Walter Reed had come to Johns Hopkins in 1876 to study with Newell Martin and then returned in 1890 to work with Welch, Abbott, Councilman, Simon Flexner, and George Nuttall. By the time he left in October 1891, Reed was exceptionally well trained in pathological and bacteriological methods. He had undertaken a study of typhoid in relationship to the liver[9] and also published a paper on erysipelas.[10] Reed essentially was a protégé of George Sternberg, who immediately after becoming Surgeon General established the Army Medical School in Washington, D.C., and assigned Reed to duty as curator of the Army Medical Museum and Professor of Bacteriology and Clinical Microscopy in the Medical School. Reed continued to come to Johns Hopkins and was in constant contact with Welch and Flexner with regard to their bacteriological studies, and attended conferences and meetings in the clinical departments.

James Carroll was also a regular army soldier, received his medical degree from the University of Maryland, and then took postgraduate training in pathology and bacteriology at Johns Hopkins during the winters of 1891–1892 and 1892–1893.[9] He worked in close collaboration with Walter Reed at the Army Medical School.

Jesse Lazear did his undergraduate work at Johns Hopkins, went to Columbia University in New York where he received his medical degree in 1892, spent 2 years at Bellevue Hospital, spent some time at the Pasteur Institute in Paris, and then returned to Johns Hopkins where he was Osler's assistant resident in medicine in 1895–1896. He also worked with William Sidney Thayer, the chief medical resident, on the malarial parasite and its relationship to the mosquito.[11]

Aristides Agramonte, born in Cuba, was a fellow student of Lazear and graduated in medicine at Columbia the same year. At the time of his appointment, he was already working on yellow fever in Havana, as was Lazear, both being appointed Contract Surgeons. Only Agramonte had not received some of his training at Johns Hopkins. The task as specified in a letter to Reed by Sternberg was as follows:

> You will naturally give special attention to questions relating to the etiology and prevention of yellow fever. As you are familiar with what has already been done by other bacteriologists in this field of investigation, I do not consider it necessary to give you any suggestions or detailed instructions. But it is evident that the most important question which will occupy your attention is that which relates to the etiology of this disease.[12]

The first meeting of the group was on the afternoon of June 25, 1900, on the veranda of the Officer's quarters at Columbia Barracks Hospital. After deciding on the first steps to be taken, they unanimously agreed that whatever the results of their studies would be, the results would be considered the work of the board as a body and never as an outcome of any particular individual, although each member had reasonable freedom in carrying out his individual methods of research. Reed, Carroll, and Lazear were to remain at the Barracks Hospital, and Agramonte was to be in charge of the laboratory at the Military Hospital in Havana where he was to study the yellow fever cases sent there. They set to work immediately since there was an epidemic in the town of Quemados near Camp Columbia. Agramonte performed autopsies on the victims and Carroll obtained material for cultures, while Lazear examined the tissues. Shortly thereafter, a severe outbreak occurred in the interior city of Santa Clara with the death of some American soldiers; it was assumed that the disease had been brought from Havana. But as Agramonte said years later:

> as to the actual cause of the disease, we were still entirely at sea; it helped us little to know that a man could be infected in Havana, take a train for a town in the interior and start an outbreak there in the course of time. [13]

Then in June, reports came from Pinar del Rió at the extreme western part of the island that great mortality from "pernicious malarial fever" was occurring and Reed sent Agramonte to investigate. He found that the disease was yellow fever. Reed rushed to Pinar del Rió, and they both made the same observations that had been made for past generations — that soldiers who had slept in the same beds occupied by others who had died of yellow fever did not contract the disease. And most remarkably a soldier who had been confined to the guardhouse since June 6, came down with the disease on the 12th and died on the 18th while eight other solders confined to the same cell never contracted the illness. As Reed wrote in one of his later classic papers:

> It was conjectured at the time that, perhaps, some insect capable of conveying the infection, such as the mosquito, had entered through the cell window, bitten this particular prisoner and then passed out.[14]

Reed considered this only as a supposition, because although Ronald Ross had shown a few years earlier that the mosquito was the vector in the transmission of malaria, Carlos Finlay, a Cuban physician who believed that the mosquito *Aedes egypti* was the carrier of yellow fever, had carried out experiments that definitely seemed to disprove his own theory. During the years, 1881–1885, Finlay had attempted to produce yellow fever in as many as 100 individuals by allowing an Aedes mosquito to feed on a patient who had showed symptoms of yellow fever for two to four days and then having the same mosquito bite an uninfected person.[15] In these experiments there resulted no cases of severe yellow fever and only a few which Finlay called "mild." Finlay explained his lack of success primarily on the basis that most of the individuals were probably already immune from a prior infection. However, now we know that the lack of success was Finlay's lack of knowledge of the extrinsic period, which is the period of time that must elapse after the mosquito bites an infected individual and is able to bite and infect another individual. This period is a minimum of 12 days, and in Finlay's protocol, the interval was a maximum of 4 days. This was the key to the problem. It was first suspected by Henry R. Carter of the Marine Hospital Service, who had received his medical degree from the University of Maryland in 1879. He was investigating an 1898 epidemic in two small communities in Mississippi, Taylor and Orwood, where the farm houses were as much as one mile apart and there was an interval of approximately 14-21 days between the first infection in one community and a secondary one in the second community. Specifically, Carter came to the following conclusion:

> 1. If a visitor to the home of the first victim of yellow fever visits before 12 days have elapsed since the person became ill, and returns to his home and does not return, he will not contract yellow fever.
> 2. If the visitor comes to the home of the patient, more than 12 days after the person became ill, even if the patient has died and been buried, it is likely that the visitor will become ill with yellow fever.
> 3. If the visitor in (2) returns to his home community where there have been no cases of yellow fever, and becomes sick there, his family members do not become ill until another 12 days have passed.

Carter published his findings in May of 1900[16] and it was unlikely that the Yellow Fever Board had read it. By a stroke of luck, Carter was stationed in Cuba as a quarantine officer and spoke to Jesse Lazear on June 25th about the "extrinsic period" and the next day sent him a copy of his May article. This information, together with their experience at Pinar del Rió, made the Board rethink their ideas. On August 1st, the Board met again and Reed stated that

> at this stage of our investigation it seemed to me, and I so expressed the opinion to my colleagues, that the time had arrived when the plan of our work should be radically changed; that the search for the specific agent of yellow fever, while not abandoned, should be given secondary consideration, until we had first definitely learned something about the way or ways in which the disease was propagated from the sick to the well. I felt well nigh convinced that we could obtain no light whatever upon the task that had been set before us, unless we substituted this line of work for the one we had been pursuing, and that in view of the splendid work of Ross, Bignami and others with regard to the propagation of malarial fever, together with the well known thermal influences intimately connected not only with the epidemiology of the disease in the United States, but also . . . on the island of Cuba, it was of the highest importance that the agency of an intermediate host, such as that of the mosquito, should either be proven or disproven.[17]

Because Lazear was the only one with experience with mosquitoes (as a result with his work with William Thayer at Johns Hopkins), Reed assigned him to this part of the investigation. They also visited Carlos Finlay, who was elated to hear that the Board proposed to evaluate his theory. He offered his help in addition to supplying eggs of *Aedes egypti*, which was the mosquito that was most prominently found around houses in which there were yellow fever cases and were bred as "wigglers" in pots, cisterns, tin cans, and old bottles that caught rain water. The young female mosquitoes that resulted were allowed to feed on yellow fever patients during the early days of August and then before 12 days had elapsed, fed on healthy volunteers. None became ill, the Board was discouraged and Finlay was devastated.

Then a break came when James Carroll was bitten August 27th by a mosquito which had fed twelve days before on a severe case of yellow fever victum on the second day of the illness; on August 30th, he developed a violent case of the disease. Carroll then told Agramonte that he must have contracted the disease while performing an autopsy on a yellow fever victim. Although Lazear knew about Carter's "extrinsic period" all through the month of July, he evidently did not give much credence to the work because the early experiments with volunteers did not take it into consideration. This illustrates again the difficulty the human mind has in accepting new ideas.

The next experiment was done on William H. Dean, a soldier of the Seventh Cavalry, who said he "ain't scared of 'em" (mosquitoes), and allowed, on August 31st, Lazear to place four different mosquitoes on his arm, which had previously bitten yellow fever patients from 2 to 16 days before. Five days later Dean developed a severe case of yellow fever, but recovered as did James Carroll. Agramonte and Lazear sent a cable to Reed, who had been called back to Washington, that on the basis of the cases of Carroll and Dean the theory of the transmission of yellow fever by mosquitoes had been confirmed although further work would continue. Then on September 13th, Jesse Lazear, while collecting blood from yellow fever patients, was bitten by a mosquito that had settled on the back of his hand. Because he had already been bitten by an experimental mosquito that had feasted on a yellow fever patient 10 days before and he had not become ill, Lazear assumed he had achieved some immunity and was not concerned. However five days after this accidental bite, Lazear developed a severe case of yellow fever, with the extremely high fever, albuminuria, jaundice, black vomitus, and as described by Agramonte:

> Tuesday, the 25th of September saw the end of the life full of promise; one more name, that of Jesse W. Lazear, was graven upon the portals of immortality. And we may feel justly proud for having had it, in any way, associated with our own.[18]

However, upon Reed's return to Cuba, more comprehensive studies[19] and more volunteers were required to give definitive proof not only to whether mosquitoes transmitted yellow fever but also to the conditions under which this occurred. It was paramount to carry out the experiments in the best traditions of those being carried out at the Johns Hopkins. Therefore on November 20th, an experimental station named Camp Lazear was established in an open remote area a few miles from the hospital. It consisted of seven army tents, guarded by soldiers chosen because of their interest in the project. In addition to attempting to provide unequivocal proof of the mosquito vector, it was decided to disprove, once and for all, that fomites or the soiled bed clothes and bedding of victims of yellow fever are not infectious. Consequently, two wooden structures 14 × 20 feet were erected eight yards apart. One was called the Infected Mosquito Building and was divided near the middle with a permanent wire screen partition and had good ventilation. The other structure was called the Infected Clothing Building and was built with air tight walls and ceilings, screened doors and windows, and was not only insect proof but had poor ventilation. The experimental protocol was as follows:

> 1. Three non-immune men entered the Infected Clothing Building on November 30th where they encountered three beds, some boxes and a trunk which were filled with pillows, underwear, pajamas, towels, sheets and blankets soiled with the blood and discharges of yellow fever patients. They had instructions to unpack the trunk and boxes, handle and shake the clothing so that if any yellow fever germs were present they would surely be released. The men were nauseated and repelled by the fomites, but they stayed and slept there for twenty nights, although they were allowed to spend their days in a nearby tent.
> 2. In the Infected Mosquito Building, one young soldier, John R. Kissinger, who refusing any monetary reward, allowed himself to be bitten by five mosquitoes which had previously bitten yellow fever patients during the early stages of the disease, two, fifteen, nineteen and twenty one days before. In three days Kissinger was ill with yellow fever but recovered. The experiment was repeated with three more volunteers (who accepted payment for their participation) who also became ill. By this time other volunteers, seeing the results of the study, changed their minds and withdrew from the project. But not all. John J. Moran, a civilian employee, also with a stipulation that he would not accept any remuneration, entered the Infected Mosquito Building and allowed himself to be bitten by infected mosquitoes, well beyond the "extrinsic period" which was now almost definitely proven, and confined himself to one half of the room. The other half divided by a mosquito proof wire screen, was occupied by two other volunteers who

> slept there for three weeks. Although Moran developed yellow fever on the fourth day, the other two men on the other side of the room remained healthy proving that only the bite of infected mosquitoes can transmit the disease. But because of the chance that the two men on the mosquito-less side of the room could have been immune, one of the men, Warren Jernegan, volunteered to be injected with blood taken from a yellow fever patient in the second day of his disease. Jernigan developed yellow fever four days later, which showed that although the mosquito is nature's way of transmitting the disease, the microorganism does not go through a metamorphosis in the mosquito but can be transmitted directly from blood to blood.

Thus in a series of elegant experiments in the best tradition of the new Johns Hopkins Medical School, which were published in 1901, the mystery of the transmission of yellow fever that had mystified physicians for more than two hundred years was solved. Walter Reed expressed his thoughts on the matter in a letter written to his wife at the conclusions of the studies of the Board:

> Columbia Barracks
> Quemados, Cuba
> 11: 50 PM, Dec. 31, 1900
> Only ten minutes of the old century remain. Here I have been sitting, reading that most wonderful book, "La Roche on Yellow Fever", written in 1853. Forty seven years later it has been permitted to me and my assistants to lift the impenetrable veil that has surrounded the causation of this most wonderful, dreadful pest of humanity and to put it on a rational and scientific basis. I thank God that this had been accomplished during the latter days of the old century. May its cure be wrought out in the early days of the new! The prayer that has been mine for twenty years, that I might be permitted in some way or at some time to do something to alleviate human suffering has been granted! A thousand Happy New Years . . . Hark, there go the twenty four hour buglers in concert, all sounding "Taps" for the old year.[20]

The three Johns Hopkins men of the Army Board were not able to bask long in their victory, Lazear dying in Cuba before the final experiments, Reed in 1902 from a perforated appendix, and Carroll in 1907

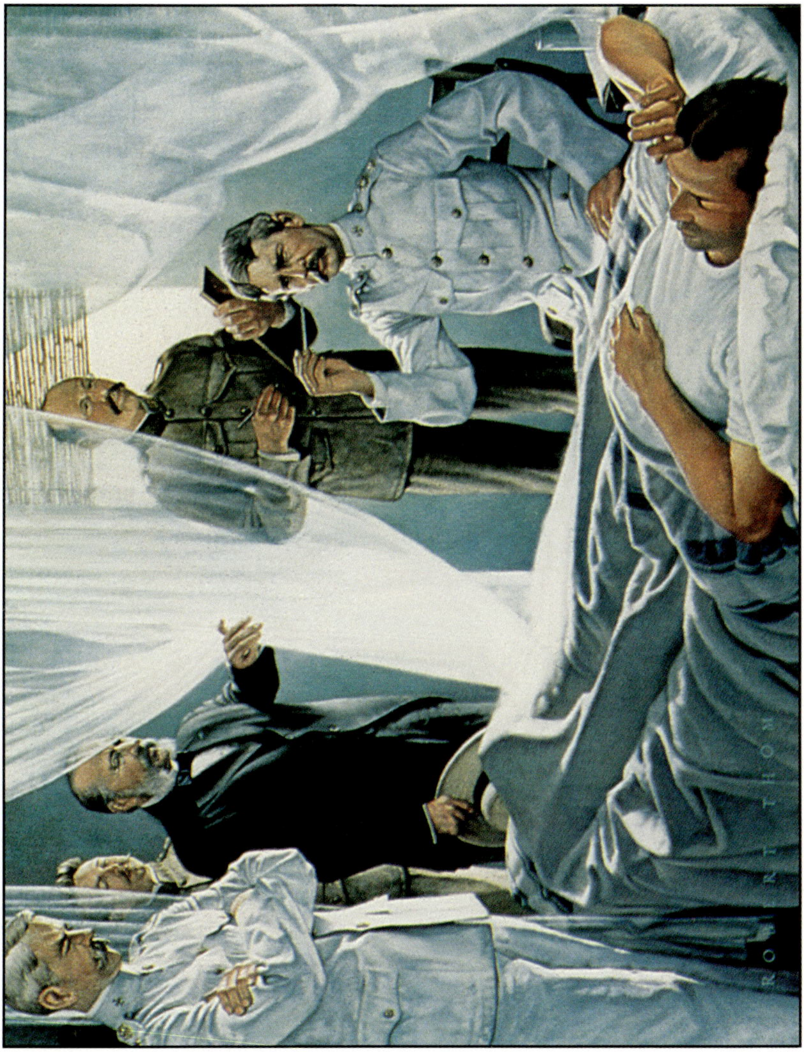

Left to right: Major W. C. Gorgas, A. Agramonte, Carlos Finlay, James Carroll, Major W. Reed. Patient was J. Kissinger.

THE CONQUEST OF YELLOW FEVER

from residual effects of his severe case of yellow fever. But their work was the first great American conquest in the annals of medical progress, a result of the Johns Hopkins Renaissance, and one of the factors that caused Osler's Minerva Medica to shortly after move to the New World.

Bibliography

1. Reed, W., and Carroll, J., The Prevention of Yellow Fever, *Medical Record*, **60**, No. 17, 1901.
2. Gilbert, C.N.P., *Histoire Médicale de l'armée Francaise a Saint-Domingue, ou mémoire sur la fievre jaune.* Gabon and Co. Paris , 1803.
3. Hirsch, A., *Handbook of Geographical and Historical Pathology*, Vol. 1, p. 336. Translated by Charles Creighton, The New Sydenham Society, London, 1883.
4. Ibid, p. 369.
5. Sternberg, M., *George Miller Sternberg*, AMA Press, Chicago, 1920.
6. Ibid, p. 292.
7. Ibid, p. 110
8. Sanarelli, J., Etiologie et pathologie de la fièvre jaune. *Ann. Inst. Pasteur*, **11**, p. 433, 1897.
9. Reed, W., An investigation into the so-called lymphoid nodules of the liver in typhoid fever. *Johns Hopkins Hosp*. Rep., **5**, p. 379, 1895.
10. Reed, W., The contagiousness of erysipelas. *Boston Med. and Surg. Jour.*, **126**, p. 237, 1892.
11. Kelly, H.A., *Walter Reed and Yellow Fever*, p. 265, McClure Phillips and Co., New York, 1906.
12. Gibson, J. M., *Soldier in White*, p. 222. Duke Univ. Press, Durham, 1958.
13. Agramonte, A., *The Inside History of a Great Medical Discovery*, p. 12. Havana, 1915.
14. Reed, W., The propagation of yellow fever; observations based on recent researches, *Med. Rec.*, **60**, No. 6, p. 202, 1901.
15. Ibid, p. 204.
16. Carter, H.R., A note on the interval between infecting and secondary cases of yellow fever from the records of the yellow fever at Orwood and Taylor, Miss. in 1898. *New Orleans Med. and Surg. Jour.*, **52**, p. 617, 1900.
17. Ref. 14, p. 203.
18. Ref. 13, p. 21.
19. Ref. 14, p. 204.
20. Ref. 11, p. 152.

Epilogue

With the advent of the twentieth century, there was a quantum jump in scientific and medical knowledge as more financial and human resources were poured into these areas. The Western World and particularly the United States essentially made science the new religion, although it gave "lip service" to its professed Judaic–Christian traditions. Science promoted progress, and the promise of the Enlightenment that this progress, by achieving control over Nature, would solve the problems of the world and increase man's happiness was looked upon by society with an essentially uncritical optimism. But as the twenty-first century is approached, there is a deep sense of disillusionment with the rewards of progress and Shelley's optimistic thought that "happiness and science dawn late upon the earth" (*The Daemon of the World*). Of the scourges of mankind, science has produced the ability to alleviate most of the pestilences of the world, and Man has gained the knowledge to prevent famine. Under optimum conditions, these advances could allow each child on earth a statistically longer life than was ever before possible.

But ominous shadows have also been cast by scientific advancement, and William Osler, who had shared Shelley's optimism during his early career, began to become more cautious during the last decade of the nineteenth century. Osler was enthralled with the great scientific institutions of Germany and so wanted to emulate them in North America and wrote in 1894:

> Germany will be our model. She is great because she has a large group of men pursuing pure science with unflagging industry, with self denying zeal and with high ideals. No secondary motives sway their minds, but unhampered by social or theological prejudices, they have been enabled to cherish "the truth which has never been deceived — that complete truth carries with it the antidote against bane and danger which follow in the train of half knowledge" (Helmholtz).[1]

But Osler also saw a danger:

> Science has done much, and will do more, to alleviate the unhappy condition in which so many millions of our fellow

> creatures live, and in no way more than in mitigating some of the horrors of disease; but we are too apt to forget that apart and beyond her domain lie those irresistible forces which alone sway the hearts of men. With reason, science never parts company but with feeling, emotion, passion — what has she to do? They are not of her; they owe her no allegiance. She may study, analyze, and define — she can never control them, and by no possibility can their ways be justified to her. . . . Listen to the words of a student of the heart of man, a depiction of his emotions. "In all ages the reason of the world has been at the mercy of brute force. The reign of law has never had more than a passing reality, and never can have more so long as man is human. The individual intellect and the aggregate intelligence of nations and races, have alike perished in the struggle of mankind, to revive again, indeed, but as surely to be again put to the edge of the sword. Look where you will throughout the length and breadth of all that was the world, 5000 or 500 years ago; everywhere passion has swept thought before it, and belief, reason. Passion rules the world and rules alone. And passion is neither of the head or the hand, but of the heart. Love, hate, ambition, anger, avarice, either make a slave of intelligence to serve their impulses, or break down its impotent opposition with the unanswerable argument of brute force, and tear it to pieces with iron hands." (Marion Crawford)[2]

Osler was to experience first hand the realization of his warning when as Professor of Medicine at Oxford, with the outbreak of World War I, he was soon to see not only his beloved son die on the battlefield but also millions of other young men on both sides. It resulted in a disillusionment from which he never recovered and was undoubtedly a factor in his death in 1920.

In 1915 with the war in France raging he said that:

> The explanation of this (war) is that we are still in the childhood of civilization. Some millions of years divide the Tertiary period, when man broke away from the great ape stock, and the dawn of our modern era, when " iron, cold iron" became master of the world. Only with the working of metals did progress become possible. In Time our civilization is but

> a thin fringe like the layer of living polyps on the coral reef, capping the dead generations on which it rests. The lust of war is still in the blood, we cannot help it. There was, and there is as yet, no final appeal but to the ordeal of battle. Only let us get the race in its true perspective in which a thousand years are but as yesterday, and in which we are contemporaries of the Babylonians and Egyptians and all together within Plato's year. Let us remember, too, that war is a human development, unknown to other animals. Though Nature is ruthless "in tooth and claw", collective war between members of the same species is not of her weapons . . . and yet in what a fool's paradise many have been living, flaunting in the face of history our wish for peace — seeking it, ensuing it, with the war drums throbbing in our ears.[3]

Since Osler's death in 1920, his warnings and insights have long since been forgotten by his fellow men. By 1945, with one of the most brilliant breakthroughs in scientific knowledge — the discoveries and the ability to release the vast energies within the atomic nucleus — the atomic bomb was built after which it was realized with certainty that science had indeed created a Frankenstein monster. The means were then available and would always remain in the future for the destruction of all life on the planet.

A similar warning came from perhaps an unlikely source, General Douglas MacArthur, who after the disaster of Hiroshima and Nagasaki, said at the signing of the surrender of Japan in 1945:

> Men since the beginning of time have sought peace. Various methods through the ages have attempted to devise an international process to prevent or settle disputes between nations. From the very start workable methods were found insofar as individual citizens were concerned, but the mechanics of an instrumentality of larger international scope have never been successful. Military alliances, balances of power, leagues of nations, all in turn failed, leaving the only path to be by the way of the crucible of war. We have had our last chance. If we do not now devise some greater and more equitable system, Armageddon will be at our door. The problem is basically theological and involves a spiritual recrudescence and improvement of human character that will synchronize with our almost matchless advances in science, art, literature and all

> material and cultural developments of the past two thousand years. It must be of the spirit if we are to save the flesh.[4]

The great advances made in medical science, which essentially started in the nineteenth century, and expanded during the twentieth, will be for naught if man-made dangers to the earth's environment cannot be avoided. Although the major concern over the last half of the twentieth century has been the danger of a nuclear holocaust, comparatively little attention has been given to the adverse effects of excessive population growth. It took four million years for humanity to reach a population of two billion people but only 30 years to add a third billion; and it is predicted that there will be an additional billion for each decade during the next century. The lack of awareness by mankind that humans are not the owners of the planet, but merely custodians, has catastrophic potential. There must be self-imposed limits on the extent the custodians be allowed to pollute and ravage that which sustains them. The civilization that has evolved over thousands of years is equally threatened by the seeking of temporary power or security (for or by any country or groups of people) by means of weapons of destruction or by population encouragement. Both of these threats must be prevented or discouraged. Mankind's deepest obligation is to future generations—the past and present are simply prologue.

Bibliography

1. Osler, W., The Leaven of Science, p. 92, in *Equanimitas with Other Addresses*. Blakiston Co. Philadelphia, 1951
2. Ibid, p. 93
3. Osler, W., *Science and War*, p. 6. Clarendon Press, Oxford, 1915
4. MacArthur, D., *Reminiscences*, p. 276. McGraw-Hill, New York, 1964

Pathology Index

A

Abbe: Ernst 133, 214
Abbott: A.C. 357, 363, 388, 389
Abel: John Jacob 378
Abernethy: John 85, 331
Ackerknecht: Erwin 51, 196, 201
Acland: Sir Henry 77, 78, 95
Adams: Robert 97
Addison 321; Thomas 80, 87, 91, 348; William 190, 313
Agassiz: L. 367
Agramonte: Aristide 389, 390, 391, 393, 394
Albury: W. 54
Alibert: Jean 67
Amici: G. 133
Andral: Gabriel 63, 113, 121, 129, 173, 308, 309, 331
Andrus: E. Cowles 379
Armstrong: George 368
Arrhenius: S. 175
Aschoff: Ludwig 192
Asher: Leon 380
Ashford: B.K. 272
Astruc: Jean 33, 328
Auenbrugger: Leopold 58
Aurelius: Marcus 6
Avicenna 20

B

Bacon: Francis 25, 40, 47, 160, 328
Baer: William 372
Baetjer: F.H. 372
Baeumler: Christian 152
Baillie: Mathew 85
Balard: A. 202
Bancroft: Joseph 273; Thomas 274
Bang: Bernhard 237; Ivar 309
Barcroft: J. 8

Barker: Lewellys 357
Barlow: Claude H. 270
Bateman: Thomas 80
Baumes: J.B.T. 40
Baumgarten: Paul 299
Bayle: Gaspard Laurent 58, 61, 62, 113, 330
Bayliss: W.M. 8
Bayne-Jones: Stanhope 357
Beale: Lionel 134
Beckmann: Otto 152
Behring: Emil von 236, 239
Bell: Benjamin 80; Charles 80, 101; John 80, 101
Beneke: R. 137
Benivieni: Antonio 21, 327
Bennett: J. 102, 133, 134, 314
Benninghoff: A. 6
Bentley: C.A. 271
Bernard: Claude 8, 11, 67, 163, 166, 169, 175, 179, 208, 303, 307, 308
Bernheim: Bertram 351, 371
Bert: P. 67
Berthold: A. 308
Berzelius: J. 124
Bichat: M. Xavier 9, 13, 43, 45, 47, 52, 95, 113, 346, 348
Biermayer: Lorenz 113
Bignami: A. 278, 393
Bilharz: T. 264, 268, 269, 270
Billings: J. 356, 360, 361, 363, 369
Billroth: T. 110, 210, 221, 373
Biot: J. 202, 207
Birch-Hirschfeld: A. 217, 220
Bismarck: Otto von 144
Bizzozero: G. 194, 310, 318, 320, 367
Black: Joseph 78
Blizard: William 85
Bloodgood: Joseph 372
Blumer: George 357
Boë: de le 29, 31, 33
Boerhaave: Hermann 12, 31, 39, 348
Bonaparte: Napoleon 50, 64, 268, 387
Bonet: Theophile 33
Booker: William D. 357
Bordet: Jules 301

Bordeu: Theophile de 40
Borelli: Giovanni 39
Bostock: John 130
Botkin: Sergei 152
Bouillaud: Jean 66
Boveri: T. 137
Bowditch: H.P. 348, 362, 379
Bowman: W. 134
Boyle: Robert 25–33, 26, 29, 328
Braconnot: H. 124
Bretonneau: Pierre 64, 147, 159, 234
Brie: Johan de 263
Bright: Richard 80, 87, 348
Brock: G.S. 269
Broussais 64
Brown: John 40; Robert 146, 267
Brown-Sequard: C.E. 175
Bruce: David 236, 285, 286, 287, 288, 289
Brücke: Ernst 135, 174
Budd: William 225
Bumm: Ernst von 227
Burnet: McFarlane 302
Burns: Robert 78
Burton-Sanderson: John 175

C

Cabanis: George 47
Cagniard-Latour: C. 205
Cannon: Walter 8, 187
Carnegie: Andrew 344
Carroll: J. 389, 390, 391, 393, 394, 396
Carswell: Robert 103, 331
Carter: Henry R. 392, 394
Castellani: Aldo 287
Catto: J. 269
Cayol: J.B. 62, 330
Celsus: A. Cornelius 189
Chamberland: Charles 251
Chaussier: Francois 50
Cheselden: William 81
Cheyne: John 80, 97
Chiari: Hans 363

Chomel: August 67
Christison: Robert 80, 102
Christy: Cuthbert 287
Chrzonszczewsky: N. 137
Clark 375; Alonzo 348; James 80
Clift: William 85
Cobbold: T.S. 264, 271, 273, 274
Cohn: Ferdinand 183
Cohnheim: Julius 10, 137, 144, 152, 155, 179, 189, 192–196, 196, 229, 296, 310, 314, 317, 336, 339, 340, 348, 356, 357, 359, 360, 363
Coiter: Volcher 33
Colbert: Jean Baptise 48
Cole: Rufus 357
Colles: Abraham 80, 97
Colombo: Realdo 22
Columella 199
Comte: Auguste 48
Condillac: Etienne de 47
Cooper: Astley 77, 80, 85, 86, 348
Cornil: Andre 137, 152
Corrigan: John 76, 97, 101
Corvisart: Jean Nicolas 43, 50, 52, 58, 114, 348
Councilman: William 152, 192, 227, 276, 277, 355, 361, 363, 389
Craigie: David 80, 102
Crawford: Marion 402
Crick: F. 2
Crowe: Samuel 372, 380
Cruikshank: William 80
Cruveilhier: Jean 63, 117, 334
Cullen: Thomas 357, 375; William 39, 42, 79
Cushing: Harvey 367, 372, 373, 379–380
Czermak: Johann 152

D

Daland: J. 312
Dale: William 77
Darwin: C. 295, 345
Davaine: Casimir 214, 264
Dean: William H. 394
Deiters: Otto 152
Delafield: Francis 359

Demarquay: Jean 272
Desault: Pierre Joseph 50
Descartes: R. 2, 5, 25, 47
Dobell: Clifford 130
Donaldson: H.H. 362
Donato: Marcella 33
Donné: A. 135, 367
Dubini: Angelo 270
Dubois-Reymond: E. 135, 174
Duchenne: Guillaume 67
Duclaux: Emile 208, 218
Dujardin: F. 264
Dumas: J.B. 202, 207, 208
Dupuytren: Guillaume 54, 63, 67
Durham: Herbert 226, 240, 301
Dutton: J.E. 287

E

Eberth: Carl 225
Edison: Thomas 344
Ehrenberg 133
Ehrlich: P. 137, 175, 183, 195, 229, 236, 278, 285, 301, 303, 309, 314–319, 319, 356, 364, 367, 377
Erigena: Johannes Scotus 19
Erlanger: Joseph 379
Eustachi: Bartolomeo 22
Evans: Alice 237; Griffith 286; Herbert M. 383

F

Falloppio: Gabriele 22, 327
Felix: Francois 48
Fergusson: Robert 78
Fernel: Jean 22, 33
Fick: Adolf 175
Finlay: Carlos 391
Fitz: R.H. 152
Flemming: W. 137, 333
Flexner: Simon 357, 358, 389, 390
Flint: Austin 214, 309, 320, 360
Flourens: M.J.P. 175
Flügge: C. 300
Folin: Otto 309

Forbes: John 80
Foreest: Pieter van 33
Foster: M. 175, 264, 308, 361
Fourcroy: Antoine 49, 202
Fox: Wilson 152
Fracastoro: Girolamo 199, 200, 201
Fraenkel: Albert 224
Frank: Johann Peter 32, 113
Franklin: Benjamin 80
Frederich William III 108
Frerichs: F. 317, 319, 348, 367
Frey: M. von 137, 378
Friedländer: Carl 223, 224, 225
Friedreich: Nikolaus 152
Frobenius: Wilhelm 360
Froriep: Robert 143

G

Gaertner: August 240
Gaffky: Georg 221, 225, 233, 234, 235, 238
Galen 1, 17–33, 39, 155, 327
Galileo 25, 160
Garden: Alexander 80
Garrison: W. 21, 234
Garrod: A. 308
Gatch: Willis 372
Gates: Frederick 383, 384
Gavarret: J. 63, 309
Gegenbaur: Karl 152
Gengou: O. 301
Gentron: Charles Deshais 328
Gerard 20
Gerhard: W.W. 348
Gerhardt: Carl 152
Gerlach: Joseph 135
Gilman: D.C. 184, 356, 361, 363
Goethe: J. 108
Goeze: Johan 263
Goltz: F. 175
Goodsir: John 102, 147
Gowers: William 311
Graaf: de 25, 29

Grafenberg: Johann Schenck von 33
Gram: Hans 223, 224, 227
Grassi: Giovanni 271, 284
Graves: Robert James 80, 97
Gravitz: Paul 152
Greisinger: W. 268, 271
Grew: Nehemiah 146
Gross: Samuel 346
Gruber: M. 226, 301
Grüby: David 135, 285
Guldberg: C.M. 175
Guy-Lussac: J.L. 202

H

Haeckel: Ernst 144, 152
Haën: Anton de 32; de 12
Hali Abbas 20
Hall: Marshall 80
Haller: Albrecht von 54
Halsted: William S. 351, 358, 371, 371–373, 372, 375, 377, 379, 380
Hansen: Armauer 226
Harrison: Ross 362
Harvey: W. 22–33, 26, 155, 328, 348, 356
Hawkins: Caesar 80
Hayem: G. 314, 320, 367
Hebra: F. 174, 217, 348
Hedin: S. 312
Heidenhain: Rudolf 137, 175, 317
Helmholtz: Herman 135, 175
Helmont: J. van 39, 331
Henderson: L.J. 8
Henle: Jacob 108, 135, 145, 146, 148, 185, 189, 201, 202, 337
Henry: William 343
Herbst: G. 267
Hering: Ewald 175
Hertwig: Oscar 137, 333; Richard 137
Hesse: Walter 222
Heurnius: Jan 29, 31; Otto 31
Hewson: William 313
Hill: John 329
Hippocrates 17, 31, 47, 58, 327
Hirsch: A. 388

His 378; Wilhelm 152, 175, 376
Hodgkin: Thomas 80, 87, 95, 130, 331, 348
Hoff: J van't 175
Hoffman: Christoph Ludwig 39
Holmes: Oliver Wendell 113, 217, 348
Holt: L. Emmett 379
Home: Francis 80
Hooke: Robert 146
Hope: James 80, 86, 103
Hoppe-Seyler: F. 152, 175, 311, 359, 378
Horner: William E. 346
Horsley: Victor 372
Hosak: David 346
Howard: W.T. 357
Howell: William Henry 362, 378
Hueppe: Ferdinand 152
Humboldt: W. 108, 109
Hume: David 78
Hunter 155; John 13, 73, 81, 130, 187, 189, 331, 346, 348, 356; William 73, 81, 113
Huxley: T. 313, 361, 367

J

Jackson: James 346
Jacobi: Abraham 359
Jahn: Jena 173
Jenner: Edward 85, 249
Jensen: Zacharias 129
Jones 314; T.W. 313

K

Kampf: Johann 39
Kelly: H. 351, 357, 373–375, 376
Kerckring: Theodore 33
Key: Aston 87; Axel 152
King: Lester 12
Kitosato: Shibasaburo 228, 238
Klebs: E. 144, 148, 152, 217, 234, 275, 337
Koch: R. 10, 159, 176, 183, 210–214, 219, 220, 221, 224, 228, 229, 230, 233, 234, 235, 236, 238, 240, 249, 252, 271, 303, 320, 336, 348, 356, 360, 364, 377, 388

Kocher: Theodore 380
Kohlraush 124
Kölliker: R.A. 129, 135, 146, 179, 332
Kronecker: Hugo 175, 380
Kruif: Paul de 236, 288
Kühne: Willy 175, 180
Kupffer: Karl 135
Kussmaul: A. 117, 152, 378

L

La Mettrie: Julian de 47
Laennec: R. 13, 43, 45, *52*, 54, 64, 95, 113, 114, 174, 348
Lafleur: H.A. 369
Lancisi: G. 33, 275
Langenbeck: B. 334
Langerhans: Robert 152
Lannelongue: M. 218
Laplace: P.S. 1
Laveran: C.A. 275, 276, 277, 278, 287
Lavoisier: A.L. 1, 202
Lazarus: A. 319
Lazear: Jesse 389, 390, 391, 393, 394, 396
Lebert: Hermann 135
Lee: Frederic Schiller 362
Leeuwenhoek: A. van 25, 29, 30, 129, 313
Legallois: J.J.C. 175
Lehman: Carl 122
Leidy: J. 267, 367
Leiper: R.T. 270
Lesch: J. 54
Leuckart: R. 264, 267, 271
Lewis: T. 286; T.R. 273
Lichtheim: Ludwig 183
Lieberkuhn: J. 137
Liebig: Justus 122, 124, 205
Lieutaud: Joseph 33, 50
Linnaeus. *See* Linné: Carl von
Linné: Carl von 41
Lister 210; Joseph 97, 146
Lobstein: J.F. 331
Locke: John 25, 43, 47

Loeffler: Friedrich 221, 226, 235, 238
Loos: Arthur 271
Louis: P.C.A. 13, 65, 114, 348
Lower: R. 25
Ludwig: C. 174, 175, 307, 348, 359, 360, 376, 378

M

MacArthur: Douglas 403
Macartney: James 97
MacCallum: W.C. 357
MacConkey: A.J. 226
Magendie: F. 10, 54, 63, 67, 121, 129, 159, 159–165, 173, 175, 179, 187, 303, 307, 308
Malgaigne: Joseph 67
Mall: F.P. 358, 373, 376–378
Mallory: F.B. 227
Malpighi: M. 25, 33, 39, 313
Mandl: Louis 135
Manson: P. 201, 269, 273, 274, 278, 284
Marchand: Felix 152
Marchiafava: E. 278
Mareschal: Georges 49
Martin: H.N. 355, 356, 361, 363, 376, 378
Martius: Friedrich 152
McKee: Alexander 184
Mesmer: Franz 40
Metchnikoff: E. 295, 300, 301, 302, 303, 336
Mettrie: de la 2
Miescher: F. 175
Minot: G. 321, 379
Monro: Alexander 31, 79
Montaigne: Michel de 12
Morgagni: G.B. 9, 32, 43, 44, 50, 328
Morton: Richard 33
Müller: Johannes 13, 107, 108, 133, 135, 145, 146, 147, 152, 159, 173, 174, 189, 263, 332, 333, 340, 348

N

Nabarro: D.N. 287
Nageli: Carl von 210
Naunyn: B. 378

Needham: John 207; Joseph 2
Neisser: Albert 180, 226
Neumann 310; E. 194, 318
Newton: I. 25, 26, 160
Nicolaier: A. 238
Niemeyer: Paul 174
Nocard: M. 233
Nuttall: George 300, 357, 389

O

Obermeier: Otto 210
Ogata: M. 228
Ogston: Alexander 220
Opie: E. 357
Orth: J. 152, 234, 375
Osler: W. 8, 11, 12, 14, 26, 31, 118, 125, 154, 155, 179, 202, 210, 225, 276, 278, 320, 345, 351, 355, 357, 361, 364–369, 373, 378, 379, 383, 384, 390, 399, 401
Owen: R. 264

P

Paget: James 264, 268; Stephen 335
Papanicolaou: G.N. 135
Paracelsus 20, 39, 327, 331
Parkinson: James 85
Pasteur: Louis 10, 67, 68, 103, 155, 159, 176, 200, 202, 205, 208, 249, 295, 301, 303, 314, 336, 344, 356, 364, 377, 388, 389
Perkin: William 137
Petit: Marc Antoine 52
Petri: Richard 222
Pettenkofer: Max von 234, 360
Peyronie: François de la 49
Pfeiffer: Richard 300
Pflueger: Eduard 135, 175, 307
Physick: Philip Syng 85, 346
Pinel: Philippe 43, 47
Piorry: Pierre 67
Planck: Max 199
Pliny the Elder 199
Pollender: Franz 214
Ponfick: Emil 152

Pott: Percivall 329
Pouchet: Felix 207
Prudden: T. Mitchell 345, 360

Q

Quekett: John 134

R

Ranvier: L.A. 137
Raspail: F.V. 135
Rather: Leland 191, 338
Rayer: Pierre 66, 214
Recamier: J.C.A. 333
Recklinghausen: F.D. von 152, 191, 192, 217, 223, 363, 378
Redi: Francesca 206, 263
Reed: Walter 201, 344, 374, 389, 389–391, 390, 391
Reichert: Karl 135, 337
Reil: Johann Christian 40
Reinhardt: Benno 135, 145
Remak: Robert 135, 147, 333, 336
Remsen: Ira 356
Rich: Arnold 379
Richard: E. 276
Ricord: Phillippe 66
Rindfleisch: Georg Eduard 152, 217
Ringer: Sidney 175
Risse: G. 42
Rockefeller: John D. 383; John T. 344
Rokitansky: K. 9, 13, 108, 113–126, 129, 151, 185, 217, 307, 308, 331, 335, 348
Rollet: A. 175
Romanovsky: D. 320
Rosenbach: Friedrich 222; Ottomar 183
Ross: R. 133, 201, 263, 274, 278, 279, 280, 282, 283, 284, 391, 393
Rostan: Leon 67
Roux: E. 206, 218, 233, 235, 236, 251, 252, 295
Rowntree: Leonard G. 378
Roy: Charles 183
Rubner: Max 175
Rudolphi 108; Karl 263
Rusch: Benjamin 80

Russell: Bertrand 302
Rutherford: John 31, 79
Ruysch: Frederik 33

S

Salmon: D.E. 240
Salomonsen: Carl 183, 229
Sanarelli: Giuseppe 389
Sanderson: Burton 367
Sandifort: Eduard 33
Sargent: John Singer 351
Sauvages: Francois Boissier de 41
Schelling: F. von 107
Schleiden: M.S. 146
Schmiedeberg: O. 378
Schoenheimer: Rudolf 7
Schottmuller: Hugo 240
Schultze: M. 133, 135, 313, 320, 367
Schwann: T. 133, 135, 146, 189, 332
Scudamore: Charles 80
Sedgwick: William Thompson 362
Semmelweis: I.P. 217
Senac: Jean Baptiste 33
Senn: Nicholas 374, 375
Severino: Marco 33
Sewell: Henry 362, 376
Sharpey: William 175
Sharpey-Schafer: E. 175, 308
Sherrington: C.S. 8, 372
Shiga: K. 239, 301
Shippen: William Jr. 80
Simpson: James Young 102
Skoda: J. 13, 58, 114, 217, 348
Smith: Adam 78, 133, 343; Theobald 201, 240
Soemmerring: Samuel von 329
Spallanzani: L. 207, 307
Spinoza: B. 25, 30, 47
Stahl: Georg 39
Stannius: Hermann 135
Stark: K.W. 173
Starling: E. 8, 175, 308
Steenstrup: Johannes 264

Sternberg: G. 224, 276, 277, 363, 388, 389, 390
Stiles: Charles W. 271
Stillé: Alfred 348
Stokes: William 80, 97, 101
Stoll: Maximilien 32
Störck: Anton 32
Strasburger: Eduard 333
Straus: M. 233
Swammerdam: J. 25, 29, 30, 313
Sweiten: Gerhard van 12, 32, 113
Sydenham: Thomas 9, 25, 31, 40, 43, 47, 147, 159, 169, 200
Sylvius: J. 22, 331
Syme: James 101

T

Thayer: W.S. 357, 370, 390
Thenard: L.S. 202
Thiersch: C. 335, 336
Thoma: Richard 311
Thomson: John 80, 101
Thuillier: L. 233
Todd: R.B. 134
Tommasi-Crudeli: C. 152
Traube: L. 10, 64, 169, 173, 179, 180, 348, 367
Travers: Benjamin 87
Trousseau: Armand 65, 67

V

Valentin: G. 133, 135, 285
Valsalva: A 33
Van Slyke: Donald 309
Vanderbilt: Cornelius 344
Varro 199
Vauquelin: L.N. 202
Velpeau: Alfred 65
Vesalius: A. 22, 26, 155, 199, 348, 356
Vetter: A. 32, 113
Vicq-d'Azyr: Felix 49
Vierordt: K. 175, 310
Vieussens: Raymond de 33
Villemin: Jean 228

Virchow: R. 9, 10, 13, 63, 64, 85, 86, 102, 107, 117, 118–119, 135, 143, 144, 146, 151, 152, 152–153, 159, 165, 169, 174, 179, 183, 184, 185, 190, 191, 195, 196, 210, 234, 268, 275, 296, 300, 302, 303, 314, 332, 333, 334, 336, 339, 348, 356, 359, 361, 367, 375
Vogel: Julius 331
Voit: Carl 175
Voltaire: Jean Francois Marie 47
von Schelling 108

W

Waage: P. 175
Wagner: E. 113, 133, 359
Waldeyer: W. 137, 192, 217, 317, 337, 338, 359
Waller: A. 190
Waterhouse: Benjamin 346
Watson: J. 2
Weichselbaum: Anton 224, 227
Weigert: C. 137, 152, 183, 219, 299, 314, 317, 363
Welch: H.W. 155, 180, 184, 345, 351, 357–359, 363, 367, 369, 370, 372, 373, 379, 380, 388, 389, 390
Welcher: H. 311
Whipple: George 357
Widal: F. 226
Wilks: S. 96
Williams: John Whitridge 357
Willis: Thomas 25, 29, 33
Winternitz: Milton 357
Wintrobe: M. 321
Wistar: Caspar 80
Wöhler: F. 317
Woodhead: Sims 237
Wright: Almroth 237; J.H. 227, 320
Wucherer: O. 271, 272
Wunderlich: Carl 64, 169, 173, 179

Y

Yersin: Alexander 228, 235
Young: Hugh 372

Z

Zeigler: E. 299
Zeiss: Carl 311
Zenker: F. 267
Ziemmsen: Hugo 152
Zimmermann: G. 190